Advancements in Sports Medicine

Advancements in Sports Medicine

Editors

Jiwu Chen
Yaying Sun

MDPI • Basel • Beijing • Wuhan • Barcelona • Belgrade • Manchester • Tokyo • Cluj • Tianjin

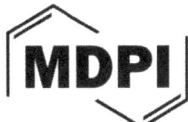

Editors
Jiwu Chen
Shanghai Jiaotong University
Shanghai, China

Yaying Sun
Fudan University
Shanghai, China

Editorial Office
MDPI
St. Alban-Anlage 66
4052 Basel, Switzerland

This is a reprint of articles from the Special Issue published online in the open access journal *Journal of Clinical Medicine* (ISSN 2077-0383) (available at: https://www.mdpi.com/journal/jcm/special_issues/Advancements_Sports_Medicine).

For citation purposes, cite each article independently as indicated on the article page online and as indicated below:

LastName, A.A.; LastName, B.B.; LastName, C.C. Article Title. *Journal Name* **Year**, *Volume Number*, Page Range.

ISBN 978-3-0365-8024-1 (Hbk)
ISBN 978-3-0365-8025-8 (PDF)

Cover image courtesy of Yaying Sun

© 2023 by the authors. Articles in this book are Open Access and distributed under the Creative Commons Attribution (CC BY) license, which allows users to download, copy and build upon published articles, as long as the author and publisher are properly credited, which ensures maximum dissemination and a wider impact of our publications.

The book as a whole is distributed by MDPI under the terms and conditions of the Creative Commons license CC BY-NC-ND.

Contents

About the Editors vii

Yaying Sun and Jiwu Chen
Advancements in Sports Medicine
Reprinted from: *J. Clin. Med.* **2023**, *12*, 3489, doi:10.3390/jcm12103489 1

Xiangwei Li, Yujia Xiao, Han Shu, Xianding Sun and Mao Nie
Risk Factors and Corresponding Management for Suture Anchor Pullout during Arthroscopic
Rotator Cuff Repair
Reprinted from: *J. Clin. Med.* **2022**, *11*, 6870, doi:10.3390/jcm11226870 3

**Logan W. Gaudette, Molly M. Bradach, José Roberto de Souza Junior, Bryan Heiderscheit,
Caleb D. Johnson, Joshua Posilkin, et al.**
Clinical Application of Gait Retraining in the Injured Runner
Reprinted from: *J. Clin. Med.* **2022**, *11*, 6497, doi:10.3390/jcm11216497 17

Xianshan Guo, Shizhe Guo, Hongmei Zhang and Zhen Li
Does Aerobic plus Machine-Assisted Resistance Training Improve Vascular Function in Type 2
Diabetes? A Systematic Review and Meta-Analysis of Randomized Controlled Trials with Trial
Sequential Analysis
Reprinted from: *J. Clin. Med.* **2022**, *11*, 4257, doi:10.3390/jcm11154257 31

Yuhan Zhang, Shaohua Liu, Yaying Sun, Yuxue Xie and Jiwu Chen
Knee Cartilage Change within 5 Years after Aclr Using Hamstring Tendons with Preserved
Tibial-Insertion: A Prospective Randomized Controlled Study Based on Magnetic Resonance
Imaging
Reprinted from: *J. Clin. Med.* **2022**, *11*, 6157, doi:10.3390/jcm11206157 43

Mei Ma, Bowen Zhang, Xinxin Yan, Xiang Ji, Deyu Qin, Chaodong Pu, et al.
Adaptive Posture-Balance Cardiac Rehabilitation Exercise Significantly Improved Physical
Tolerance in Patients with Cardiovascular Diseases
Reprinted from: *J. Clin. Med.* **2022**, *11*, 5345, doi:10.3390/jcm11185345 63

**Cordula Leonie Merle, Lisa Richter, Nadia Challakh, Rainer Haak, Gerhard Schmalz,
Ian Needleman, et al.**
Associations of Blood and Performance Parameters with Signs of Periodontal Inflammation in
Young Elite Athletes—An Explorative Study
Reprinted from: *J. Clin. Med.* **2022**, *11*, 5161, doi:10.3390/jcm11175161 75

**Francisco Martins, Krzysztof Przednowek, Cíntia França, Helder Lopes,
Marcelo de Maio Nascimento, Hugo Sarmento, et al.**
Predictive Modeling of Injury Risk Based on Body Composition and Selected Physical Fitness
Tests for Elite Football Players
Reprinted from: *J. Clin. Med.* **2022**, *11*, 4923, doi:10.3390/jcm11164923 89

**Karsten Keller, Katharina Hartung, Luis del Castillo Carillo, Julia Treiber, Florian Stock,
Chantal Schröder, et al.**
Exercise Hypertension in Athletes
Reprinted from: *J. Clin. Med.* **2022**, *11*, 4870, doi:10.3390/jcm11164870 103

Youfeng Guo, Haihong Zhao, Haowei Xu, Huida Gu, Yang Cao, Kai Li, et al.
Albumin-to-Alkaline Phosphatase Ratio as a Prognostic Biomarker for Spinal Fusion in Lumbar
Degenerative Diseases Patients Undergoing Lumbar Spinal Fusion
Reprinted from: *J. Clin. Med.* **2022**, *11*, 4719, doi:10.3390/jcm11164719 121

Shuang Cong, Jianying Pan, Guangxin Huang, Denghui Xie and Chun Zeng
The Modified Longitudinal Capsulotomy by Outside-In Approach in Hip Arthroscopy for Femoroplasty and Acetabular Labrum Repair—A Cohort Study
Reprinted from: *J. Clin. Med.* **2022**, *11*, 4548, doi:10.3390/jcm11154548 . . . . **133**

Ian J. Wellington, Lukas N. Muench, Benjamin C. Hawthorne, Colin L. Uyeki, Christopher L. Antonacci, Mary Beth McCarthy, et al.
Clinical Outcomes following Biologically Enhanced Demineralized Bone Matrix Augmentation of Complex Rotator Cuff Repair
Reprinted from: *J. Clin. Med.* **2022**, *11*, 2956, doi:10.3390/jcm11112956 . . . . **143**

About the Editors

Jiwu Chen

Professor Jiwu Chen, Ph.D, currently works in Shanghai General Hospital, Shanghai Jiaotong University, China. He has focused on clinical and basic research into sports injuries for a long time, and has been funded by the National Natural Science Foundation of China six times. He has more than 100 publications, among which several have been published in *The American Journal of Sports Medicine*, *Bioactive Materials*, *Small*, etc. Currently, Prof. Chen serves as the chairman-elect of the Sports Medicine Specialty Branch of the Shanghai Medical Association, the vice chairman of the Sports Medicine Branch of the Chinese Research Hospital Association, and the deputy leader of the Sports Medicine Group of the Orthopedic Branch of the Chinese Medical Doctor Association, as well as being a member of the ISAKOS Shoulder Joint Committee, etc. Prof. Chen's achivements in arthroscopic surgery are substantial, with 500–1000 surgeries per year. At the 2017 ISAKOS Biennial Conference, he served as the only invited Chinese expert to give a demonstration of arthroscopic surgery of a massive rotator cuff tear.

Yaying Sun

Dr. Yaying Sun, Ph.D, currently works in Huashan Hospital, Fudan University, Shanghai, China. He serves as the member of various editorial boards, including the *International Journal of Nanomedicine*, *Burns & Trauma*, *Journal of Clinical Medicine*, etc., and the reviewer of several scientific journals. In 2021, Dr. Sun received funding from the National Natural Science Foundation of China. His ongoing research interests are regenerative medicine of skeletal muscle and tendons/ligaments and the mechanism of aging of the musculoskeletal system, as well as multi-discipline research regarding the crosstalk between the musculoskeletal system, sports activity and exercise, and other disorders, especially cancer and chronic diseases.

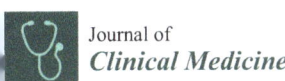

Editorial

Advancements in Sports Medicine

Yaying Sun [1] and Jiwu Chen [2,*]

1. Huashan Hospital, Fudan University, Shanghai 200040, China
2. Department of Sports Medicine, Shanghai General Hospital, Shanghai Jiaotong University, Shanghai 200080, China
* Correspondence: jeevechen@gmail.com

Sports medicine has developed rapidly in recent years. Countless advancements have been achieved regarding the mechanism, repair, and recovery of sports injuries. The interaction between sports medicine and other disciplines is also a trending topic. Multi-disciplinary outcomes are being increasingly yielded. In this Special Issue, we have collected several clinical advancements in sports medicine.

Rotator cuff tear is a common shoulder disorder in clinical practice. Based on tear size, treatment methods can be divided into direct repair using suture anchors or repair with augmentation due to a massive tear size. Li et al. conducted a review of the current literature and reported that bone quality, insertion depth, insertion angle, size of rotator cuff tear, preoperative corticosteroid injections, anchor design, and the materials used to produce anchors may influence the anchor pullout strength, leading to a poor recovery [1]. Regarding massive rotator cuff tear that cannot be fixed directly, Wellington et al. used a biologically enhanced demineralized bone matrix for the augmentation and found that 10 of 20 patients who received this treatment still suffered from a retear at follow-up [2]. This outcome suggested that there is still a long way to go to enhance the repair of rotator cuff.

For trunk, spinal fusion is usually applied for patients with lumbar degeneration with overall good results. However, some may still experience failure. Guo et al. noticed that the albumin-to-alkaline phosphatase ratio can be used as a prognostic biomarker for measuring clinical outcomes after spinal fusion [3]. Regarding lower limb, Cong et al. reported a modified capsulotomy approach to facilitate the arthroscopic femoroplasty and acetabular labrum repair, with the clinical data supporting its popularization [4]. Regarding knee, Zhang et al. found that anterior cruciate ligament reconstruction using an insertion preservation technique has a protective effect on cartilage degeneration in long-term follow-up [5].

In addition to the general population, novel advancements have also been achieved regarding injuries in athletes. Martins established a predictive model for injury risk in football players [6], while Keller et al. pointed out some divergences in terms of exaggerated blood pressure response in athletes [7]. Gaudette et al. studied runner injuries and emphasized the importance of gait retaining for post-injury recovery [8]. Merle et al. focused on the oral health of young athletes and revealed an association of blood/performance indexes and periodontal inflammation [9].

Some interesting multi-disciplinary research is also included in this Issue. Guo et al. conducted a systematic review and found that aerobic plus machine-assisted resistance training may improve the vascular function in patients with type 2 diabetes [10], while Ma et al. found that adaptive posture-balance cardiac rehabilitation exercise could remarkably restore physical tolerance in a population suffering from cardiovascular diseases [11]. The interaction between sports medicine and other subjects will no doubt make this discipline more meaningful in the future.

Author Contributions: Y.S. organized the paper and J.C. revised the paper. All authors have read and agreed to the published version of the manuscript.

Citation: Sun, Y.; Chen, J. Advancements in Sports Medicine. *J. Clin. Med.* **2023**, *12*, 3489. https://doi.org/10.3390/jcm12103489

Received: 3 April 2023
Accepted: 22 April 2023
Published: 16 May 2023

Copyright: © 2023 by the authors. Licensee MDPI, Basel, Switzerland. This article is an open access article distributed under the terms and conditions of the Creative Commons Attribution (CC BY) license (https://creativecommons.org/licenses/by/4.0/).

Conflicts of Interest: The authors declare no conflict of interest.

References

1. Li, X.; Xiao, Y.; Shu, H.; Sun, X.; Nie, M. Risk Factors and Corresponding Management for Suture Anchor Pullout during Arthroscopic Rotator Cuff Repair. *J. Clin. Med.* **2022**, *11*, 6870. [CrossRef] [PubMed]
2. Wellington, I.J.; Muench, L.N.; Hawthorne, B.C.; Uyeki, C.L.; Antonacci, C.L.; McCarthy, M.B.; Connors, J.P.; Kia, C.; Mazzocca, A.D.; Berthold, D.P. Clinical Outcomes Following Biologically Enhanced Demineralized Bone Matrix Augmentation of Complex Rotator Cuff Repair. *J. Clin. Med.* **2022**, *11*, 2956. [CrossRef] [PubMed]
3. Guo, Y.; Zhao, H.; Xu, H.; Gu, H.; Cao, Y.; Li, K.; Li, T.; Hu, T.; Wang, S.; Zhao, W.; et al. Albumin-to-Alkaline Phosphatase Ratio as a Prognostic Biomarker for Spinal Fusion in Lumbar Degenerative Diseases Patients Undergoing Lumbar Spinal Fusion. *J. Clin. Med.* **2022**, *11*, 4719. [CrossRef] [PubMed]
4. Cong, S.; Pan, J.; Huang, G.; Xie, D.; Zeng, C. The Modified Longitudinal Capsulotomy by Outside-In Approach in Hip Arthroscopy for Femoroplasty and Acetabular Labrum Repair-A Cohort Study. *J. Clin. Med.* **2022**, *11*, 4548. [CrossRef] [PubMed]
5. Zhang, Y.; Liu, S.; Sun, Y.; Xie, Y.; Chen, J. Knee Cartilage Change within 5 Years after Aclr Using Hamstring Tendons with Preserved Tibial-Insertion: A Prospective Randomized Controlled Study Based on Magnetic Resonance Imaging. *J. Clin. Med.* **2022**, *11*, 6157. [CrossRef] [PubMed]
6. Martins, F.; Przednowek, K.; França, C.; Lopes, H.; de Maio Nascimento, M.; Sarmento, H.; Marques, A.; Ihle, A.; Henriques, R.; Gouveia, É.R. Predictive Modeling of Injury Risk Based on Body Composition and Selected Physical Fitness Tests for Elite Football Players. *J. Clin. Med.* **2022**, *11*, 4923. [CrossRef] [PubMed]
7. Keller, K.; Hartung, K.; Del Castillo Carillo, L.; Treiber, J.; Stock, F.; Schröder, C.; Hugenschmidt, F.; Friedmann-Bette, B. Exercise Hypertension in Athletes. *J. Clin. Med.* **2022**, *11*, 4870. [CrossRef] [PubMed]
8. Gaudette, L.W.; Bradach, M.M.; de Souza Junior, J.R.; Heiderscheit, B.; Johnson, C.D.; Posilkin, J.; Rauh, M.J.; Sara, L.K.; Wasserman, L.; Hollander, K.; et al. Clinical Application of Gait Retraining in the Injured Runner. *J. Clin. Med.* **2022**, *11*, 6497. [CrossRef] [PubMed]
9. Merle, C.L.; Richter, L.; Challakh, N.; Haak, R.; Schmalz, G.; Needleman, I.; Rüdrich, P.; Wolfarth, B.; Ziebolz, D.; Wüstenfeld, J. Associations of Blood and Performance Parameters with Signs of Periodontal Inflammation in Young Elite Athletes-An Explorative Study. *J. Clin. Med.* **2022**, *11*, 5161. [CrossRef] [PubMed]
10. Guo, X.; Guo, S.; Zhang, H.; Li, Z. Does Aerobic plus Machine-Assisted Resistance Training Improve Vascular Function in Type 2 Diabetes? A Systematic Review and Meta-Analysis of Randomized Controlled Trials with Trial Sequential Analysis. *J. Clin. Med.* **2022**, *11*, 4257. [CrossRef] [PubMed]
11. Ma, M.; Zhang, B.; Yan, X.; Ji, X.; Qin, D.; Pu, C.; Zhao, J.; Zhang, Q.; Lowis, H.; Li, T. Adaptive Posture-Balance Cardiac Rehabilitation Exercise Significantly Improved Physical Tolerance in Patients with Cardiovascular Diseases. *J. Clin. Med.* **2022**, *11*, 5345. [CrossRef] [PubMed]

Disclaimer/Publisher's Note: The statements, opinions and data contained in all publications are solely those of the individual author(s) and contributor(s) and not of MDPI and/or the editor(s). MDPI and/or the editor(s) disclaim responsibility for any injury to people or property resulting from any ideas, methods, instructions or products referred to in the content.

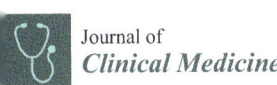

Review

Risk Factors and Corresponding Management for Suture Anchor Pullout during Arthroscopic Rotator Cuff Repair

Xiangwei Li [†], Yujia Xiao [†], Han Shu, Xianding Sun and Mao Nie *

Center for Joint Surgery, Department of Orthopaedics, The Second Affiliated Hospital of Chongqing Medical University, Chongqing 400010, China
* Correspondence: 302218@cqmu.edu.cn
† These authors contributed equally to this work.

Abstract: Introduction: Due to the aging of the population, the incidence of rotator cuff tears is growing. For rotator cuff repair, arthroscopic suture-anchor repair has gradually replaced open transosseous repair, so suture anchors are now considered increasingly important in rotator cuff tear reconstruction. There are some but limited studies of suture anchor pullout after arthroscopic rotator cuff repair. However, there is no body of knowledge in this area, which makes it difficult for clinicians to predict the risk of anchor pullout comprehensively and manage it accordingly. Methods: The literature search included rotator cuff repair as well as anchor pullout strength. A review of the literature was performed including all articles published in PubMed until September 2021. Articles of all in vitro biomechanical and clinical trial levels in English were included. After assessing all abstracts ($n = 275$), the full text and the bibliographies of the relevant articles were analyzed for the questions posed ($n = 80$). Articles including outcomes without the area of interest were excluded ($n = 22$). The final literature research revealed 58 relevant articles. Narrative synthesis was undertaken to bring together the findings from studies included in this review. Result: Based on the presented studies, the overall incidence of anchor pullout is not low, and the incidence of intraoperative anchor pullout is slightly higher than in the early postoperative period. The risk factors for anchor pullout are mainly related to bone quality, insertion depth, insertion angle, size of rotator cuff tear, preoperative corticosteroid injections, anchor design, the materials used to produce anchors, etc. In response to the above issues, we have introduced and evaluated management techniques. They include changing the implant site of anchors, cement augmentation for suture anchors, increasing the number of suture limbs, using all-suture anchors, using an arthroscopic transosseous knotless anchor, the Buddy anchor technique, Steinmann pin anchoring, and transosseous suture repair technology. Discussion: However, not many of the management techniques have been widely used in clinical practice. Most of them come from in vitro biomechanical studies, so in vivo randomized controlled trials with larger sample sizes are needed to see if they can help patients in the long run.

Keywords: rotator cuff tear; rotator cuff repair; bone quality; osteopenia; osteoporosis; anchor pullout; pullout strength

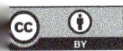

1. Introduction

Due to the aging of the population, the incidence of rotator cuff tears is growing [1,2]. For rotator cuff repair, arthroscopic suture-anchor repair has gradually replaced open transosseous repair, so suture anchors are now considered increasingly important in rotator cuff tear reconstruction [3]. The majority of patients with rotator cuff tears are over 60 years old, and osteoporosis is very common among them [4,5]. This means that their proximal humeral bone quality is often poor, which will increase the incidence of anchor pullout [6,7] (Figure 1). Anchor pullout is one of the mechanisms of suture anchor failure. It occurs at the anchor-bone interface during arthroscopic rotator cuff repair, resulting in pullout of the anchors from the bone [8]. In terms of biomechanics, pullout strength is the pullout force measured when anchor pullout occurs at the anchor-bone interface. Studies have attempted to find new methods to improve pullout strength, thus reducing the risk of anchor pullout.

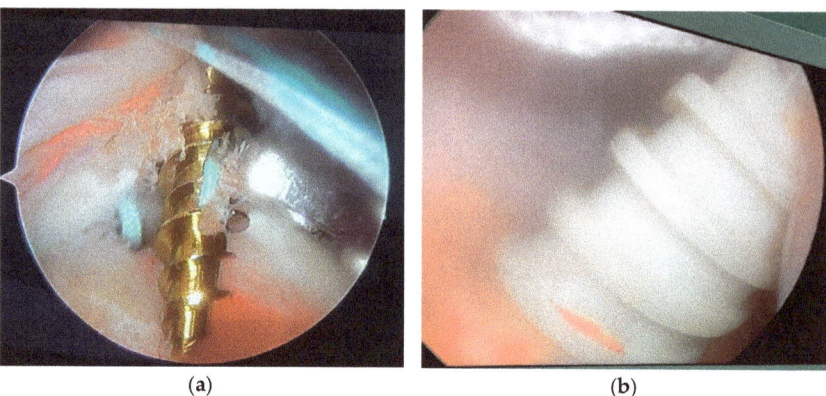

Figure 1. (a) Intraoperative metallic suture anchor pullout; (b) intraoperative polyetheretherketone suture anchor pullout.

The purpose of this review is to summarize the body of knowledge on suture anchor pullout during arthroscopic rotator cuff repair. We will first briefly introduce the incidence of anchor pullout before discussing the reason why the suture anchor pulls out. Lastly, we will describe in detail the different technologies and studies that have been used to solve the problem of anchor pullout, and we will compare their pros and cons to help future practice.

2. Method

The literature search included rotator cuff repair as well as anchor pullout strength. A review of the literature was performed, including all articles published in PubMed until September 2021. The following search terms were used alone and in combination: "Rotator cuff repair", "anchor pullout", and "pullout strength". The articles were assessed considering the following research aspects: definition, incidence of anchor pullout, risk factor for anchor pullout, and anchor pullout management.

Articles of all in vitro biomechanical and clinical trial levels in English were included. After assessing all abstracts ($n = 275$), the full text and the bibliographies of the relevant articles were analyzed for the questions posed ($n = 80$). Articles including outcomes without the area of interest were excluded ($n = 22$). Specifically, publications from 1990 to 2021 were included because of the advancements in biomechanics, surgical treatments, and improved understanding of pullout strength for suture anchors. The final literature research revealed 58 relevant articles. Narrative synthesis was undertaken to bring together the findings from studies included in this review.

3. Results

3.1. Total Incidence of Anchor Pullout

The incidence of anchor pullout varies depending on the circumstances. The incidence of early anchor pullout after arthroscopic rotator cuff repair is approximately 0.1%–3.1%, while the incidence of anchor pullout during surgery is higher, approximately 3.3%–5.4%. Anchor pullout is one of the three mechanical mechanisms of revision surgery failure, with an incidence of approximately 4.5%.

3.1.1. Early Anchor Pullout

A retrospective, monocentric study [9] by Skaliczki et al., showed that early anchor pullout was observed in six patients out of 5327 (0.1%).

Earlier studies found much higher rates of early anchor pullout. Benson et al. [10] investigated 269 patients who underwent arthroscopic rotator cuff repair and found six cases of early anchor pullout (2.4%). In their study of 127 patients, Dezaly et al. [11] reported a 3.1% prevalence of early anchor displacement. The difference may be caused by the different time points of the radiographic evaluation: The time period considered in the latter two studies also included part of the rehabilitation, while the observation time of Skaliczki et al. [9] was immediately after surgery. That is, early anchor pullout in the series of Skaliczki et al. [9] is mainly attributed to surgical intervention, while the results of Benson et al. [10] and Dezaly et al. [11] are at least partly due to the rehabilitation process.

3.1.2. Anchor Pullout during Surgery

The incidence of anchor pullout during surgery has not been investigated, and only a few articles [9–11] have reported the incidence of early postoperative anchor failure.

A retrospective study [12] by Jung and colleagues showed that of 1076 patients who underwent arthroscopic rotator cuff repair, 483 were treated with screw-in-type bioabsorbable or biocomposite anchors, and 593 were treated with soft anchors. In the screw-in-type anchor group, 16 patients (3.3%, 16/483) experienced anchor pullout during surgery. Of the 593 patients treated by soft anchor insertion, 32 (5.4%, 32/593) experienced anchor pullout. These rates are not significantly different. Intraoperative anchor pullout was much more likely to happen in patients with larger rotator cuff tears, women, older people, or those who had shoulder stiffness before surgery.

3.1.3. Anchor Pullout Has a Relatively Low Incidence

Cummins et al. [8] found three mechanisms by which rotator cuff repairs fail mechanically at the time of revision surgery: rotator cuff suture pullout from the repaired tendon (86.3% of cases), new tears in a different place (9.1% of cases), and complete anchor displacement, or pullout, from the bone (4.5% of cases).

3.2. Risk Factors for Suture Anchor Pullout

The reason why the suture anchor pulls out is the poor stability of anchor fixation in arthroscopic rotator cuff repair. The stability is determined by bone quality, insertion depth, insertion angle, anchor design, the materials used to produce anchors [13–19] and so on.

3.2.1. Bone Quality

Pullout strength depends on bone mineral density [4,20,21].

Suture anchors have better pullout characteristics when placed in areas of higher bone mineral density (BMD) [4,20,22,23]. However, the use of anchors in patients who are elderly and who may be osteoporotic [24] can potentially increase the likelihood of anchor pullout. The bone quality of the greater tuberosity is one of the factors affecting repair integrity [6]. In patients with poor bone quality, the failure rate after rotator cuff repair is as high as 68% [4,25]. The quality of the proximal humerus bone also deteriorates with age and is more pronounced in patients who have RCT. Djurasovic et al. [7] reviewed 80 cases of failed rotator cuff repair and showed that 10% of them had anchor migration or loosening. Anchor migration is a state between anchor loosening and pullout, and it is incomplete anchor pullout. From these results, we can see that the lower the bone mineral density, the more easily the anchor will cut out of the humerus [4]. These studies provide a theoretical basis for various augmentation technologies.

3.2.2. Anchor Material and Design

The mechanical fixation (pullout strength) of suture anchors is determined by their design, such as the pitch and number of threads, length, size, and overall shape [4,10,26]. Anchors of various designs, materials, and sizes have been invented. The pullout strength can differ according to the material and design of suture anchors [27–29].

Anchors made of different materials have different incidences of anchor pullout. Tingart et al. [4] found that the pullout strength of metal screw-type anchors is higher than that of biodegradable hook-type anchors. In addition, most studies using radiotransparent (RT) anchors have reported complications caused by bioabsorbable anchors resulting in bone lysis, defects, and sometimes fractures [30–32], which may lead to late pullout. However, osteolysis has no effect on clinical outcomes [33]. Polyetheretherketone (PEEK) anchors, although non-absorbable, also enlarge the peripheral bones significantly more laterally than medially in double-row (DR) repairs [34], which may be the reason why they pull out. In short, the use of anchors of different materials will produce different pullout strengths, which is the reason why anchor pullout occurs under specific circumstances.

A study by Chae and colleagues [35] indicated that high pullout strength was primarily attributed to geometric design factors of the suture anchors, such as greater contact surface area between the anchor threads and surrounding bone, overall length, number of threads, and height of the thread. It is possible that the contact surface area between the anchor threads and surrounding bone is related to other geometric design factors of the suture anchor, such as the overall length, diameter, number of threads, height of the thread, pitch, and helix angle. Chae et al., found that the number and height of threads were positively correlated with the pullout strength among suture anchors of several geometric designs. In fact, the number and height of threads are the most important geometric design factors for increasing the contact surface area between suture anchors and surrounding bone. Their results support the points of view that greater thread-to-bone surface contact leads to greater pullout strength and that screw threads impart improved holding strength due to the increased through contact with the surface of the bone [36–38]. Kang et al. [39] reported that a micropore bioabsorbable suture anchor had higher pullout strength, which may have been related to the bone growth induced by the micropore bioabsorbable anchor. Even though more clinical trials need to be conducted to confirm the above assumptions, there is no doubt that these research results point us in a new direction when it comes to anchor design.

Therefore, the clinical application of anchors with different designs will often bring about different pullout strengths and lead to different incidences of anchor pullout. Anchor design determines the stability of anchor fixation, which is one of the reasons why anchor design affects the incidence of anchor pullout.

3.2.3. Number of Anchors (Distance between Anchors)

The relationships of the pullout strength to the anchor material, anchor design, insertion angle, insertion depth, and bone mineral density have been investigated [3,15,16,20,40–42]. However, these studies only focused on the pullout strength of one anchor. One study investigated the pullout strength of two anchors instead of one [43], finding that the pullout strength of two anchors was higher. Kawakami and colleagues [44] showed that in polyurethane and porcine models, the minimum distance between anchors to not reduce the pullout strength was 6 mm, which was less than the previously determined 10-mm separation, and this result was not affected by the different bone qualities, even when applied to osteoporotic bone. When two anchors are placed 4 mm apart, there are two possible reasons for the decrease in pullout strength. First, when two anchors are very close, the cancellous bone around the anchors is not strong enough to support both. Second, in fact, a 4-mm distance means that adjacent anchors will overlap. The contact area between the anchor thread and the cancellous bone decreases as the amount of overlap increases. The contact area of the anchor thread is closely linked to the pullout strength [37,45]. When calculating the distance between two anchors, we mean from center to center, so the minimum distance without decreasing the pullout strength may be different for suture anchors with different diameters. However, due to financial constraints, only two types of suture anchors were examined in this study, compared to the ideal situation of testing all commercially available anchors.

All-suture anchors are biomechanically inferior to screw-in-type anchors [46]. However, Ntalos et al. [47] reported that all-suture anchors and traditional anchors had similar average pullout strengths in an unlimited cyclic model. Moreover, compared with traditional anchors, all-suture anchors have a smaller volume, which allows more of them to be implanted in the same volume of bone [48]. The overall biomechanical performance is improved by sharing the load at multiple fixation points. However, the minimum distance between all-suture anchors seems not to have been reported.

3.2.4. Insertion Angle

Accidental anchor pullout is a common mechanism of repair failure, and its occurrence is affected by bone quality and the implantation technique [49,50]. The relationship between anchor pullout and anchor insertion angle has also been studied. It was widely accepted and understood that placing the anchor at 45° to the insertion surface would display the strongest pullout strength [4,15,18–20,51] after Burkhart's proposal of the deadman theory in 1995 [52].

In 2009, Strauss et al., used cadaveric shoulders to study the effects of anchor insertion angle and rotator cuff tendon repair [49]. The torn supraspinatus tendons were repaired by single suture anchor with an insertion angle of 45° or 90°. The results showed that the rotator cuff repair with the anchor inserted at 90° to the bone surface was stronger than the repair with the anchor inserted at 45°. However, compared with the whole repaired construct, the effect of insertion angle on just anchor pullout strength was of more interest to the researchers.

In 2014, Clevenger et al., tested the pullout strength of anchors with insertion angles from 45° to 135° in 15° increments [14]. According to the findings, anchors set at an acute angle to the pulling axis were substantially weaker than those positioned at an obtuse angle. It did not appear to necessarily match the clinical settings, though, as just one type of synthetic cancellous bone was used and no cortical bone. In 2016, Nagamoto et al., conducted a biomechanical test of anchor insertion angle using the greater tuberosity of porcine humeri and three different densities of synthetic cancellous bones with a 2-mm-thick cortical bone connected to one side. Their findings showed that regardless of bone density, the pullout strength of the anchors implanted at 90° to the bone surface was higher than the anchors inserted at 45° [16].

In the same year, Itoi et al., comprehensively evaluated their laboratory data against previous data and concluded that insertion angles of 45° and 90° were the strongest for threadless and threaded anchors, respectively [53,54]. So, whether threaded or threadless anchors are used should also affect the choice of insertion angle. Threadless anchors provide less friction. In this case, inserting an anchor at 45° had a higher pullout strength than inserting an anchor at 90° or more. In contrast, threaded anchors can provide substantial friction. Therefore, the maximum pullout strength can be obtained by inserting the anchor at 90°.

In 2018, Ntalos et al.'s [47] biomechanical study demonstrated that the maximal force in all-suture and traditional anchors could be detected at a 90° insertion angle. Regardless of the kind, the pullout strength was decreased when they were inserted at more acute (45°) or obtuse (110°) angles. Those differences were not statistically significant, though. They thought that the angle at which the anchor was inserted was not as important in the clinic as people had thought [47].

3.2.5. Size of Rotator Cuff Tear

The retrospective cohort study by Benson and colleagues provided conclusive evidence that patients with larger rotator cuff tears have a significantly higher incidence of anchor pullout. They found [10] that among 251 patients who used metallic suture anchor for rotator cuff repair, six had early anchor pullout, with an overall incidence of about 2.4%. The incidence of rotator cuff tears less than or equal to 3 cm was 0.5%, and the incidence in tears greater than 3 cm was 11%. In large tears, the suture anchor bears higher tension, so the incidence of anchor pullout will also be higher.

3.2.6. Insertion Depth

In a biomechanical study, Bynum et al. [15] showed that changing the insertion depth of the suture anchor affected the mechanical properties and the failure modes of suture anchor constructs. Suture anchors inserted with the suture eyelet deep had premature failure because of construct elongation.

Kirchhof et al. [55] reported that screwing the anchor deeper did not increase the pullout strength. This is because the deep bone mineral density of the greater tuberosity is relatively low. For patients with osteoporosis, this is of no help. Osteoporosis usually involves the patient's cancellous bone first, resulting in a decrease in cancellous bone quality, followed by cortical bone. Therefore, the deep bone mineral density of the greater tuberosity for patients with osteoporosis is relatively low, and screwing the anchor deeper cannot improve the pullout strength.

Therefore, there is no consistent conclusion on whether increasing the insertion depth of the anchor improves the pullout strength.

3.2.7. The Effect of Corticosteroid Injections on Anchor Pullout Strength

Because RCT patients usually have obvious pain symptoms, corticosteroid injections (CSIs) into the subacromial space have been an important treatment for RCT patients. Puzzitiello et al. [56] showed that for patients who had received CSIs within two weeks, their suture anchor pullout strength decreased significantly after arthroscopic rotator cuff repair. There was no significant decrease after 3 or 4 weeks. These findings suggest that for patients who have received CSIs before surgery, we should ensure that they receive surgery after a certain interval of time.

3.3. Anchor Pullout Management

As mentioned above, rotator cuff repair has a high retear rate, and the risk of failure increases with the age of the patient [57] and with the size of the tear [58]. The quality of the proximal humerus also deteriorates with age, and this phenomenon is more common in RCT patients. With the continuous development and popularity of arthroscopic rotator cuff repair, the practice of open rotator cuff repair in the new generation of surgeons is becoming rarer. This section focuses on various management techniques and biomechanical principles for anchor pullout during arthroscopic rotator cuff repair.

3.3.1. Changing the Implant Site of Anchors

For arthroscopic rotator cuff repair, the suture anchor is implanted in the proximal humerus, usually into the greater tuberosity. Many studies have analyzed the bone quality distribution of the greater tuberosity.

In 2003, an in vitro biomechanical study by Tingart et al. [4] demonstrated that, within the proximal part of the greater tuberosity, trabecular bone mineral density of the posterior region and cortical bone mineral density of the middle region were highest, respectively. However, loads to failure in the anterior and middle regions were, on average, 62% higher than the load to failure in the posterior region. They came to the conclusion that cortical bone mineral density was a stronger predictor of pullout strength in the proximal region of the tuberosity than trabecular bone mineral density. The pullout strength might be improved by placing suture anchors in the proximal-anterior and proximal-middle regions of greater tuberosity [20].

Kirchhof et al. [5] performed high-resolution peripheral quantitative CT scanning on 36 cadaver specimens, finding that the volume of highest bone quality was found at the posteromedial aspect. Sakamoto et al. [59] used multidetector row computed tomography to successfully perform an in vivo evaluation of the bone microstructure of the humeral greater tuberosity in patients with rotator cuff tears. They also obtained the same results as Kirchhof et al. According to the findings of both studies, the posterior medial region of the greater tuberosity was the best location for anchor insertion in terms of bone quality. This contradicted the results of Tingart et al. [4].

3.3.2. Cement Augmentation for Suture Anchors

Bone grafting or using bone cement to fill the void caused by osteoporotic bone resorption or large cystic changes within the subchondral plate can effectively improve the bone quality of patients undergoing arthroscopic rotator cuff repair. It is very difficult to perform structural bone grafting under arthroscopy, and the pullout strength will not be improved immediately, so it is clinically more feasible to inject bone cement to enhance bone quality and improve pullout strength.

Oshtory and colleagues [60] reported that the pullout strength of suture anchors injected with tricalcium phosphate cement increased by 29%. Giori and colleagues [61] reported a 71% gain in pullout strength with anchor augmentation by polymethyl methacrylate (PMMA) cement. Although the pullout strength was improved, PMMA cement is not bioabsorbable, which may make revision surgery harder. Moreover, PMMA cement produces a thermal effect during the curing process, which may also cause bone necrosis, making the pullout strength uncontrollable in specific cases.

Postl and colleagues [62] reported that the pullout strength of suture anchors injected with bioabsorbable and fiber-reinforced calcium phosphate cement increased by 66.8%. This fiber-reinforced calcium phosphate cement can reach a pullout strength similar to that of PMMA cement but also retains the properties of calcium phosphate cement; that is, it does not produce a thermal effect and is bioabsorbable [63]. This new bone cement combines the advantages of calcium phosphate cement and PMMA cement and is a promising reinforcing material. To be applied in the clinic, it needs to be evaluated in further in vivo experiments.

The biomechanical results above show that it is theoretically tenable to improve the pullout strength of different materials by bone cement augmentation (Table 1).

Table 1. Pullout strength increment for augmentation with different types of bone cement.

Study	Types of Bone Cement	Testing Model	Anchor Type	Percentage Increase (%)	p Value
Giori et al. [61]	PMMA bone cement	Cadaveric humerus	Metal screw-like suture anchors (5-mm Fastin RC; Mitek, Norwood, MA, USA)	71	$p = 0.02$
Oshtory et al. [60]	Bioabsorbable tricalcium phosphate cement	Cadaveric humerus	Metal screw-like suture anchors (5-mm Fastin RC; Mitek, Norwood, MA, USA)	29	$p = 0.027$
Postl et al. [62]	The bio-absorbable and fiber-reinforced calcium phosphate cement	Cadaveric humerus	titanium suture anchors (Corkscrew FT 1 Suture Anchors, Arthrex, Naples, FL, USA)	66.8	$p < 0.001$

In fact, not only the material of the bone cement but also the injection method of bone cement has a great impact on the final biomechanical results. Braunstein et al. [64] drilled a hole first, then injected bone cement, and finally implanted an anchor. However, this method can easily lead to the extrusion of bone cement, which is not feasible in an arthroscopic setting. Aziz and colleagues [65] introduced a new bone cement injection method that used an open architecture-type anchor. This method allowed the operator to implant the anchor first and then directly inject bone cement through a cannulated in situ suture anchor with fenestrations. This anchor can make the bone cement interlace and bond with the surrounding bone better, increasing the surface area in contact with the bone, so it may have higher pullout strength. At the same time, we can limit the bone cement injection to the distal end of the anchor, which can effectively reduce the occurrence of bone cement extrusion and the thermal effect on the healing surface, thereby reducing the incidence of bone necrosis. In this way, the method can help to retain the bone quality and improve the pullout strength.

The experimental results of in vitro biomechanical studies also confirm the hypothesis above. Aziz and colleagues [65] reported that the pullout strength increased by 167% when bone cement was injected through an open architecture-type anchor, which was much higher than the pullout strength obtained by using the injection method of Braunstein et al. [64], which was only 45% to 47%, depending on the anatomic location.

3.3.3. Using All-Suture Anchors

The pullout strength of an all-suture anchor mainly depends on the thickness of cortical bone [66]. Therefore, preoperative cortical bone thickness evaluation and no decortication during operation are particularly important to improve the pullout strength of all-suture anchors.

There is controversy about comparisons of pullout strength between all-suture anchors and traditional anchors. Negra and colleagues found that the failure load of all-suture anchors is less than that of traditional anchors, and they also have a significantly greater rate of anchor pullout by various failure mechanisms than traditional anchors [46]. However, this conclusion still needs to be further verified in a representative repair model. On the contrary, Ntalos et al. [47] confirmed that all-suture anchors and conventional anchors have no significant difference in biomechanical effects, and their pullout strength is also similar.

All-suture anchors have a much smaller volume than the traditional screw-in anchors, which allows us to enhance the pullout strength of the repaired construct by implanting more all-suture anchors in the limited bone [67].

3.3.4. Increasing the Number of Suture Limbs

Shi et al. [68] found that when controlling for the number of sutures, using more suture limbs will result in a higher ultimate failure load. Conversely, when controlling for the number of sutured limbs, they found no significant differences among SR anchored, DR anchored, TOE, and transosseous repairs. In fact, they found that the number of sutures, the number of suture limbs, and the number of mattress stitches were more important in determining the overall strength than the suture structure.

3.3.5. Buddy Anchor Technique

As we know, in patients with osteoporosis, the inserted suture anchors are likely to be unstable. Thus, Brady and Burkhart [36] introduced the buddy anchor technique as a salvage technique: a second anchor is inserted adjacent to the loose anchor to create an interference fit and subsequent higher pullout strength [36,38]. As reported by Denard and Burkhart, the essential mechanism of the buddy anchor system is reinforcement of the pull-out strength by interference fit [69].

One biomechanical study by Horoz et al., supported this technique [38]. They found that in osteoporotic bone, two interlocking suture anchors were stronger than a single anchor. The pullout strength was increased by interlocking a second suture anchor with the first. However, another study contradicted this finding [44]. The opposing view was that placing the two anchors to overlap would reduce the anchor bone contact area and thus reduce the pullout strength [44]. However, the effectiveness of the buddy anchor technique was for the original loose anchor, and the study did not evaluate whether the use of the buddy anchor technique helped to enhance the fixation of the original loose anchor. These two studies were in vitro biomechanical, and more in vivo clinical studies are needed to demonstrate the effect of buddy screwing in the future.

Jung et al. [12] used the buddy screwing technique to augment repair in 16 patients who experienced intraoperative anchor pullout. Three patients had early postoperative failure after buddy screwing. They thought that placing another anchor in an enlarged area tended to result in instability. However, this study was not strictly a randomized controlled trial. The number of cases was also limited since intraoperative anchor pullout was uncommon.

3.3.6. Steinmann Pin Anchoring

Jung et al., invented a new anchor pullout management technique, bar anchoring with a threaded Steinmann pin (BASP) [12]. Using a threaded Steinmann pin (S-pin) (2.3 mm) and sutures, BASP was used to anchor pullouts during surgery. A threaded S-pin was trimmed to a length of 25–30 mm, and the center two-fifths of the S-pin were wrapped with three strands of a No. 2 high-strength suture and tied. A grasper was used to move the S-pin to the pullout site after its short part had been inserted through the anchor insertion portal. A specially made impactor was then attached to the end of the S-pin while being held below the cortical bone of the GT. The suture strands were then withdrawn to cause the S-pin to flip into the cancellous bone of the GT. Firm tension was gradually applied to the strands while observing the S-pin through the GT hole to ensure fixation. The three strands were attached to the S-pin using the Revo knot, a non-sliding knot, and were then used to repair the ruptured tendon.

In this study, the success rate of pullout management was 100% (13/13) for the BASP technique. At 6 months postoperatively, the tendon healing rate in patients undergoing BASP was 92.3% (12/13).

We can say that the BASP technique achieves satisfactory results both in terms of preventing suture anchor re-pullout and improving the tendon healing rate.

3.3.7. Using an Arthroscopic Transosseous Knotless Anchor

For arthroscopic rotator cuff repair, the most commonly used technology is TOE repair technology. It is not a real transosseous repair technology, and suture anchors are still needed, which means that this technology still brings a risk of anchor pullout, especially in elderly patients and patients with osteoporosis.

Therefore, some surgeons have developed an arthroscopic transosseous knotless (ATOK) anchor to realize true transosseous repair through arthroscopic technology. A noninferiority trial by Sandow and colleagues [70] showed that none of the 15 patients who received the ATOK anchor for rotator cuff repair had anchor displacement or anchor pullout.

Compared with the widely used TOE repair technology, ATOK anchor repair can potentially reduce the incidence of anchor pullout. The effect of this technology also needs to be validated by randomized controlled trials with larger sample sizes.

3.3.8. Transosseous Suture Repair Technology

The advent of suture anchors helped popularize arthroscopic rotator cuff repair due to the ease and speed of operation and their facilitation of instrumentation [20]. However, arthroscopic rotator cuff repair with suture anchors is not reliable for patients with osteoporosis, so some scholars have readopted transosseous suture repair. Of course, the current transosseous suture repair is not the same as the earlier arthrotomy but is performed under arthroscopy.

Randelli et al. [71] conducted a randomized controlled trial to compare the effectiveness of arthroscopic transosseous repair to single-row suture anchor repair. The two procedures produced equal results in terms of functional and radiological outcomes. Moreover, transosseous repair was found to reduce pain more quickly in the first month after surgery.

A matched cohort study by Srikumaran et al. [72] showed that in terms of patient-reported results, shoulder range of motion, and structural integrity, there are no differences between transosseous and transosseous equivalent suture-bridge rotator cuff repair procedures. The operating time was the same for all procedures. However, future randomized controlled trials are still needed to further demonstrate the equivalence of the two techniques.

These results demonstrate that arthroscopic transosseous repair can achieve the same results as arthroscopic rotator cuff repair with suture anchor in all aspects, and as a repair technique using only sutures without anchors, it can be used as an alternative treatment option for patients with anchor pullout. However, in patients with osteoporosis, suture cutting of the bone may also lead to failure of the repair.

In order to avoid bone cutting, some authors advise using a broader suture, such as a 2 mm tape, rather than the thinner No2 wire [73]. Due to its ideal viscoelastic properties [74] and broader contact surface with bone and soft tissue, this tape would exert the same force but less pressure at the contact region.

A cohort study by Beauchamp et al. [75] showed that arthroscopic transosseous repair using 2 mm tape material achieved significant mid-term functional improvement in this group of patients, with results statistically unaffected by larger tear size (>3 cm) or older age ($\geq$65 years), which also happen to be risk factors for anchor pullout after rotator cuff repair with suture anchor. Therefore, arthroscopic transosseous repair using 2 mm braided suture tape could be an alternative surgical option to reduce the risk of anchor pullout for these two types of patients.

4. Discussion and Clinical Inspirations

This review organizes the body of knowledge on anchor pullout through a literature review. However, there are still some issues that need to be addressed in this area.

There are very few studies on the incidence of anchor pullout. Although the overall incidence of anchor pullout is not too high [8–12], studies of pullout rates under certain conditions, such as in patients with poor bone quality, needed, which are important for clinicians' preoperative decision making.

Additionally, we present the risk factors for anchor pullout. The effect of bone quality on pullout strength is relatively well established, and clinical studies with larger sample sizes would provide stronger support for the existing view. For anchor material and design, anchor insertion angle and depth, the existing findings are mainly from in vitro biomechanical studies [30–40,46–48], which do not fully simulate the clinical situation, and more in vivo clinical studies are needed to confirm the existing findings in the future. The minimum distance (center-to-center) of suture anchors without decreasing the pullout strength varies with anchor diameter [44]. The available studies only tested two types of suture anchors rather than all commercially available suture anchors. The minimum distance between all suture anchors has not been reported yet. Since the level of evidence from existing studies is low, future randomized controlled trials are needed to evaluate the effect of rotator cuff tear size and CSIs on pullout strength [10,56].

The focus of this review is corresponding management for suture anchor pullout. For the anchor implantation site, Kirchhof and Sakamoto only evaluated the distribution of total bone mineral density in the greater tuberosity without performing the corresponding biomechanical tests, and their findings cannot be used as predictors of anchor pullout strength [5,59]. From this point of view, the conclusions of Tingart et al. [4] seem to be more credible. Their study showed that placing the anchor in the anterior and middle regions proximal to the GT resulted in an average load to failure 62% higher than placing it in the posterior region [20]. Prospective clinical trials are necessary to understand whether the available managements can reduce anchor pullout rates and improve patient prognosis. By comparing the in vitro biomechanical data, we found that PMMA bone cement provides greater pullout strength compared to various new bone cements, despite its various drawbacks [60,62,63]. For the bone cement injection method, the injection of bone cement through an open architecture-type anchor is also superior to the traditional method of drilling a hole first, then injecting bone cement, and finally implanting the anchor [64,65]. However, the arthroscopic application of this technique still needs to overcome some technical difficulties, which require additional in vivo clinical studies. When a patient is at high risk for anchor pullout, we can assess their cortical bone thickness preoperatively, and if the cortical bone quality is good, we can use all suture anchors for rotator cuff repair because they are small and can be implanted in greater numbers, which can improve the overall pullout strength [66,67]. Buddy screwing, BASP, and ATOK are three relatively new techniques. They are not only theoretically valid but have also been demonstrated in several studies. In fact, buddy anchor technique is a controversial technique. In the case of a small sample size, its in vivo application has a failure rate of 19% (3/16) [12], but it remains one of the few means of remedy in the event of intraoperative anchor pullout. In contrast, better pullout strength was achieved using the BASP technique and the ATOK anchor, and neither in vivo study reported anchor displacement or pullout [12,70]. However, these two techniques are more complex to perform, and in practice, buddy screwing remains a trusted and relatively simple remedy. However, neither of these studies were strict randomized controlled trials, nor was the sample size large enough [1,36,38,44,69,70]. Relatively speaking, arthroscopic transosseous suture repair is a more established technique. Its equivalence to suture anchor repair was also confirmed by a randomized controlled trial [71]. Arthroscopic transosseous suture repair does not involve the use of suture anchors at all, which is very suitable for patients at high risk of anchor pullout. However, this technique also presents a new problem; that is, the sutures may cut the osteoporotic bone, leading to repair failure. However, there are no studies on the probability of anchor pullout and bone cutting with suture anchor repair and transosseous suture repair for the same bone quality, respectively. Some cohort studies suggest that the use of wider sutures may reduce the risk of transosseous suture repair failure [73–75]. However, due to the uncertainty about the incidence of bone cutting, in vitro biomechanical studies using a severe osteoporosis model may help to increase positive results and thus help us better evaluate the effectiveness of this approach.

In conclusion, not many of the management techniques have been widely used in clinical practice. Since most are derived from in vitro biomechanical studies, in vivo randomized controlled trials with larger sample sizes are needed to confirm whether they can ultimately benefit patients.

Author Contributions: Conceptualization, X.L. and M.N.; methodology, X.L.; writing—original draft preparation, X.L. and Y.X.; writing—review and editing, X.L., Y.X., H.S., X.S. and M.N. All authors have read and agreed to the published version of the manuscript.

Funding: This work is supported by research funding from the National Natural Science Foundation of China (No.82002307), Natural Science Foundation of Chongqing (cstc2021jcyj-msxmX0121). Mao Nie and Xianding Sun was supported by the Kuanren Talents Program of the second affiliated hospital of Chongqing Medical University.

Institutional Review Board Statement: Not applicable.

Informed Consent Statement: Not applicable.

Data Availability Statement: No new data were created or analyzed in this study. Data sharing is not applicable to this article.

Conflicts of Interest: The authors declare no conflict of interest.

References

1. Colvin, A.C.; Egorova, N.; Harrison, A.K.; Moskowitz, A.; Flatow, E.L. National Trends in Rotator Cuff Repair. *J. Bone Jt. Surg.* **2012**, *94*, 227–233. [CrossRef] [PubMed]
2. Harryman, D.T., 2nd; Hettrich, C.M.; Smith, K.L.; Campbell, B.; Sidles, J.A.; Matsen, F.A., 3rd. A prospective multipractice investigation of patients with full-thickness rotator cuff tears: The importance of comorbidities, practice, and other covariables on self-assessed shoulder function and health status. *J. Bone Jt. Surg. Am.* **2003**, *85*, 690–696. [CrossRef]
3. Barber, F.A.; Herbert, M.A. Cyclic Loading Biomechanical Analysis of the Pullout Strengths of Rotator Cuff and Glenoid Anchors: 2013 Update. *Arthrosc. J. Arthrosc. Relat. Surg.* **2013**, *29*, 832–844. [CrossRef] [PubMed]
4. Tingart, M.J.; Apreleva, M.; Lehtinen, J.; Zurakowski, D.; Warner, J.J. Anchor design and bone mineral density affect the pull-out strength of suture anchors in rotator cuff repair: Which anchors are best to use in patients with low bone quality? *Am. J. Sports Med.* **2004**, *32*, 1466–1473. [CrossRef] [PubMed]
5. Kirchhoff, C.; Braunstein, V.; Milz, S.; Sprecher, C.M.; Fischer, F.; Tami, A.; Ahrens, P.; Imhoff, A.B.; Hinterwimmer, S. Assessment of bone quality within the tuberosities of the osteoporotic humeral head: Relevance for anchor positioning in rotator cuff repair. *Am. J. Sports Med.* **2010**, *38*, 564–569. [CrossRef] [PubMed]
6. Tingart, M.J.; Bouxsein, M.L.; Zurakowski, D.; Warner, J.P.; Apreleva, M. Three-dimensional distribution of bone density in the proximal humerus. *Calcif. Tissue Res.* **2003**, *73*, 531–536. [CrossRef]

7. Djurasovic, M.; Marra, G.; Arroyo, J.S.; Pollock, R.G.; Flatow, E.L.; Bigliani, L.U. Revision Rotator Cuff Repair: Factors Influencing Results. *J. Bone Jt. Surg.* **2001**, *83*, 1849–1855. [CrossRef]
8. Cummins, C.A.; Murrell, G.A. Mode of failure for rotator cuff repair with suture anchors identified at revision surgery. *J. Shoulder Elb. Surg.* **2003**, *12*, 128–133. [CrossRef]
9. Skaliczki, G.; Paladini, P.; Merolla, G.; Campi, F.; Porcellini, G. Early anchor displacement after arthroscopic rotator cuff repair. *Int. Orthop.* **2015**, *39*, 915–920. [CrossRef]
10. Benson, E.C.; MacDermid, J.C.; Drosdowech, D.S.; Athwal, G.S. The Incidence of Early Metallic Suture Anchor Pullout After Arthroscopic Rotator Cuff Repair. *Arthrosc. J. Arthrosc. Relat. Surg.* **2010**, *26*, 310–315. [CrossRef]
11. Dezaly, C.; Sirveaux, F.; Philippe, R.; Wein-Remy, F.; Sedaghatian, J.; Roche, O.; Molé, D. Arthroscopic treatment of rotator cuff tear in the over-60s: Repair is preferable to isolated acromioplasty-tenotomy in the short term. *Orthop. Traumatol. Surg. Res.* **2011**, *97*, S125–S130. [CrossRef] [PubMed]
12. Jung, W.; Kim, D.O.; Kim, J.; Kim, S.H. Novel and reproducible technique coping with intraoperative anchor pullout during arthroscopic rotator cuff repair. *Knee Surg. Sports Traumatol. Arthrosc.* **2020**, *29*, 223–229. [CrossRef] [PubMed]
13. Pietschmann, M.F.; Fröhlich, V.; Ficklscherer, A.; Gülecyüz, M.F.; Wegener, B.; Jansson, V.; Müller, P.E. Suture anchor fixation strength in osteopenic versus non-osteopenic bone for rotator cuff repair. *Arch. Orthop. Trauma Surg.* **2009**, *129*, 373–379. [CrossRef] [PubMed]
14. Clevenger, T.A.; Beebe, M.J.; Strauss, E.J.; Kubiak, E.N. The Effect of Insertion Angle on the Pullout Strength of Threaded Suture Anchors: A Validation of the Deadman Theory. *Arthrosc. J. Arthrosc. Relat. Surg.* **2014**, *30*, 900–905. [CrossRef]
15. Bynum, C.K.; Lee, S.; Mahar, A.; Tasto, J.; Pedowitz, R. Failure mode of suture anchors as a function of insertion depth. *Am. J. Sports Med.* **2005**, *33*, 1030–1034. [CrossRef]
16. Nagamoto, H.; Yamamoto, N.; Sano, H.; Itoi, E. A biomechanical study on suture anchor insertion angle: Which is better, 90° or 45°? *J. Orthop. Sci.* **2017**, *22*, 56–62. [CrossRef]
17. Barber, F.A.; Hapa, O.; Bynum, J.A. Comparative Testing by Cyclic Loading of Rotator Cuff Suture Anchors Containing Multiple High-Strength Sutures. *Arthrosc. J. Arthrosc. Relat. Surg.* **2010**, *26*, S134–S141. [CrossRef]
18. Bisbinas, I.; Magnissalis, E.A.; Gigis, I.; Beslikas, T.; Hatzokos, I.; Christoforidis, I. Suture anchors, properties versus material and design: A biomechanical study in ovine model. *Eur. J. Orthop. Surg. Traumatol.* **2010**, *21*, 95–100. [CrossRef]
19. Mahar, A.T.; Tucker, B.S.; Upasani, V.V.; Oka, R.S.; Pedowitz, R.A. Increasing the insertion depth of suture anchors for rotator cuff repair does not improve biomechanical stability. *J. Shoulder Elbow Surg.* **2005**, *14*, 626–630. [CrossRef]
20. Tingart, M.J.; Apreleva, M.; Zurakowski, D.; Warner, J.J. Pullout strength of suture anchors used in rotator cuff repair. *J. Bone Jt. Surg.* **2003**, *85*, 2190–2198. [CrossRef]
21. Brand, J.C., Jr.; Pienkowski, D.; Steenlage, E.; Hamilton, D.; Johnson, D.L.; Caborn, D.N. Interference screw fixation strength of a quadrupled hamstring tendon graft is directly related to bone mineral density and insertion torque. *Am. J. Sports Med.* **2000**, *28*, 705–710. [CrossRef] [PubMed]
22. Poukalova, M.; Yakacki, C.M.; Guldberg, R.E.; Lin, A.; Saing, M.; Gillogly, S.D.; Gall, K. Pullout strength of suture anchors: Effect of mechanical properties of trabecular bone. *J. Biomech.* **2010**, *43*, 1138–1145. [CrossRef] [PubMed]
23. Yakacki, C.M.; Poukalova, M.; Guldberg, R.E.; Lin, A.; Saing, M.; Gillogly, S.; Gall, K. The effect of the trabecular microstructure on the pullout strength of suture anchors. *J. Biomech.* **2010**, *43*, 1953–1959. [CrossRef]
24. Yamada, M.; Briot, J.; Pedrono, A.; Sans, N.; Mansat, P.; Mansat, M.; Swider, P. Age- and gender-related distribution of bone tissue of osteoporotic humeral head using computed tomography. *J. Shoulder Elb. Surg.* **2007**, *16*, 596–602. [CrossRef] [PubMed]
25. Martinel, V.; Bonnevialle, N. Contribution of postoperative ultrasound to early detection of anchor pullout after rotator cuff tendon repair: Report of 3 cases. *Orthop. Traumatol. Surg. Res.* **2020**, *106*, 229–234. [CrossRef] [PubMed]
26. Yamakado, K.; Katsuo, S.-I.; Mizuno, K.; Arakawa, H.; Hayashi, S. Medial-Row Failure After Arthroscopic Double-Row Rotator Cuff Repair. *Arthrosc. J. Arthrosc. Relat. Surg.* **2010**, *26*, 430–435. [CrossRef]
27. Barber, F.A.; Coons, D.A.; Ruiz-Suarez, M. Cyclic Load Testing of Biodegradable Suture Anchors Containing 2 High-Strength Sutures. *Arthrosc. J. Arthrosc. Relat. Surg.* **2007**, *23*, 355–360. [CrossRef] [PubMed]
28. Deakin, M.; Stubbs, D.; Bruce, W.; Goldberg, J.; Gillies, R.M.; Walsh, W.R. Suture Strength and Angle of Load Application in a Suture Anchor Eyelet. *Arthrosc. J. Arthrosc. Relat. Surg.* **2005**, *21*, 1447–1451. [CrossRef]
29. Meyer, D.C.; Fucentese, S.F.; Ruffieux, K.; Jacob, H.A.; Gerber, C. Mechanical testing of absorbable suture anchors. *Arthrosc. J. Arthrosc. Relat. Surg.* **2003**, *19*, 188–193. [CrossRef]
30. Dhawan, A.; Ghodadra, N.; Karas, V.; Salata, M.J.; Cole, B.J. Complications of Bioabsorbable Suture Anchors in the Shoulder. *Am. J. Sports Med.* **2011**, *40*, 1424–1430. [CrossRef]
31. Park, A.Y.; Hatch, J.D. Proximal humerus osteolysis after revision rotator cuff repair with bioabsorbable suture anchors. *Am. J. Orthop.* **2011**, *40*, 139–141. [PubMed]
32. Glueck, D.; Wilson, T.C.; Johnson, D.L. Extensive Osteolysis after Rotator Cuff Repair with a Bioabsorbable Suture Anchor: A Case Report. *Am. J. Sports Med.* **2005**, *33*, 742–744. [CrossRef] [PubMed]
33. Park, J.-Y.; Jang, S.-H.; Oh, K.-S.; Li, Y.J. Radiolucent rings around bioabsorbable anchors after rotator cuff repair are not associated with clinical outcomes. *Arch. Orthop. Trauma Surg.* **2017**, *137*, 1539–1546. [CrossRef] [PubMed]

34. Haneveld, H.; Hug, K.; Diederichs, G.; Scheibel, M.; Gerhardt, C. Arthroscopic double-row repair of the rotator cuff: A comparison of bio-absorbable and non-resorbable anchors regarding osseous reaction. *Knee Surg. Sports Traumatol. Arthrosc.* **2013**, *21*, 1647–1654. [CrossRef]
35. Chae, S.-W.; Kang, J.-Y.; Lee, J.; Han, S.-H.; Kim, S.-Y. Effect of structural design on the pullout strength of suture anchors for rotator cuff repair. *J. Orthop. Res.* **2018**, *36*, 3318–3327. [CrossRef]
36. Brady, P.C.; Arrigoni, P.; Burkhart, S.S. What do you do when you have a loose screw? *Arthroscopy* **2006**, *22*, 925–930. [CrossRef]
37. Yakacki, C.M.; Griffis, J.; Poukalova, M.; Gall, K. Bearing area: A new indication for suture anchor pullout strength? *J. Orthop. Res.* **2009**, *27*, 1048–1054. [CrossRef]
38. Horoz, L.; Hapa, O.; Barber, F.A.; Hüsemoğlu, B.; Özkan, M.; Havitçioğlu, H. Suture Anchor Fixation in Osteoporotic Bone: A Biomechanical Study in an Ovine Model. *Arthroscopy* **2017**, *33*, 68–74. [CrossRef]
39. Kang, Y.G.; Kim, J.-H.; Shin, J.-W.; Baik, J.-M.; Choo, H.-J. Induction of bone ingrowth with a micropore bioabsorbable suture anchor in rotator cuff tear: An experimental study in a rabbit model. *J. Shoulder Elb. Surg.* **2013**, *22*, 1558–1566. [CrossRef]
40. Green, R.N.; Donaldson, O.W.; Dafydd, M.; Evans, S.L.; Kulkarni, R. Biomechanical study: Determining the optimum insertion angle for screw-in suture anchors-is deadman's angle correct? *Arthroscopy* **2014**, *30*, 1535–1539. [CrossRef]
41. Sano, H.; Takahashi, A.; Chiba, D.; Hatta, T.; Yamamoto, N.; Itoi, E. Stress distribution inside bone after suture anchor insertion: Simulation using a three-dimensional finite element method. *Knee Surg. Sports Traumatol. Arthrosc.* **2012**, *21*, 1777–1782. [CrossRef] [PubMed]
42. Pietschmann, M.F.; Gülecyüz, M.F.; Fieseler, S.; Hentschel, M.; Rossbach, B.; Jansson, V.; Müller, P.E. Biomechanical stability of knotless suture anchors used in rotator cuff repair in healthy and osteopenic bone. *Arthroscopy* **2010**, *26*, 1035–1044. [CrossRef]
43. Gülecyüz, M.; Bortolotti, H.; Pietschmann, M.; Ficklscherer, A.; Niethammer, T.; Roßbach, B.; Müller, P. Primary stability of rotator cuff repair: Can more suture materials yield more strength? *Int. Orthop.* **2016**, *40*, 989–997. [CrossRef]
44. Kawakami, J.; Yamamoto, N.; Nagamoto, H.; Itoi, E. Minimum Distance of Suture Anchors Used for Rotator Cuff Repair Without Decreasing the Pullout Strength: A Biomechanical Study. *Arthrosc. J. Arthrosc. Relat. Surg.* **2018**, *34*, 377–385. [CrossRef] [PubMed]
45. Chapman, J.R.; Harrington, R.M.; Lee, K.M.; Anderson, P.A.; Tencer, A.F.; Kowalski, D. Factors affecting the pullout strength of cancellous bone screws. *J. Biomech. Eng.* **1996**, *118*, 391–398. [CrossRef] [PubMed]
46. Nagra, N.S.; Zargar, N.; Smith, R.D.J.; Carr, A.J. Mechanical properties of all-suture anchors for rotator cuff repair. *Bone Jt. Res.* **2017**, *6*, 82–89. [CrossRef] [PubMed]
47. Ntalos, D.; Sellenschloh, K.; Huber, G.; Briem, D.; Püschel, K.; Morlock, M.M.; Frosch, K.-H.; Fensky, F.; Klatte, T.O. Conventional rotator cuff versus all-suture anchors—A biomechanical study focusing on the insertion angle in an unlimited cyclic model. *PLoS ONE* **2019**, *14*, e0225648. [CrossRef]
48. Fleischli, J.E. Editorial Commentary: Biomechanics of All Suture Anchors: What We Know So Far. *Arthrosc. J. Arthrosc. Relat. Surg.* **2018**, *34*, 2796–2798. [CrossRef]
49. Strauss, E.; Frank, D.; Kubiak, E.; Kummer, F.; Rokito, A. The effect of the angle of suture anchor insertion on fixation failure at the tendon-suture interface after rotator cuff repair: Deadman's angle revisited. *Arthroscopy* **2009**, *25*, 597–602. [CrossRef]
50. Barber, F.A.; Cawley, P.; Prudich, J.F. Suture anchor failure strength—An in vivo study. *Arthrosc. J. Arthrosc. Relat. Surg.* **1993**, *9*, 647–652. [CrossRef]
51. De Carli, A.; Vadalà, A.; Monaco, E.; Labianca, L.; Zanzotto, E.; Ferretti, A. Effect of cyclic loading on new polyblend suture coupled with different anchors. *Am. J. Sports Med.* **2005**, *33*, 214–219. [CrossRef] [PubMed]
52. Burkhart, S.S. The deadman theory of suture anchors: Observations along a south Texas fence line. *Arthroscopy* **1995**, *11*, 119–123. [CrossRef]
53. Itoi, E.; Nagamoto, H.; Sano, H.; Yamamoto, N.; Kawakami, J. Deadman theory revisited12. *Bio-Med. Mater. Eng.* **2016**, *27*, 171–181. [CrossRef] [PubMed]
54. Nagamoto, H.; Yamamoto, N.; Itoi, E. Effect of anchor threads on the pullout strength: A biomechanical study. *J. Orthop.* **2018**, *15*, 878–881. [CrossRef] [PubMed]
55. Kirchhoff, C.; Kirchhoff, S.; Sprecher, C.M.; Ahrens, P.; Imhoff, A.B.; Hinterwimmer, S.; Milz, S.; Braunstein, V. X-treme CT analysis of cancellous bone at the rotator cuff insertion in human individuals with osteoporosis: Superficial versus deep quality. *Arch. Orthop. Trauma. Surg.* **2012**, *133*, 381–387. [CrossRef] [PubMed]
56. Puzzitiello, R.N.; Patel, B.H.; Forlenza, E.M.; Nwachukwu, B.U.; Allen, A.A.; Forsythe, B.; Salzler, M.J. Adverse Impact of Corticosteroids on Rotator Cuff Tendon Health and Repair: A Systematic Review of Basic Science Studies. *Arthrosc. Sports Med. Rehabilitation* **2020**, *2*, e161–e169. [CrossRef]
57. Boileau, P.; Brassart, N.; Watkinson, D.J.; Carles, M.; Hatzidakis, A.M.; Krishnan, S.G. Arthroscopic repair of full-thickness tears of the supraspinatus: Does the tendon really heal? *J. Bone Jt. Surg. Am.* **2005**, *87*, 1229–1240. [CrossRef]
58. Duquin, T.R.; Buyea, C.; Bisson, L.J. Which method of rotator cuff repair leads to the highest rate of structural healing? A systematic review. *Am. J. Sports Med.* **2010**, *38*, 835–841. [CrossRef]
59. Sakamoto, Y.; Kido, A.; Inoue, K.; Sakurai, G.; Hashiuchi, T.; Munemoto, M.; Tanaka, Y. In vivo microstructural analysis of the humeral greater tuberosity in patients with rotator cuff tears using multidetector row computed tomography. *BMC Musculoskelet. Disord.* **2014**, *15*, 351. [CrossRef]
60. Oshtory, R.; Lindsey, D.P.; Giori, N.J.; Mirza, F.M. Bioabsorbable Tricalcium Phosphate Bone Cement Strengthens Fixation of Suture Anchors. *Clin. Orthop. Relat. Res.* **2010**, *468*, 3406–3412. [CrossRef]

61. Giori, N.J.; Sohn, D.H.; Mirza, F.M.; Lindsey, D.P.; Lee, A.T. Bone Cement Improves Suture Anchor Fixation. *Clin. Orthop. Relat. Res.* **2006**, *451*, 236–241. [CrossRef] [PubMed]
62. Postl, L.K.; Ahrens, P.; Beirer, M.; Crönlein, M.; Imhoff, A.B.; Foehr, P.; Burgkart, R.; Braun, C.; Kirchhoff, C. Pull-out stability of anchors for rotator cuff repair is also increased by bio-absorbable augmentation: A cadaver study. *Arch. Orthop. Trauma. Surg.* **2016**, *136*, 1153–1158. [CrossRef] [PubMed]
63. Kafchitsas, K.; Geiger, F.; Rauschmann, M.; Schmidt, S. Zementverteilung bei Vertebroplastieschrauben unterschiedlichen Designs [Cement distribution in vertebroplasty pedicle screws with different designs]. *Orthopade* **2010**, *39*, 679–686. [CrossRef] [PubMed]
64. Braunstein, V.; Ockert, B.; Windolf, M.; Sprecher, C.M.; Mutschler, W.; Imhoff, A.; Postl, L.K.L.; Biberthaler, P.; Kirchhoff, C. Increasing pullout strength of suture anchors in osteoporotic bone using augmentation—A cadaver study. *Clin. Biomech.* **2015**, *30*, 243–247. [CrossRef]
65. Aziz, K.; Shi, B.Y.; Okafor, L.C.; Smalley, J.; Belkoff, S.M.; Srikumaran, U. Pullout strength of standard vs. cement-augmented rotator cuff repair anchors in cadaveric bone. *Clin. Biomech.* **2018**, *54*, 132–136. [CrossRef]
66. Ntalos, D.; Huber, G.; Sellenschloh, K.; Saito, H.; Püschel, K.; Morlock, M.M.; Frosch, K.H.; Klatte, T.O. All-suture anchor pullout results in decreased bone damage and depends on cortical thickness. *Knee Surg. Sports Traumatol. Arthrosc.* **2020**, *29*, 2212–2219. [CrossRef]
67. Oh, J.H.; Jeong, H.J.; Yang, S.H.; Rhee, S.-M.; Itami, Y.; McGarry, M.H.; Lee, T.Q. Pullout Strength of All-Suture Anchors: Effect of the Insertion and Traction Angle—A Biomechanical Study. *Arthrosc. J. Arthrosc. Relat. Surg.* **2018**, *34*, 2784–2795. [CrossRef]
68. Shi, B.Y.; Diaz, M.; Binkley, M.; McFarland, E.G.; Srikumaran, U. Biomechanical Strength of Rotator Cuff Repairs: A Systematic Review and Meta-regression Analysis of Cadaveric Studies. *Am. J. Sports Med.* **2018**, *47*, 1984–1993. [CrossRef]
69. Denard, P.J.; Burkhart, S.S. Techniques for Managing Poor Quality Tissue and Bone During Arthroscopic Rotator Cuff Repair. *Arthrosc. J. Arthrosc. Relat. Surg.* **2011**, *27*, 1409–1421. [CrossRef]
70. Sandow, M.J.; Schutz, C.R. Arthroscopic rotator cuff repair using a transosseous knotless anchor (ATOK). *J. Shoulder Elb. Surg.* **2019**, *29*, 527–533. [CrossRef]
71. Randelli, P.; Stoppani, C.A.; Zaolino, C.; Menon, A.; Randelli, F.; Cabitza, P. Advantages of Arthroscopic Rotator Cuff Repair With a Transosseous Suture Technique: A Prospective Randomized Controlled Trial. *Am. J. Sports Med.* **2017**, *45*, 2000–2009. [CrossRef]
72. Srikumaran, U.; Huish, E.G.; Shi, B.Y.; Hannan, C.V.; Ali, I.; Kilcoyne, K.G. Anchorless Arthroscopic Transosseous and Anchored Arthroscopic Transosseous Equivalent Rotator Cuff Repair Show No Differences in Structural Integrity or Patient-reported Outcomes in a Matched Cohort. *Clin. Orthop. Relat. Res.* **2020**, *478*, 1295–1303. [CrossRef] [PubMed]
73. Chillemi, C.; Mantovani, M.; Osimani, M.; Castagna, A. Arthroscopic transosseous rotator cuff repair: The eight-shape technique. *Eur. J. Orthop. Surg. Traumatol.* **2017**, *27*, 399–404. [CrossRef] [PubMed]
74. Taha, M.E.; Schneider, K.; Clarke, E.C.; O'Briain, D.E.; Smith, M.M.; Cunningham, G.; Cass, B.; Young, A.A. A Biomechanical Comparison of Different Suture Materials Used for Arthroscopic Shoulder Procedures. *Arthrosc. J. Arthrosc. Relat. Surg.* **2020**, *36*, 708–713. [CrossRef] [PubMed]
75. Beauchamp, J.; Beauchamp, M. Functional outcomes of arthroscopic transosseous rotator cuff repair using a 2-mm tape suture in a 137-patient cohort. *JSES Int.* **2021**, *5*, 1105–1110. [CrossRef]

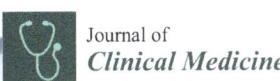

Review

Clinical Application of Gait Retraining in the Injured Runner

Logan W. Gaudette [1], Molly M. Bradach [1], José Roberto de Souza Junior [1,2], Bryan Heiderscheit [3], Caleb D. Johnson [1,4], Joshua Posilkin [1], Mitchell J. Rauh [5], Lauren K. Sara [1], Lindsay Wasserman [1], Karsten Hollander [6] and Adam S. Tenforde [1,*]

1. Spaulding Rehabilitation Hospital, Spaulding National Running Center, Department of Physical Medicine and Rehabilitation, Harvard Medical School, Boston, MA 02138, USA
2. Graduate Program of Sciences and Technologies in Health, University of Brasilia, Brasilia 72220-275, DF, Brazil
3. Department of Orthopedics and Rehabilitation, University of Wisconsin, Madison, WI 53706, USA
4. United States Army Research Institute for Environmental Medicine, Military Performance Division, Natick, MA 01760, USA
5. Doctor of Physical Therapy Program, San Diego State University, San Diego, CA 92182, USA
6. Institute of Interdisciplinary Exercise Science and Sports Medicine, Faculty of Medicine, MSH, Medical School Hamburg, 20457 Hamburg, Germany
* Correspondence: atenforde@mgh.harvard.edu; Tel.: +1-617-952-6804

Abstract: Despite its positive influence on physical and mental wellbeing, running is associated with a high incidence of musculoskeletal injury. Potential modifiable risk factors for running-related injury have been identified, including running biomechanics. Gait retraining is used to address these biomechanical risk factors in injured runners. While recent systematic reviews of biomechanical risk factors for running-related injury and gait retraining have been conducted, there is a lack of information surrounding the translation of gait retraining for injured runners into clinical settings. Gait retraining studies in patients with patellofemoral pain syndrome have shown a decrease in pain and increase in functionality through increasing cadence, decreasing hip adduction, transitioning to a non-rearfoot strike pattern, increasing forward trunk lean, or a combination of some of these techniques. This literature suggests that gait retraining could be applied to the treatment of other injuries in runners, although there is limited evidence to support this specific to other running-related injuries. Components of successful gait retraining to treat injured runners with running-related injuries are presented.

Keywords: gait retraining; running-related injuries; kinetics; kinematics; rehabilitation

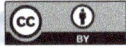

1. Background

The sport of running has positive effects on both physical [1] and mental [2] wellbeing. Unfortunately, runners experience a high rate of running-related injuries (RRIs). While reports of incidence rate vary depending on the population, up to 79% of recreational runners suffer a RRI each year [3]. In addition, RRIs have a high rate of recurrence. For example, female youth runners with a history of bone stress injury (BSI) have a 5 times elevated risk of sustaining a subsequent BSI [4]. Similar rates of injury reoccurrence were found in high school cross country runners [5].

Prior research has characterized risk factors for RRI. Of those that are modifiable, risk factors include neuromuscular, kinetic, kinematic, and spatiotemporal variables. While muscle weakness and imbalance may contribute to RRIs [6], strengthening alone may be insufficient for modifying biomechanical abnormalities that contribute to RRI [7]. Several variables related to running mechanics are thought to be related to injury and are frequent targets of intervention, including hip adduction [8,9], trunk lean [10,11], vertical loading rates [12–18], and step rate [19–22].

Gait retraining has been described as a method to change running biomechanics contributing to a given RRI [23]. Gait retraining using external feedback was first described in patients following stroke [24]. It used concepts of motor learning for both acquisition and transfer phases and resulted in sustained improvements in hemiparetic gait. These concepts have since been applied to the management of RRIs by addressing a variety of aspects related to gait mechanics. Gait retraining typically involves the use of devices to measure the targeted biomechanical variable and provide external visual, verbal, or auditory cues to facilitate change. These external cues are described as biofeedback, and a faded biofeedback design refers to gradual reduction in external cues to promote learning of a new desired movement pattern without further feedback [24].

For gait retraining to be effective, biomechanical risk factors associated with RRI must be properly identified, and, if possible, addressed appropriately during treatment. The results of a recent systematic review and meta-analysis, which evaluated different forms of gait retraining [23], suggest that the literature surrounding gait retraining is occasionally inconsistent and largely inconclusive. There is need for a more easily digestible guide for clinicians seeking to implement gait retraining in the treatment of injured runners. The purpose of this narrative review is to provide a practical overview of what is known on biomechanical risk factors for RRI, gait retraining strategies to alter these risk factors, and provide clinical practical application of this knowledge.

2. Methods

This narrative review included studies related to the following topics: (I) Biomechanical risk factors for RRI, and (II) Gait retraining for runners with RRI. No restrictions were placed on language, publication date, participant age, gender, and duration of symptoms or stage of disease. Articles were excluded if: (I) running was not the primary focus of the study; (II) there was not a clear description of the gait retraining protocol used; (III) feedback was not removed after gait retraining to determine if gait adjustments could be maintained; (IV) the protocol did not use multiple sessions to allow for motor learning to occur. Additionally, studies that were not presented as a full manuscript (i.e., abstracts) were excluded. PubMed and EMBASE were the databases used. The date of the last search was 30 June 2022. Subject headings, synonyms, relevant terms, and variant spellings of three concepts (running biomechanics; gait retraining; running-related injuries) were used for the searches on each database. This strategy was used for each database with the appropriate truncation. All references were imported into Mendeley Reference Manager (Version 2.65.0), and duplicates were removed. The screening of eligible studies was performed in two steps: (I) screening the titles and abstracts, and (II) screening the full texts. List of references of the retrieved studies were searched to identify additional publications. Eligibility assessment was performed by two reviewers (LWG and MB). Disagreements were resolved by discussion between the two review authors. If no agreement could be reached, a final arbitration was performed by a third independent reviewer (AST). Relevant information was organized using the following topics: (I) Biomechanical risk factors for RRI; (II) Gait retraining overview; (III) Interventions characterizing gait retraining variables; (IV) Clinical application of gait retraining; (V) Limitation of current gait retraining strategies.

3. Biomechanical Risk Factors for Running-Related Injury (RRI)

Two recent systematic reviews of prospective studies have examined potential biomechanical risk factors for RRI [25,26]. Both reviews concluded that there was not strong evidence for a single biomechanical variable as a risk factor for all RRIs. The lack of an association between biomechanical variables and grouped RRI indicates the importance of investigating injury-specific biomechanical risk factors for RRI.

A recent systemic review examined biomechanical risk factors for several common RRIs including hamstring tendinopathy, patellofemoral pain syndrome (PFPS), patellar tendinopathy, iliotibial band syndrome, medial tibial stress syndrome, tibial stress fractures, Achilles tendinopathy, and plantar fasciitis [27]. Criteria for inclusion of a biomechanical risk factor in the study was a significant difference from a control group in one prospective study or two retrospective studies [27]. Levels of evidence for biomechanical risk factors for specific RRIs varied from conflicting evidence to moderate evidence.

The strongest evidence supported decreased braking impulse [28,29] and increased ground contact time [28,29] for PFPS, increased duration of rearfoot eversion angle [30,31] and increased contralateral pelvic drop angle [30,32] for medial tibial stress syndrome, and increased average [33,34] and instantaneous loading rate [33,35] of vertical ground reaction force for plantar fasciitis. Each biomechanical variable was observed to have moderate evidence as risk factors for specific RRIs. More limited evidence was found for biomechanical risk factors for Achilles tendinopathy and tibial stress fractures, and very limited evidence was found for iliotibial band syndrome. No biomechanical variables met the study criteria for inclusion for patellar tendinopathy and hamstring tendinopathy. Definitions of potential biomechanical risk factors can be found below in Table 1.

Table 1. Definitions of key biomechanical variables.

Variable Name	Variable Definition
Vertical Impact Peak (VIP)	The local maximum found between initial foot strike and the maximum ground reaction force [12]
Vertical Average Loading Rate (VALR)	Slope of the ground reaction force curve from 20% to 80% of the vertical impact peak, measured in body weights per second (BW/s) [12]
Vertical Instantaneous Loading Rate (VILR)	Maximum slope of the ground reaction force curve from 20% to 80% of the vertical impact peak, measured in BW/s [12]
Braking Impulse	A measure of the total force applied in the posterior direction during stance phase. Area under the anteroposterior ground reaction force curve from initial contact until midstance [36]
Peak Tibial Acceleration	Maximum tibial acceleration at time of initial contact (also known as "impacts") [12]

4. Gait Retraining Overview

A narrative review published in 2020 evaluated the use of gait retraining as an intervention for PFPS [37]. The review included mostly case series or studies that did not contain a control group. Most biomechanical interventions included in the review, specifically decreasing hip adduction, increasing trunk lean, transitioning from a rearfoot strike (RFS) to a forefoot strike pattern, and increasing cadence, resulted in a reduction of pain [37]. The review also concluded that greater gait retraining session volume and a faded feedback design resulted in better outcomes compared to studies without a faded feedback design.

While a previous systematic review conducted in 2015 found foot strike manipulation had the greatest effect on kinematic measures and live feedback of tibial acceleration had the greatest effect on kinetic measures [38], a more recent systematic review and meta-analysis of gait retraining by Doyle et al. [23], which included only randomized controlled trials, concluded that the best evidence for gait retraining for runners supported step rate-based gait retraining. Though it achieved only moderate evidence, step rate-based gait retraining was shown to increase step rate, decrease stride length, decrease peak hip adduction (HADD) during stance, increase footstrike angle at initial contact and decrease VALR and VILR. Moderate evidence was also found for the ability of tibial acceleration based gait retraining to lower VILR.

While some gait retraining studies have reported a decrease in pain and improvement in functional outcomes in patients that underwent gait retraining, an insufficient number of studies reported pain measurements or clinical outcomes compared to a control group for inclusion in the systematic review and meta-analysis for conclusions regarding the effectiveness of gait retraining on patient pain or clinical outcomes to be made [23]. A summary of gait retraining studies and their effect on various clinical and biomechanical outcome variables can be seen in Table 2.

Table 2. Overview of Gait Retraining Studies.

	Adjusted Variable	Feedback	Subjects	Retraining Design	Outcomes
Noehren et al., 2011 [8]	HADD	Visual display and verbal cues	10 female runners with PFPS and high HADD	Faded, 8 sessions over 2 weeks	86% reduction in pain with 11-point increase in LEFI. Significant reduction in HADD and contralateral pelvic drop. All changes persisted at 1-month follow-up
Willy et al., 2012 [9]	HADD	Visual feedback from mirror and verbal cues	10 female runners with PFPS	Faded, 8 sessions over 2 weeks	Reduced HADD, thigh adduction and contralateral pelvic drop. All changes persisted at the 1- and 3-month follow-ups, although HADD increased from post-trial to 1- and 3-month follow-ups
Esculier et al., 2018 [19]	Step rate	Not clear	69 runners with PFPS	Not faded, 5 sessions over 8 weeks	No difference in KOS-ADLS scores between runners who received both education and gait retraining compared to runners who only received education on load management
Willy et al., 2016 [20]	Step rate	Visual feedback from Garmin Forerunner	30 healthy runners with high loading rates	Faded, 8 runs, no feedback on 4th, 6th or 8th run	Significant increase in step rate, significant reduction in VALR, VILR, HADD and knee eccentric work
Baumgartner et al., 2019 [21]	Step rate	Visual feedback from watch	38 healthy runners, step rate <170	Not faded	Significant increase in step rate from 79.9 +/− 4.8 to 86.8 +/− 5.7 strides per leg per minute
Crowell and Davis 2011 [12]	Tibial acceleration	Visual feedback	10 healthy RFS runners with high tibial acceleration	Faded, 8 sessions over 2 weeks	Significant reductions in tibial acceleration, VALR, VILR that persisted at 1-month follow-up
Clansey et al., 2014 [13]	Tibial acceleration	Visual feedback	22 healthy RFS male runners with high tibial accelerations	Not faded, 6 sessions over 3 weeks	Significant reductions in tibial acceleration, VALR, VILR at post-trial. Only tibial acceleration remained significant at the 1-month follow-up
Bowser et al., 2018 [14]	Tibial acceleration	Visual feedback	19 healthy RFS runners with high tibial acceleration	Faded, 8 sessions over 2 weeks	Significant reductions in tibial acceleration, VIP, VALR, VILR, at follow-up timepoints of 1, 6, and 12 months
Cheung et al., 2018 [39]	Tibial acceleration	Visual feedback	16 healthy runners with high tibial accelerations	Faded, 8 sessions over 2 weeks	In the post-trial participants were distracted but still had significant reduction in VALR, VILR and tibial acceleration compared to pre-trial

Table 2. *Cont.*

	Adjusted Variable	Feedback	Subjects	Retraining Design	Outcomes
Ching et al., 2018 [15]	Tibial acceleration	Audio feedback	16 healthy runners with high tibial acceleration	Faded, 8 sessions over 2 weeks	In the post-trial participants were distracted but still had significant reduction in VALR, VILR and tibial acceleration compared to pre-trial. Additional feedback did not change loading rates in runners that had already undergone gait retraining
Zhang et al., 2019 [17]	Tibial acceleration	Visual feedback	13 healthy runners with high tibial acceleration	Faded, 8 sessions over 2 weeks	37.3% reduction in peak tibial acceleration, runners maintained lower tibial accelerations at +/− 10% of their self-selected pace
Zhang et al., 2019 [16]	Tibial acceleration	Visual feedback	12 healthy runners with high tibial acceleration	Faded, 8 sessions over 2 weeks	Runners were able to maintain lower tibial accelerations during overground running and treadmill slope running, but not overground slope running
Sheerin et al., 2020 [18]	Tibial acceleration	Haptic feedback through watch	18 healthy runners with high tibial acceleration	Faded, 8 sessions over 2 weeks	41% reduction in average tibial acceleration on a treadmill. 17% reduction in tibial acceleration during overground running
da Silva Neto et al., 2022 [40]	Vertical ground reaction force	Visual feedback	24 healthy RFS runners	Not faded, 8 sessions over 2 weeks	Reduced maximum force in the midfoot and medial rearfoot. Showed gait retraining can be performed overground rather than with a treadmill
Cheung and Davis 2011 [41]	Forefoot strike pattern	Audio feedback from buzzer in shoe	3 female runners with PFPS	Faded, 8 sessions over 2 weeks	All 3 participants had decreased VALR and VILR by 10.9–35.1%. Pain scores were improved by 10.4–19.5 points
Roper et al., 2016 [42]	Forefoot strike pattern	Visual feedback from mirror and verbal cues	16 RFS runners with running-related knee pain	Faded, 8 sessions over 2 weeks	Significant reduction in pain from 5.3 to 1.0 at post-trial and 1-month follow-up
Chan et al., 2020 [43]	Midfoot strike pattern	Visual display of footstrike pattern	20 healthy RFS male runners	Faded, 8 sessions over 2 weeks	Only 40% of participants successfully transitioned to midfoot strike pattern, those who did displayed no difference in vertical loading rate
Yang et al., 2020 [44]	Forefoot strike pattern	Audio feedback from mobile app	17 healthy RFS runners	Not faded	Significantly lower loading rates, significantly higher ankle joint moment from pre- to post-study. Significantly lower loading rates in participants who underwent gait retraining and switched to minimalist shoes compared to those who just switched to minimalist shoes

Table 2. *Cont.*

	Adjusted Variable	Feedback	Subjects	Retraining Design	Outcomes
Chan et al., 2021 [45]	Forefoot strike pattern	Audio feedback	16 healthy runners	Faded, 8 sessions over 2 weeks	75% of participants switched to non rearfoot striking over level ground, 94% over uphill running and 88% over downhill running
Teng et al., 2020 [10]	Trunk lean	Visual display of trunk lean	12 healthy RFS runners	Faded, 5 sessions over 8 weeks	Significant reduction in PFJ stress, knee extensor moment, peak ankle plantar flexor moment, significant increase in peak hip extensor moment
Helmhout et al., 2015 [46]	Forefoot strike pattern and step rate	Education and audio feedback from verbal cues	19 military members with chronic exertional compartment syndrome for at least 2 months	Not faded	Significant increase in running distance, significant increase in SANE and LLOS, significant decrease in PSC
Futrell et al., 2020 [47]	Forefoot strike pattern and step rate	Audio feedback from metronome for step rate group, audio feedback for footstrike pattern group	39 healthy RFS runners without a history of bone stress injuries and with step rates below 170	Faded, 8 sessions over 2 weeks	41% reduction in VALR in the footstrike pattern group compared to 14% reduction in VALR in the step rate group at 1-week post-trial. Changes were maintained at 6 months post-trial
Miller et al., 2021 [48]	Forefoot strike pattern and step rate	Audio feedback from metronome and verbal cues	9 injured military service members	Not faded	Significant reduction in VALR, increase in step rate, significant improvement in patient SANE scores. All participants remained injury free at 6-month follow-up
Bonacci et al., 2018 [49]	Footwear and step rate	Audio feedback from metronome	14 RFS runners with PFPS	Faded, 10 sessions over 6 weeks	All subjects in gait retraining had reduction in pain and improvement in function. Significantly lower anterior knee pain compared to orthotics group
Molina-Molina et al., 2022 [50]	Footwear and step rate	Audio feedback from a metronome for step rate group, removal of shoes for barefoot group	70 healthy runners	Not faded, 30 sessions over 3 weeks	Significant decrease in rearfoot strike angle in barefoot group and step rate group. Significant increase in step rate at comfortable speed for step rate group. At a high speed, step rate increased for the barefoot group and decreased for the step rate group.
dos Santos et al., 2019 [11]	Forefoot strike pattern, step rate and forward trunk lean	Audio feedback from clinician for footstrike and forward trunk lean groups, audio feedback from metronome for step rate group	18 runners with PFPS	Faded, 8 sessions over 2 weeks	All 3 groups had decreased pain, increased functionality and decreased LEFS scores from pre- to post-trial. All changes were maintained at a 6-month follow-up. AKPS scores decreased from pre-trial to post-trial in the footstrike and trunk lean groups and between pre-trial and 6-month follow-up in all groups

Clinical Outcomes: LEFI- Lower Extremity Functional Index (same as LEFS), KOS-ADLS- Knee Outcome Survey–Activities of Daily Living Scale, SANE- Single Assessment Numeric Evaluation, LLOS- Lower Leg Outcome Survey, PSC- Patient Specific Complaints questionnaire, LEFS- Lower Extremity Functional Scale, AKPS- Anterior Knee Pain Scale, VAS- Visual Analog Scale.

5. Interventions Characterizing Gait Retraining Variables

Biomechanical targets of gait retraining studies (shown above in Table 2) include degree of hip adduction [8,9], step rate [19–21], tibial acceleration [12,14–18,39,45], footstrike pattern [41–44] and trunk lean [10]. The outcome measures of each study varied and included pain and functionality in injured runners, joint angles, and measures of loading rates (such as VALR and VILR) in healthy runners.

While the literature supporting hip adduction as a risk factor for PFPS is inconsistent [27], two studies have reported beneficial outcomes related to reduced hip adduction in runners with PFPS [8,9]. One study used a real time display generated by motion capture technology to display hip adduction [8], while the other study used visual feedback with a full-length mirror [9]. Both studies reported decreases in pain and increases in functionality, exceeding the minimal clinically important difference, at the end of the trial and at a 1- or 3-month follow-up.

Increases in step rate by 5% or 10% have been shown to lower COM vertical excursion, decrease breaking impulse and transition runners towards a more anterior footstrike pattern [36]. Three gait retraining studies have shown that step rate can be altered through gait retraining outside of a laboratory setting, including while runners continue with their training [20,21,50]. Willy et al. [20] found that this increase in step rate was also associated with a decrease in VALR, VILR and HADD [20]. A decrease in pain and increase in functionality was seen at the 6-month follow-up in runners that underwent gait retraining to increase their step rate by 10% [11]. The changes in step rate seen after gait retraining may not be constant at faster speeds, however [50]. One prospective study found no difference in KOS-ADLS scores between runners who received education on load management and underwent gait retraining based on step rate compared to those who only received education on load management [19]. A possible side effect of step rate-based gait retraining is calf muscle soreness. In one study, 43% of participants mentioned calf muscle soreness [49]. However, this did not affect running volume.

Tibial acceleration is a common variable of interest in gait retraining studies as a surrogate measure of loading rate. While a variety of techniques can be used to decrease tibial acceleration, some studies have found that runners are capable of lowering their tibial accelerations with visual feedback combined with instruction to land "softly" and "quietly" [14,39,41]. A study that used visual feedback of accelerometer data for gait retraining found significant reductions in tibial acceleration, VIP, VALR and VILR at post-training compared to pre-training [14]. Tibial acceleration, VIP, VALR and VILR all remained significantly reduced at 1-month, 6-month, and 12-month follow-ups.

Transitioning from a rearfoot strike to a forefoot strike has been shown to decrease loading rates while running [41]. Improvements in clinical outcomes that reach minimal clinically important difference in patients with PFPS that switch to a forefoot strike have been reported in a case series study [11]. These improvements remained at a 6-month follow-up. One randomized controlled trial found a significant reduction in pain in runners with PFPS that underwent gait retraining while the control group did not experience any significant changes in pain. However, subjects that underwent gait retraining reported calf soreness while undergoing gait retraining. Twenty-five percent of participants from the retraining group also reported ankle soreness at the 1-month follow-up when running more than 4 miles in a single session [42]. Chan et al. also found that runners who transitioned to a midfoot striking pattern did not display significantly different load rates compared to rearfoot strikers [43].

While fewer studies involving trunk lean were found, improvements in functional outcomes and decreases in pain were reported immediately upon the completion of gait retraining and at a 6-month follow-up [11]. Changes in functionality between pre-training and post-training reached minimal clinically important difference. These changes were similar to the changes seen in the treatment group that transitioned to a forefoot strike pattern.

6. Clinical Application of Gait Retraining

Sports injuries are complex and result from a combination of intrinsic and extrinsic factors [51]. Although biomechanics play a role in RRIs [27], it is important to highlight that a multifactorial perspective is required, and clinicians must identify the non-linear interactions between biomechanics and other aspects that may be related to injuries [51]. Gait retraining expands upon traditional approaches of addressing impairments in strength and flexibility to address abnormal biomechanics and motor control and should be considered as an aspect of a multimodal approach.

Most research on gait retraining strategies identified in this review (Table 2) focus on changing lower extremity mechanics to address knee pain. In PFPS, best evidence guidelines include exercises to improve hip and knee strength [52]. In the basics of the preliminary strengthening phase, the patient can also be considered in the cognitive stages of learning, using different exercises to gain intrinsic awareness of these muscles, and using visual cues to gain greater proprioceptive awareness. The treatment program then progresses to the associative stages of learning as tasks become more challenging. At this point, the participant should not only improve strength based on exercise prescription but improve ability to modify their alignment in a variety of tasks.

After addressing the pre-gait guidelines for management of PFPS, patients may further benefit by participating in gait retraining programs. Changes in pain and function up to six months were seen in runners with hip adduction greater than 20° that received visual feedback and were cued to "run with your knees apart with your kneecaps pointing straight ahead" [8,9], in runners with trunk flexion of 11° that were asked to "run with an increase in flexed trunk posture" [11], in runners with step rate between 160 to 170 steps/minute that were cued via an audio metronome set at 7.5–10% above their baseline step rate [11,19,49], and in runners that adopted a forefoot strike pattern using visual feedback and cues such as "run on your toes" and/or "run on the balls of your feet" [11,42].

The programs can be done using 8–12 sessions completed over 2–4 weeks (average of 2–3 gait retraining sessions per week). In this design, the feedback is provided continually in the first week and then is gradually removed in the second week. Run time progressively increases from 15 to 30 min [8,9,11,41,42]. This faded feedback program prevents dependency on external feedback and generates long-term retention [24]. Various other gait retraining programs have been proposed for patients with PFPS [19,49,53]. These include programs using five sessions over eight weeks [19], ten sessions over six weeks [49], and or only one session of ten minutes followed by four weeks of self-administration and monitoring increased step rate [53]. Each has shown improvements in symptoms and function and thus may be considered as an alternative to the above gait retraining prescription. Considerations for type of gait retraining intervention need to account for multiple factors including type of injury being treated, injury duration, time in season, and level of competition, with the goal of developing a long-term strategy to reduce risk for new or recurrent RRI.

Gait retraining implementation must consider the role of muscle strength and fatiguability, as different strategies will have different demands of the neuromotor system. An increase in trunk flexion is associated with greater peak hip extension moment [54], and transition to a forefoot strike is associated with greater peak ankle plantarflexion moment [55]. Strengthening the calf muscles may reduce the incidence of calf soreness that was reported for the step rate [49] and forefoot strike strategies [42]. Similarly, strengthening hip extensor muscles may facilitate a better transition to a gait with increased trunk lean [56]. Further, a combination of gait retraining strategies may be used to achieve the goals of the retraining program. Previous studies based on increasing step rate instructed patients to land softly [49] or to land softly and adopt a non-rearfoot strike pattern if necessary [19].

Regardless of the benefits for injured runners, very limited evidence supports the use of gait retraining for healthy runners. Athletes with VALR greater than 70 BW/s that received visual feedback and were instructed to "run softer" presented a 62% lower occurrence of RRIs in a year [57]. Only one retrospective study provided evidence that RFS runners present higher rates of prior RRIs than non-rearfoot strikers [58] and conversely another cross-sectional study found that a non-RFS was associated with calf muscle injuries and Achilles tendinopathy. Since no prospective studies have been performed, the transition to a forefoot strike in healthy runners cannot be uniformly recommended using evidence-based treatment [59,60]. Finally, limited evidence shows that the transition to a forefoot strike does not change running economy at fast speeds and limited-to-moderate evidence shows a decrease in running economy at low-medium speeds in recreational runners [59]. Therefore, changing the foot strike pattern to improve the running economy is not recommended. The potential of the other strategies to reduce the likelihood of RRIs and improve performance was not assessed.

While gait retraining has largely been studied for those with PFPS; limited work has been conducted on addressing biomechanical risk factors in non-PFPS RRI. Examples of gait retraining strategies that may be applied to runners presenting with various injuries are illustrated in Figures 1 and 2. It is important to note that gait retraining has only been used to treat runners with PFPS and chronic exertional compartment syndrome (CECS). Studies examining the effect of gait retraining on pain and functionality in many common running injuries do not currently exist, so specific recommendations for using gait retraining in injured runners with injuries other than PFPS and CECS cannot be made. Figures 1 and 2 serve only to provide examples on how a clinician may treat an injured runner using gait retraining based on literature surrounding gait retraining studies and risk factors for specific RRIs such as medial tibial stress syndrome [30,32], tibial stress fractures [61,62], iliotibial band syndrome [63,64], PFPS [28,29,32,42,65–67], CECS [46] and plantar fasciitis [33–35].

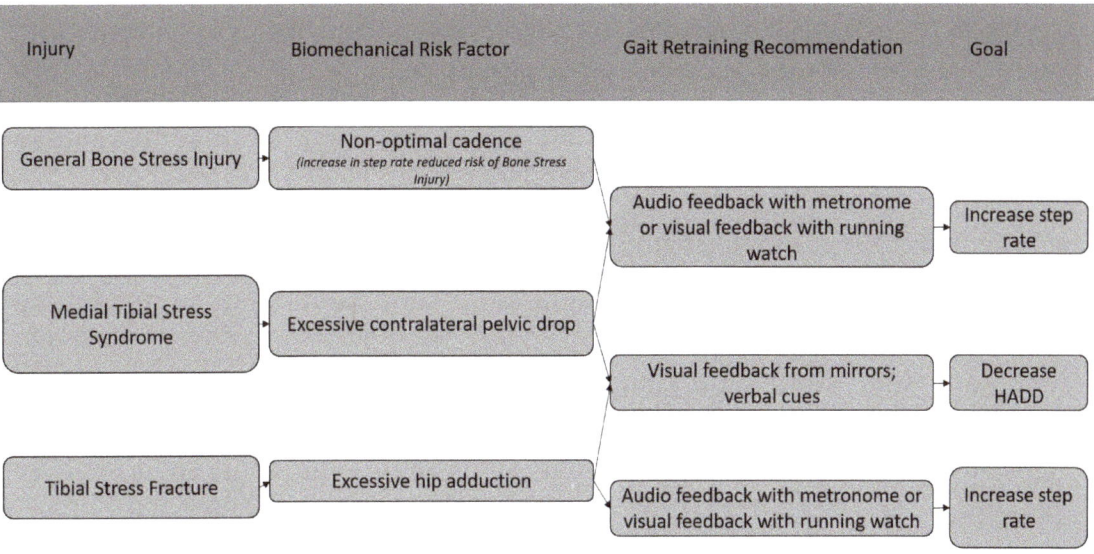

Figure 1. Examples of using gait retraining to treat bone related RRIs [22,30,32,61,62].

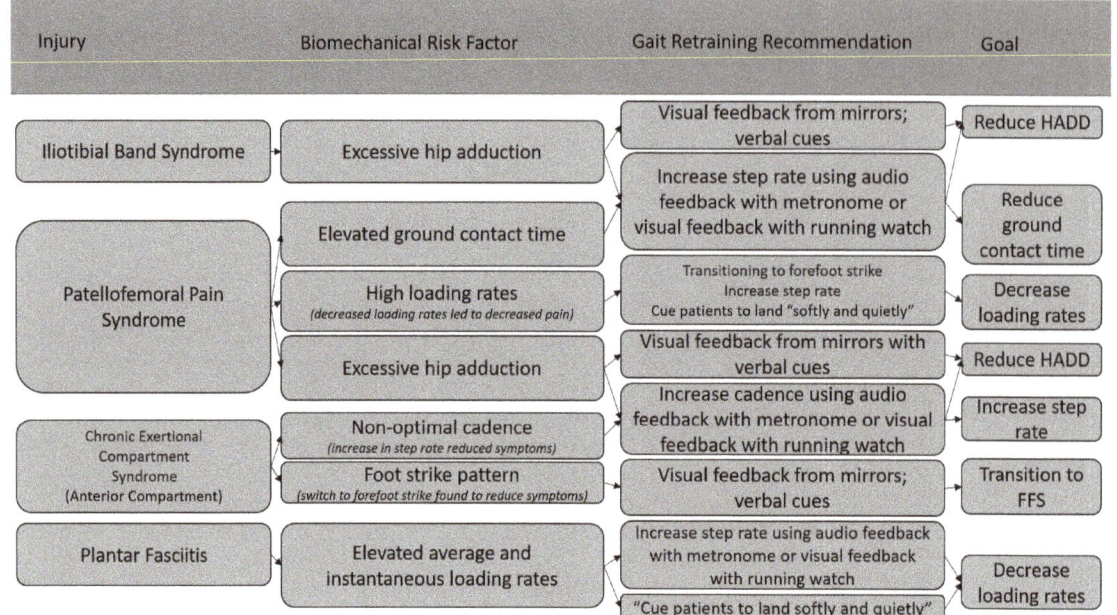

Figure 2. Examples of using gait retraining to treat other specific RRIs [28,29,32–35,42,46,63–67].

7. Limitations of Current Gait Retraining Strategies

Most studies characterizing gait retraining require participants to limit their running to gait retraining sessions in a laboratory setting [12,14]. This may discourage injured runners with an upcoming race, or those unwilling to take extended time away from running, from undergoing gait retraining. Studies that have allowed participants to continue with their own training schedules outside of gait retraining have found that runners can benefit from performing gait retraining while still participating in training outside of the laboratory [10,16,44]. Gait retraining completed outside of a laboratory setting while still continuing typical training has been observed to significantly reduce footstrike angle and increase step rate [50]. While this study did not report any negative outcomes for participants, RRI risk should be considered when allowing runners to continue with training while completing gait retraining, accounting for time for soft tissue and bone adaptations. Since this study only examined step rate manipulation, adjusting other variables may be less feasible outside of the clinical setting.

Despite the success found in gait retraining strategies employed in many of the studies examined in this review, a study conducted by Esculier et al. [19] found that education of proper training loads and education combined with gait retraining resulted in similar decreases in knee pain in runners with PFPS. Notably the session duration and frequency was lower than standard gait retraining programs and did not use a faded feedback design [8,9,11,14,18,41,42,47]. This discrepancy in results highlights that not all gait retraining protocols are equally effective, and that it is important to identify factors that may aid in the success of a gait retraining protocol.

Presently, it is unknown if gait retraining effectiveness is influenced by severity of injury. For example, improvement in pain and functionality in patients with PFPS following gait retraining only included participants that reported a pain level below a 7 out of 10 on a visual analog scale [42]. A separate investigation on gait retraining instructed PFPS patients to run only when their pain level was below a 2 out of 10 on the visual analog scale [19]. Thus, patients who report severe pain while running may benefit from undergoing other forms of treatment before beginning gait retraining.

There exists a clear gap in the literature surrounding gait retraining in terms of randomized controlled trials. Only two randomized controlled gait retraining studies have examined the effects of gait retraining as a form of injury treatment [19,42]. Both trials examined knee pain as an outcome measure and the two studies found contrasting results. While one study found a significant reduction in knee pain in the group that underwent gait retraining [42], the other study found there was no difference in knee pain in those who had undergone gait retraining and education compared to those who had underwent education alone [19]. Other studies using gait retraining did not record patient pain levels or did not include a control group. No randomized controlled trials have examined the effect of gait retraining on pain and functionality in RRIs other than PFPS. Further investigation into the effects of gait retraining as treatment for specific injuries may reveal that gait retraining is not equally effective for all types of RRIs. Identifying specific injuries that gait retraining is more effective in treating could increase the value of gait retraining as a rehabilitation tool for RRIs.

Only two studies included in this review reported adverse effects [42,49]. Both studies cited soreness of the calves that did not affect the ability of subjects to complete their training. One study reported ankle soreness at a 1-month follow-up after gait retraining. The time to achieve strength and tissue adaption must be individualized to reduce risk for RRI and gait retraining should be progressed gradually. More studies investigating potential adverse effects of gait retraining are needed before gait retraining can be fully recommended as a treatment strategy in injured runners.

8. Conclusions

While biomechanical risk factors are variable across RRIs, gait retraining may be used to modify potentially faulty running mechanics. An individualized and diagnosis-specific approach is important to address specific risk factors for the injured runner. Running mechanics can be modified using different forms of biofeedback and should use a faded feedback design for motor learning. Future studies, ideally in a randomized clinical study design, may clarify how different forms of gait retraining may be used, alone or in combination, to treat and prevent RRI.

Author Contributions: Conceptualization, L.W.G., M.M.B., A.S.T., L.W. and J.P.; formal analysis, L.W.G. and M.M.B.; writing—original draft preparation, L.W.G., M.M.B., J.P. and L.W.; writing—review and editing, J.R.d.S.J., B.H., C.D.J., L.K.S., M.J.R., K.H. and A.S.T. All authors have read and agreed to the published version of the manuscript.

Funding: This research received no external funding.

Institutional Review Board Statement: Not applicable.

Informed Consent Statement: Not applicable.

Data Availability Statement: Not applicable.

Conflicts of Interest: All authors have no disclosures related to this work. José Roberto de Souza Junior is a Fulbright visiting research student at the Spaulding National Running Center. Bryan Heiderscheit is a paid consultant to Biocore, has ownership interest in Science of Running Medicine LLC, is an advisory board member for Springbok Analytics and has received research funding (paid to institution) from the National Football League, National Basketball Association and GE Healthcare. Adam Tenforde serves as Senior editor for PM&R Journal. He gives professional talks such as grand rounds and medical conference plenary lectures and receives honoraria from conference organizers. He has participated in research funded by Arnold P. Gold Foundation (physician and patient care disparities), Football Player Health Study at Harvard (health in American-Style Football players), American Medical Society for Sports Medicine (bone density research), Uniform Health Service and Enovis (Achilles tendinopathy). He is a paid consultant for State Farm Insurance and Strava.

References

1. Lee, D.C.; Pate, R.R.; Lavie, C.J.; Sui, X.; Church, T.S.; Blair, S.N. Leisure-time running reduces all-cause and cardiovascular mortality risk. *J. Am. Coll. Cardiol.* **2014**, *64*, 472–481. [CrossRef] [PubMed]
2. Oswald, F.; Campbell, J.; Williamson, C.; Richards, J.; Kelly, P. A scoping review of the relationship between running and mental health. *Int. J. Environ. Res. Public Health* **2020**, *17*, 8059. [CrossRef] [PubMed]
3. Lun, V.; Meeuwisse, W.H.; Stergiou, P.; Stefanyshyn, D. Relation between running injury and static lower limb alignment in recreational runners. *Br. J. Sports Med.* **2004**, *38*, 576–580. [CrossRef] [PubMed]
4. Kelsey, J.L.; Bachrach, L.K.; Procter-Gray, E.; Nieves, J.; Greendale, G.A.; Sowers, M.; Brown, B.W.; Matheson, K.A.; Crawford, S.L.; Cobb, K.L. Risk factors for stress fracture among young female cross-country runners. *Med. Sci. Sports Exerc.* **2007**, *39*, 1457–1463 [CrossRef] [PubMed]
5. Rauh, M.J.; Margherita, A.J.; Rice, S.G.; Koepsell, T.D.; Rivara, F.P. High School Cross Country Running Injuries: A Longitudinal Study. *J. Clin. Sport Med.* **2000**, *10*, 110–116. [CrossRef] [PubMed]
6. Mucha, M.D.; Caldwell, W.; Schlueter, E.L.; Walters, C.; Hassen, A. Hip abductor strength and lower extremity running related injury in distance runners: A systematic review. *J. Sci. Med. Sport* **2017**, *20*, 349–355. [CrossRef]
7. Willy, R.W.; Davis, I.S. The effect of a hip-strengthening program on mechanics during running and during a single-leg squat. *J. Orthop. Sports Phys. Ther.* **2011**, *41*, 625–632. [CrossRef]
8. Noehren, B.; Scholz, J.; Davis, I. The effect of real-time gait retraining on hip kinematics, pain and function in subjects with patellofemoral pain syndrome. *Br. J. Sports Med.* **2011**, *45*, 691–696. [CrossRef]
9. Willy, R.W.; Scholz, J.P.; Davis, I.S. Mirror gait retraining for the treatment of patellofemoral pain in female runners. *Clin. Biomech.* **2012**, *27*, 1045–1051. [CrossRef]
10. Teng, H.-L.; Dilauro, A.; Weeks, C.; Odell, C.; Kincaid, H.; VanDine, B.; Wu, W.F. Short-term effects of a trunk modification program on patellofemoral joint stress in asymptomatic runners. *Phys. Ther. Sport* **2020**, *44*, 107–113. [CrossRef]
11. Dos Santos, A.F.; Nakagawa, T.H.; Lessi, G.C.; Luz, B.C.; Matsuo, H.T.; Nakashima, G.Y.; Maciel, C.D.; Serrão, F.V. Effects of three gait retraining techniques in runners with patellofemoral pain. *Phys. Ther. Sport* **2019**, *36*, 92–100. [CrossRef] [PubMed]
12. Crowell, H.P.; Davis, I.S. Gait retraining to reduce lower extremity loading in runners. *Clin. Biomech.* **2011**, *26*, 78–83. [CrossRef] [PubMed]
13. Clansey, A.C.; Hanlon, M.; Wallace, E.S.; Nevill, A.; Lake, M.J. Influence of Tibial shock feedback training on impact loading and running economy. *Med. Sci. Sports Exerc.* **2014**, *46*, 973–981. [CrossRef] [PubMed]
14. Bowser, B.J.; Fellin, R.; Milner, C.E.; Pohl, M.B.; Davis, I.S. Reducing impact loading in runners: A one-year follow-up. *Med. Sci. Sports Exerc.* **2018**, *50*, 2500–2506. [CrossRef] [PubMed]
15. Ching, E.; An, W.W.-K.; Au, I.P.H.; Zhang, J.H.; Chan, Z.Y.; Shum, G.; Cheung, R.T. Impact Loading during Distracted Running before and after Auditory Gait Retraining. *Int. J. Sports Med.* **2018**, *39*, 1075–1080. [CrossRef]
16. Zhang, J.H.; Chan, Z.Y.S.; Au, I.P.H.; An, W.W.; Cheung, R.T.H. Can runners maintain a newly learned gait pattern outside a laboratory environment following gait retraining? *Gait Posture* **2019**, *69*, 8–12. [CrossRef]
17. Zhang, J.H.; Chan, Z.Y.-S.; Au, I.P.-H.; An, W.W.; Shull, P.B.; Cheung, R.T.-H. Transfer Learning Effects of Biofeedback Running Retraining in Untrained Conditions. *Med. Sci. Sports Exerc.* **2019**, *51*, 1904–1908. [CrossRef]
18. Sheerin, K.R.; Reid, D.; Taylor, D.; Besier, T.F. The effectiveness of real-time haptic feedback gait retraining for reducing resultant tibial acceleration with runners. *Phys. Ther. Sport* **2020**, *43*, 173–180. [CrossRef]
19. Esculier, J.-F.; Bouyer, L.J.; Dubois, B.; Fremont, P.; Moore, L.; McFadyen, B.; Roy, J.-S. Is combining gait retraining or an exercise programme with education better than education alone in treating runners with patellofemoral pain? A randomised clinical trial *Br. J. Sports Med.* **2018**, *52*, 659–666. [CrossRef]
20. Willy, R.W.; Buchenic, L.; Rogacki, K.; Ackerman, J.; Schmidt, A.; Willson, J.D. In-field gait retraining and mobile monitoring to address running biomechanics associated with tibial stress fracture. *Scand. J. Med. Sci. Sports* **2016**, *26*, 197–205. [CrossRef]
21. Baumgartner, J.; Gusmer, R.; Hollman, J.; Finnoff, J.T. Increased stride-rate in runners following an independent retraining program: A randomized controlled trial. *Scand. J. Med. Sci. Sports* **2019**, *29*, 1789–1796. [CrossRef] [PubMed]
22. Kliethermes, S.A.; Stiffler-Joachim, M.R.; Wille, C.M.; Sanfilippo, J.L.; Zavala, P.; Heiderscheit, B.C. Lower step rate is associated with a higher risk of bone stress injury: A prospective study of collegiate cross country runners. *Br. J. Sports Med.* **2021**, *55*, 851–856. [CrossRef] [PubMed]
23. Doyle, E.; Doyle, T.L.A.; Bonacci, J.; Fuller, J.T. The Effectiveness of Gait Retraining on Running Kinematics, Kinetics, Performance, Pain, and Injury in Distance Runners: A Systematic Review with Meta-analysis. *J. Orthop. Sports Phys. Ther.* **2022**, *52*, 192–206. [CrossRef] [PubMed]
24. Winstein, C.J.; Gardner, E.R.; McNeal, D.R.; Barto, P.S.; Nicholson, D.E. Standing balance training: Effect on balance and locomotion in hemiparetic adults. *Arch. Phys. Med. Rehabil.* **1989**, *70*, 755–762.
25. Vannatta, C.N.; Heinert, B.L.; Kernozek, T.W. Biomechanical risk factors for running-related injury differ by sample population: A systematic review and meta-analysis. *Clin. Biomech.* **2020**, *75*, 104991. [CrossRef]
26. Ceyssens, L.; Vanelderen, R.; Barton, C.; Malliaras, P.; Dingenen, B. Biomechanical Risk Factors Associated with Running-Related Injuries: A Systematic Review. *Sports Med.* **2019**, *49*, 1095–1115. [CrossRef]

27. Willwacher, S.; Kurz, M.; Robbin, J.; Thelen, M.; Hamill, J.; Kelly, L.; Mai, P. Running-Related Biomechanical Risk Factors for Overuse Injuries in Distance Runners: A Systematic Review Considering Injury Specificity and the Potentials for Future Research. *Sports Med.* **2022**, *52*, 1863–1877. [CrossRef]
28. Duffey, M.J.; Martin, D.F.; Cannon, D.W.; Craven, T.; Messier, S.P. Etiologic factors associated with anterior knee pain in distance runners. *Med. Sci. Sports Exerc.* **2000**, *32*, 1825–1832. [CrossRef]
29. Messier, S.P.; Davis, S.E.; Curl, W.W.; Lowery, R.B.; Pack, R.J. Etiological factors associated with patellofemoral pain in runners. *Med. Sci. Sports Exerc.* **1991**, *23*, 1008–1015. [CrossRef]
30. Becker, J.; Nakajima, M.; Wu, W.F.W. Factors Contributing to Medial Tibial Stress Syndrome in Runners: A Prospective Study. *Med. Sci. Sports Exerc.* **2018**, *50*, 2092–2100. [CrossRef]
31. Becker, J.; James, S.; Wayner, R.; Osternig, L.; Chou, L. Biomechanical Factors Associated With Achilles Tendinopathy and Medial Tibial Stress Syndrome in Runners. *Am. J. Sports Med.* **2017**, *45*, 2614–2621. [CrossRef] [PubMed]
32. Bramah, C.; Preece, S.J.; Gill, N.; Herrington, L. Is There a Pathological Gait Associated with Common Soft Tissue Running Injuries? *Am. J. Sports Med.* **2018**, *46*, 3023–3031. [CrossRef] [PubMed]
33. Johnson, C.D.; Tenforde, A.S.; Outerleys, J.; Reilly, J.; Davis, I.S. Impact-Related Ground Reaction Forces Are More Strongly Associated With Some Running Injuries Than Others. *Am. J. Sports Med.* **2020**, *48*, 3072–3080. [CrossRef] [PubMed]
34. Ribeiro, A.P.; João, S.M.A.; Dinato, R.C.; Tessutti, V.D.; Sacco, I.C.N. Dynamic patterns of forces and loading rate in runners with unilateral plantar fasciitis: A cross-sectional study. *PLoS ONE* **2015**, *10*, e0136971. [CrossRef] [PubMed]
35. Pohl, M.B.; Hamill, J.; Davis, I.S. Biomechanical and Anatomic Factors Associated with a History of Plantar Fasciitis in Female Runners. *Clin. J. Sport Med.* **2009**, *19*, 372–376. [CrossRef] [PubMed]
36. Heiderscheit, B.C.; Chumanov, E.S.; Michalski, M.P.; Wille, C.M.; Ryan, M.B. Effects of step rate manipulation on joint mechanics during running. *Med. Sci. Sports Exerc.* **2011**, *43*, 296–302. [CrossRef]
37. Davis, I.S.; Tenforde, A.S.; Neal, B.S.; Roper, J.L.; Willy, R.W. Gait Retraining as an Intervention for Patellofemoral Pain. *Curr. Rev. Musculoskelet. Med.* **2020**, *13*, 103–114. [CrossRef] [PubMed]
38. Napier, C.; Cochrane, C.K.; Taunton, J.E.; Hunt, M.A. Gait modifications to change lower extremity gait biomechanics in runners: A systematic review. *Br. J. Sports Med.* **2015**, *49*, 1382–1388. [CrossRef]
39. Cheung, R.T.H.; An, W.W.; Au, I.P.H.; Zhang, J.H.; Chan, Z.Y.S.; MacPhail, A.J. Control of impact loading during distracted running before and after gait retraining in runners. *J. Sports Sci.* **2018**, *36*, 1497–1501. [CrossRef]
40. Neto, W.C.d.; Lopes, A.D.; Ribeiro, A.P. Gait Retraining with Visual Biofeedback Reduces Rearfoot Pressure and Foot Pronation in Recreational Runners. *J. Sport Rehabil.* **2022**, *31*, 165–173. [CrossRef]
41. Cheung, R.T.H.; Davis, I.S. Landing pattern modification to improve patellofemoral pain in runners: A case series. *J. Orthop. Sports Phys. Ther.* **2011**, *41*, 914–919. [CrossRef] [PubMed]
42. Roper, J.L.; Harding, E.M.; Doerfler, D.; Dexter, J.G.; Kravitz, L.; Dufek, J.S.; Mermier, C.M. The effects of gait retraining in runners with patellofemoral pain: A randomized trial. *Clin. Biomech.* **2016**, *35*, 14–22. [CrossRef] [PubMed]
43. Chan, Z.Y.S.; Zhang, J.H.; Ferber, R.; Shum, G.; Cheung, R.T.H. The effects of midfoot strike gait retraining on impact loading and joint stiffness. *Phys. Ther. Sport* **2020**, *42*, 139–145. [CrossRef] [PubMed]
44. Yang, Y.; Zhang, X.; Luo, Z.; Wang, X.; Ye, D.; Fu, W. Alterations in running biomechanics after 12 week gait retraining with minimalist shoes. *Int. J. Environ. Res. Public Health* **2020**, *17*, 818. [CrossRef] [PubMed]
45. Chan, P.P.K.; Chan, Z.Y.S.; Au, I.P.H.; Lam, B.M.F.; Lam, W.K.; Cheung, R.T.H. Biomechanical effects following footstrike pattern modification using wearable sensors. *J. Sci. Med. Sport* **2021**, *24*, 30–35. [CrossRef]
46. Helmhout, P.H.; Diebal, A.R.; van der Kaaden, L.; Harts, C.C.; Beutler, A.; Zimmermann, W.O. The effectiveness of a 6-week intervention program aimed at modifying running style in patients with chronic exertional compartment syndrome: Results from a series of case studies. *Orthop. J. Sports Med.* **2015**, *3*, 2325967115575691. [CrossRef]
47. Futrell, E.E.; Gross, K.D.; Reisman, D.; Mullineaux, D.R.; Davis, I.S. Transition to forefoot strike reduces load rates more effectively than altered cadence. *J. Sport Health Sci.* **2020**, *9*, 248–257. [CrossRef]
48. Miller, E.M.; Crowell, M.S.; Morris, J.B.; Mason, J.S.; Zifchock, R.; Goss, D.L. Gait Retraining Improves Running Impact Loading and Function in Previously Injured U.S. Military Cadets: A Pilot Study. *Mil. Med.* **2021**, *186*, E1077–E1087. [CrossRef]
49. Bonacci, J.; Hall, M.; Saunders, N.; Vicenzino, B. Gait retraining versus foot orthoses for patellofemoral pain: A pilot randomised clinical trial. *J. Sci. Med. Sport* **2018**, *21*, 457–461. [CrossRef]
50. Molina-Molina, A.; Latorre-Román, P.Á.; Mercado-Palomino, E.; Delgado-García, G.; Richards, J.; Soto-Hermoso, V.M. The effect of two retraining programs, barefoot running vs increasing cadence, on kinematic parameters: A randomized controlled trial. *Scand. J. Med. Sci. Sports* **2022**, *32*, 533–542. [CrossRef]
51. Bittencourt, N.F.N.; Meeuwisse, W.H.; Mendonça, L.D.; Nettel-Aguirre, A.; Ocarino, J.M.; Fonseca, S.T. Complex systems approach for sports injuries: Moving from risk factor identification to injury pattern recognition-Narrative review and new concept. *Br. J. Sports Med.* **2016**, *50*, 1309–1314. [CrossRef] [PubMed]
52. Willy, R.W.; Hoglund, L.T.; Barton, C.J.; Bolgla, L.A.; Scalzitti, D.A.; Logerstedt, D.S.; Lynch, A.D.; Snyder-Mackler, L.; McDonough, C.M. Patellofemoral pain clinical practice guidelines linked to the international classification of functioning, disability and health from the academy of orthopaedic physical therapy of the American physical therapy association. *J. Orthop. Sports Phys. Ther.* **2019**, *49*, CPG1–CPG95. [CrossRef] [PubMed]

53. Bramah, C.; Preece, S.J.; Gill, N.; Herrington, L. A 10% Increase in Step Rate Improves Running Kinematics and Clinical Outcomes in Runners With Patellofemoral Pain at 4 Weeks and 3 Months. *Am. J. Sports Med.* **2019**, *47*, 3406–3413. [CrossRef] [PubMed]
54. Warrener, A.; Tamai, R.; Lieberman, D.E. The effect of trunk flexion angle on lower limb mechanics during running. *Hum. Mov. Sci.* **2021**, *78*, 102817. [CrossRef]
55. Xu, Y.; Yuan, P.; Wang, R.; Wang, D.; Liu, J.; Zhou, H. Effects of Foot Strike Techniques on Running Biomechanics: A Systematic Review and Meta-analysis. *Sports Health* **2021**, *13*, 71–77. [CrossRef]
56. Teng, H.L.; Powers, C.M. Hip-extensor strength, trunk posture, and use of the knee-extensor muscles during running. *J. Athl. Train.* **2016**, *51*, 519–524. [CrossRef]
57. Chan, Z.Y.; Zhang, J.H.; Au, I.P.; An, W.W.; Shum, G.L.; Ng, G.Y.; Cheung, R.T.H. Gait Retraining for the Reduction of Injury Occurrence in Novice Distance Runners: 1-Year Follow-up of a Randomized Controlled Trial. *Am. J. Sports Med.* **2018**, *46*, 388–395. [CrossRef]
58. Daoud, A.I.; Geissler, G.J.; Wang, F.; Saretsky, J.; Daoud, Y.A.; Lieberman, D.E. Foot strike and injury rates in endurance runners: A retrospective study. *Med. Sci. Sports Exerc.* **2012**, *44*, 1325–1334. [CrossRef]
59. Anderson, L.M.; Bonanno, D.R.; Hart, H.F.; Barton, C.J. What are the Benefits and Risks Associated with Changing Foot Strike Pattern During Running? A Systematic Review and Meta-analysis of Injury, Running Economy, and Biomechanics. *Sports Med.* **2020**, *50*, 885–917. [CrossRef]
60. Hoenig, T.; Rolvien, T.; Hollander, K. Footstrike patterns in runners: Concepts, classifications, techniques, and implications for running-related injuries. *Dtsch. Z. Sportmed.* **2020**, *71*, 55–61. [CrossRef]
61. Pohl, M.B.; Mullineaux, D.R.; Milner, C.E.; Hamill, J.; Davis, I.S. Biomechanical predictors of retrospective tibial stress fractures in runners. *J. Biomech.* **2008**, *41*, 1160–1165. [CrossRef] [PubMed]
62. Milner, C.E.; Hamill, J.; Davis, I.S. Distinct hip and rearfoot kinematics in female runners with a history of tibial stress fracture. *J. Orthop. Sports Phys. Ther.* **2010**, *40*, 59–66. [CrossRef] [PubMed]
63. Ferber, R.; Noehren, B.; Hamill, J.; Davis, I. Competitive female runners with a history of iliotibial band syndrome demonstrate atypical hip and knee kinematics. *J. Orthop. Sports Phys. Ther.* **2010**, *40*, 52–58. [CrossRef] [PubMed]
64. Noehren, B.; Davis, I.; Hamill, J. ASB Clinical Biomechanics Award Winner 2006. Prospective study of the biomechanical factors associated with iliotibial band syndrome. *Clin. Biomech.* **2007**, *22*, 951–956. [CrossRef]
65. Noehren, B.; Pohl, M.B.; Sanchez, Z.; Cunningham, T.; Lattermann, C. Proximal and distal kinematics in female runners with patellofemoral pain. *Clin. Biomech.* **2012**, *27*, 366–371. [CrossRef]
66. Neal, B.S.; Barton, C.J.; Birn-jeffery, A.; Morrissey, D. Increased hip adduction during running is associated with patellofemoral pain and differs between males and females: A case-control study. *J. Biomech.* **2019**, *91*, 133–139. [CrossRef]
67. Noehren, B.; Hamill, J.; Davis, I. Prospective Evidence for a Hip Etiology in Patellofemoral Pain. *Med. Sci. Sports Exerc.* **2013**, *45*, 1120–1124. [CrossRef]

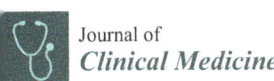

Systematic Review

Does Aerobic plus Machine-Assisted Resistance Training Improve Vascular Function in Type 2 Diabetes? A Systematic Review and Meta-Analysis of Randomized Controlled Trials with Trial Sequential Analysis

Xianshan Guo [1], Shizhe Guo [2], Hongmei Zhang [3,*] and Zhen Li [4,*]

[1] Department of Endocrinology, Xinxiang Central Hospital/The Fourth Clinical College of Xinxiang Medical University, Xinxiang 453000, China; gxs52@163.com
[2] Department of Endocrinology, Yangpu Hospital, School of Medicine, Tongji University, No. 450 Tengyue Road, Yangpu District, Shanghai 200090, China; guoshizhe@126.com
[3] Yangpu Mental Health Center, No. 585 Jungong Road, Yangpu District, Shanghai 900093, China
[4] Department of General Surgery, Yangpu Hospital, School of Medicine, Tongji University, No. 450 Tengyue Road, Yangpu District, Shanghai 200090, China
* Correspondence: 15225923683@163.com (H.Z.); lizhen3829@126.com (Z.L.)

Abstract: Type 2 diabetes mellitus (T2DM) is a chronic disease characterized by hyperglycemia, insulin resistance, and pancreatic B cell dysfunction. Hyperglycemia can cause several complications, including nephrological, neurological, ophthalmological, and vascular complications. Many modalities, such as medication, physical therapies, and exercise, are developed against vascular disorders. Among all exercise forms, aerobic plus machine-assisted resistance training is widely applied. However, whether this intervention can significantly improve vascular conditions remains controversial. In this study, an electronic search was processed for the Pubmed, Embase, and Cochrane libraries for randomized controlled trials (RCTs) comparing the efficacy of aerobic plus machine-assisted resistance training with no exercise (control) on patients with T2DM. Pulse wave velocity (PWV), the index of arterial stiffness, was chosen as primary outcome. The reliability of the pooled outcome was tested by trial sequential analysis (TSA). Secondary outcomes included systolic blood pressure (SBP) and hemoglobin A1c (HbA1c). Finally, five RCTs with a total of 328 patients were included. Compared with control, aerobic plus machine-assisted resistance training failed to provide significant improvement on PWV (MD −0.54 m/s, 95% CI [−1.69, 0.60], $p = 0.35$). On the other hand, TSA indicated that this results till needs more verifications. Additionally, this training protocol did not significantly decrease SBP (MD −1.05 mmHg, 95% CI [−3.71, 1.61], $p = 0.44$), but significantly reduced the level of HbA1c (MD −0.55%, 95% CI [−0.88, −0.22], $p = 0.001$). In conclusion, this meta-analysis failed to detect a direct benefit of aerobic plus machine-assisted resistance training on vascular condition in T2DM population. Yet the improvement in HbA1c implied a potential of this training method in mitigating vascular damage. More studies are needed to verify the benefit.

Keywords: diabetes mellitus; aerobic training; resistance training; vascular function; meta-analysis

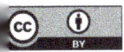

1. Introduction

The prevalence of Type 2 Diabetes Mellitus (T2DM) is increasing rapidly worldwide [1]. Characterized by hyperglycemia, insulin resistance, and pancreatic B cell dysfunction, T2DM leads to several severe complications, including but not limited to neuropathy, nephrology, and macrovascular disorders such as cardiovascular diseases [2,3]. Compared to healthy population, the risk of cardiovascular events has a twofold increase [4]. Cardiovascular event is also the leading cause of mortality in patients with T2DM [5]. Therefore, maintaining the function of vessels or retaining the damage of vessels is of vital importance.

Lifestyle modifications, such as diet control, nutrients supply, body weight regulation, and sports exercise, are well-acknowledged to improve the prognosis of T2DM [4–7]. Sports exercise can be divided into aerobic training, resistance training, or combination. As an easily accessible pattern, aerobic training helps control blood pressure, systemic inflammation, and glycemic level, et al. [8]. Way et al. found aerobic training could improve smooth muscle function, but the improvement of vascular stiffness was still questioned [9]. Alternatively, resistance training can change body composition by increasing the mass of muscle, which is important in controlling blood glucose and ameliorating insulin resistance [10]. When combined with aerobic training, this strategy may improve vascular function in healthy individuals [11]. In 2014, Li et al. found that combined aerobic and resistance training was beneficial for decreasing arterial stiffness in population with or without hypertension [12]. These findings provide the rationality of this combined training for patients with T2DM.

In recent years, clinical trials have been launched to test whether aerobic plus resistance training is beneficial to the vascular complications of T2DM. To better understand where we are now, a systematic review and meta-analysis is organized to verify the effect of aerobic plus machine-assisted resistance training on the vascular condition in patients with T2DM.

2. Materials and Methods

This systematic review was organized according to the PRISMA (Preferred Reporting Items for Systematic Reviews and Meta-analyses) checklist [13].

2.1. Search Strategy

On January 2022, the first two authors independently searched on Pubmed, Embase, and Cochrane library. Reference lists of previously published systematic reviews were also reviewed related researches. Key words used were, random *, (vessel * or cardiovascular or vascular), diabet *[title/abstract], and (exercise or training).

2.2. Study Selection

Studies focusing on the comparison of resistance plus aerobic training and no or sham training for improvement of the vascular function in T2DM population were included. The inclusion criteria were (1) randomized controlled trials (RCTs), (2) an intervention consisted of a combination of machine-assisted resistance training and aerobic training, and (3) intervention duration for at least four weeks [14]. The exclusion criteria were (1) non-randomized control trials, (2) animal studies, and (3) RCTs in which the intervention group did not have a combined training protocol, (4) combined protocol in which resistance training protocol was unclear or not machine-assisted, and (5) non-randomized clinical trials, case reports, reference abstracts, or reviews. The first two authors independently screened titles and abstracts of all searched items based on the criteria above. Once the information to make a decision was insufficient, full-text would be retrieved for further judgment. In case of debate, the senior author would decide whether to include the research.

2.3. Data Extraction

The same authors independently extracted data from eligible studies including name of first author, published year, inclusion and exclusion criteria, number of patients included, training protocols, and items of measurements, as well as conclusions. The difference of changes of central pulse wave velocity (PWV) between two groups was selected as the primary outcome, since PWV is not only an indicator arterial stiffness but also an independent predictor of cardiovascular risk [15]. Secondary outcomes included the difference of changes of systolic blood pressure (SBP) and hemoglobin A1c (HbA1c) between two group. The former reflects vasculature plasticity [16], while the latter is used for evaluating blood-glucose control over a period of time and to predict the occurrence of long-term complications due to diabetes [17].

2.4. Data Analysis

The random-effects model was applied for each comparison since patient conditions, exercise duration and modes, as well as other factors were inconsistent across RCTs. Difference in primary and secondary outcomes were measured by mean difference (MD) and 95% confidence interval (CI). For researches in which the standard deviation (SD) of pre-intervention and post-intervention difference was not reported, a correlation of 0.5 was used for dispersion estimation [18]. For researches with multiple eligible intervention groups, the control group was split equally based on the number of intervention groups, and two or more comparison pairs were input [19]. Heterogeneity was assessed by Q statistic and I^2 statistic. I^2 statistic larger than 50% were considered to have significant heterogeneity [20]. When significant heterogeneity was noticed regarding primary outcome, sensitivity analysis was conducted. One study was omitted in each turn to locate the potential source of heterogeneity. Since the number of RCTs included did not reach ten, publication bias was not detected [21]. Two-tail p value < 0.05 was considered statistically significant. Analyses were performed using Review Manager, Version 5.3 (The Nordic Cochrane Centre, The Cochrane Collaboration; Copenhagen, Denmark).

2.5. Quality Assessment

The Cochrane's risk of bias tool was used by the first two reviewers independently assess the quality of included studies [22]. Value of low, unclear or high risk of bias was assigned to the following items: random sequence generation, allocation concealment, blinding of participants and personnel, blinding of outcome assessment, incomplete outcome data, selective reporting and other bias. Disagreement was solved by discussion. The degree of inter-reviewer agreement was measured by κ value. A κ from 0.40 to 0.59 was regarded as fair, 0.60 to 0.74 as good, 0.75 or more as excellent [22].

The quality of evidence for primary outcome was rated by the Grading of Recommendations Assessment, Development, and Evaluation (GRADE) approach. The level of evidence was entitled as high, moderate, low, or very low, according to five domains: high risk of bias, imprecision, indirectness, heterogeneity, and publication bias [23–27]. Considering the limited number of studies included, publication bias could not be assessed. Instead, evidence was downgraded when heterogeneity exceeded 40% [25].

2.6. Trial Sequential Analysis

Given sparse data and repeated significance testing, the risk of type I error might be elevated by cumulative meta-analyses [28–31]. To control this potential risk, trial sequential analysis (TSA) was launched (TSA software version 0.9 Beta; Copenhagen Trial Unit, Copenhagen, Denmark) for all measurements by empirical method for the estimation of the required information size. The diversity-adjusted required information size (DIS) and the eventual breach of the cumulative Z-curve of relevant trial sequential monitoring boundaries was obtained to calculate the required information size together with a threshold for a statistically significant treatment effect [32]. An overall 5% risk of a type I error was maintained with a power of 80% [32].

3. Results

A total of 4838 titles were identified after electronic screening in three databases. After reading titles and abstracts, the full-text of seven titles were retrieved for further exclusion. The resistance training in the trial reported by Okada et al. [33] was not machine-assisted, therefore was excluded. Two studies shared the same patient cohort, so the latter one, which was a secondary analysis of the original population, was excluded [34]. One eligible study [35] was identified from a systematic review [14], and was included (Figure 1).

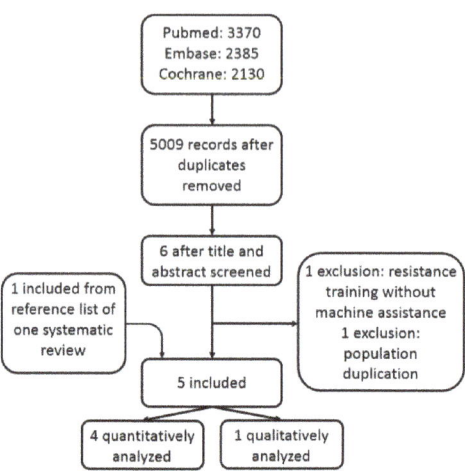

Figure 1. The flowchart of study inclusion.

Five RCTs with a total of 328 patients were included, of which four RCTs were quantitatively analyzed [35–38], while one was descriptively analyzed [39]. Basic characteristics of these studies were listed in Table 1. These researches were published from 2001 to 2019. A total of 176 patients with T2DM were allocated to aerobic plus resistance training group. The age range of the patients included in the systematic review was from about 40 to over 60 years old. In one study, only male participants were enrolled [35]. Detailed intervention, follow-up duration, and conclusions were listed in Table 2. The aerobic training consisted of cycle ergometry, walking, or treadmill et al., while resistance training focused mainly on trunk and extremities on machines. All training processes use a heart rate detector to determine the quality and quantity of exercise. Started from the beginning of exercise, two RCTs had a follow-up of 52 weeks [35,38], two had a follow-up of 26 weeks [36,37], and one had 16 weeks [39].

Table 1. Basic characteristics of included studies.

Number	Title	Authors	Year of Publication	Participants		Age	
				Exercise	Control	Exercise	Control
1	The effect of combined aerobic and resistance exercise training on vascular function in type 2 diabetes	Maiorana et al.	2001	6	16	52 ± 8 as a whole	
2	Exercise training improves baroreflex sensitivity in type 2 diabetes	Loimaala et al.	2003	24	25	53.6 ± 6.2	54 ± 5
3	A randomized trial of exercise for blood pressure reduction in type 2 diabetes: Effect on flow-mediated dilation and circulating biomarkers of endothelial function	Baron et al.	2012	49	63	58 ± 5	56 ± 6
4	Effect of exercise on blood pressure in type 2 diabetes: a randomized controlled trial	Dobrosielski et al.	2012	70	70	57 ± 6	56 ± 6
5	Effects of combined training with different intensities on vascular health in patients with type 2 diabetes: a 1-year randomized controlled trial	Magalhaes et al.	2019	28	27	59.7 ± 8.3	59.0 ± 6.5

Table 2. Measurements, exercise protocols, follow-up duration, and findings.

Number	Analyzed Measurements	Aerobic Training Protocol	Resistance Training Protocol	Follow-Up	Conclusion
1	I: Changes in forearm blood flow II: Endothelium-dependent, flow-mediated dilation of brachial artery III: Endothelium-independent glyceryl trinitrate-mediated dilation of brachial artery	A combination of cycle ergometry and treadmill walking maintained at 70% to 85% of peak heart rate.	Leg press, hip and shoulder extension, pectoral exercises, seated abdominal flexion and dual leg flexion on weight-stack machines, with an intensity 55% to 65% of pretraining maximum voluntary contraction.	16 weeks	This study supports the value of an exercise program in the management of type 2 diabetes.
2	I: Systolic blood pressure II: Pulse wave velocity III: Systemic vascular resistance index IV: HbA1c	Jog or walk twice a week at a heart rate level of 65–75% maximal oxygen consumption	Eight sessions for large muscle groups from the trunk and upper and lower extremities with three sets of 10–12 repetitions at 70–80% maximum voluntary contraction.	52 weeks	No significant changes in systemic hemodynamics were observed.
3	I: Blood pressure II: HbA1c III: Lipids IV: Endothelial biomarkers V: BMI, body and visceral fat VI: Endothelium-dependent, flow-mediated dilation of brachial artery	A 10–15 min warm-up, 45 min of aerobic exercise at a target heart rate between 60 and 90% of maximum heart rate, and a cool down.	Weight training exercises (latissimus dorsi pull down, leg extension, leg curl, bench press, leg press, shoulder press, and seated mid-rowing) for 2 sets of 12–15 repetitions at 50% of 1-repetition maximum.	26 weeks	There were no changes in endothelium-dependent flow-mediated dilation or circulating endothelial biomarkers.
4	I: Resting systolic and diastolic blood pressure II: Diabetes status III: Pulse-wave velocity IV: Body composition and fitness	45 min for treadmill, stationary cycle, or stairstepper with a target range of 60% to 90% of maximum heart rate.	Two sets of 7 exercises at 10 to 15 repetitions per exercise at 50% of 1-repetition maximum on a multistation machine	26 weeks	The lack of change in arterial stiffness suggests a resistance to exercise-induced blood pressure reduction in persons with T2DM.
5	I: Systolic and diastolic blood pressure II: HbA1c III: Conduit artery intima-media thickness IV: Carotid blood pressure V: pulse wave velocity VI: Physical activity and fitness	Continuous cycling with 40 to 60% of maximal heart rate.	10–12 repetitions of seated row, pull-down, chest press, shoulder press, leg press, one leg lunge, dead bug and regular plank, with a weight adjusted individually.	52 weeks	No effect was found for hemodynamic variables after the intervention.

Risk of bias of included studies was shown in Figure 2. Most of the studies did not mention the detail of randomization or allocation concealment. Considering the nature of exercise process, it was impossible to keep patients blinded to interventions. No studies had incomplete outcome data or selective reporting. Regarding other biases, two of the five studies had sample size calculation prior to patient enrollment, and therefore was ranked as low risk [36,38]. The κ value was 0.82, indicating an excellent consistency between two reviewers.

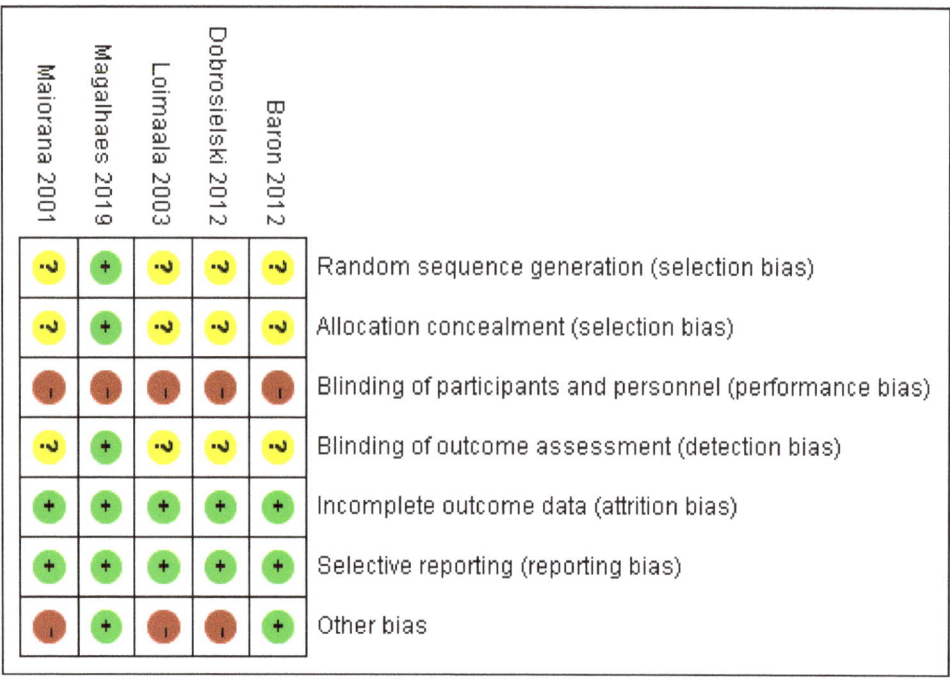

Figure 2. Risk of bias of each included study [35–39]. +: low risk; -: high risk; ?: unclear risk.

3.1. Primary Outcome

Compared with control, aerobic plus resistance training did not significantly improve PWV of patients with T2DM (MD −0.54 m/s, 95% CI [−1.69, 0.60], $p = 0.35$, three studies included [35,37,38]). The heterogeneity was not remarkable ($I^2 = 0\%$, $p = 0.86$) (Figure 3.2). Considering that study design might introduce bias and some data were calculated based on estimation, the level of evidence was low. However, this insignificance was not supported by TSA, which indicated the current outcome might be a result of limited sample size (Figure 4).

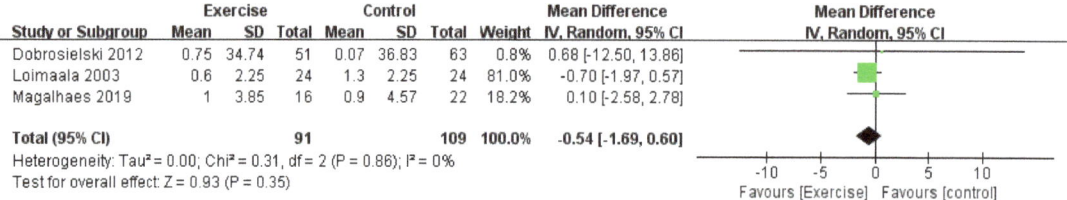

Figure 3. The pooled result of the difference of changes in pulse wave velocity between two groups [35,37,38].

3.2. Secondary Outcomes

Compared with control, aerobic plus resistance training did not significantly improve SBP of patients with T2DM (MD −1.05 mmHg, 95% CI [−3.71, 1.61], $p = 0.44$, four studies included [35–38]). The heterogeneity was not significant ($I^2 = 0\%$, $p = 0.87$) (Figure 5).

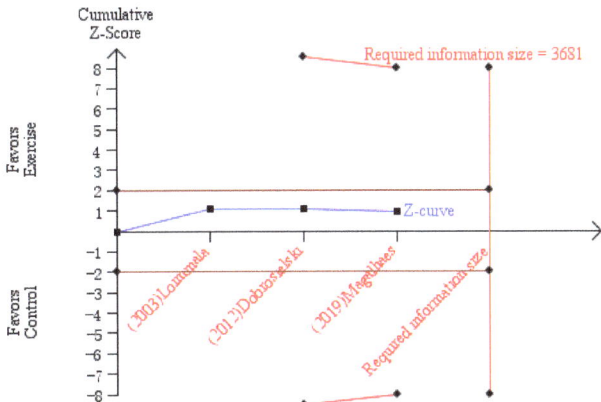

Figure 4. The result of TSA for PWV. TSA showed that the pooled results did not (z-curve, blue curve) crossed the conventional boundary of benefit (brown line) or the trial sequential monitoring boundary for benefit (upper red line), and did not reach the required sample size based on TSA (n = 3681) [35,37,38].

Study or Subgroup	Exercise Mean	SD	Total	Control Mean	SD	Total	Weight	Mean Difference IV, Random, 95% CI
Baron 2012	−2	10	49	−1	10	63	50.7%	−1.00 [−4.73, 2.73]
Dobrosielski 2012	−0.4	14.43	51	−0.7	13.39	63	26.6%	0.30 [−4.86, 5.46]
Loimaala 2003	−3	12.85	24	−1	12.91	24	13.3%	−2.00 [−9.29, 5.29]
Magalhaes 2019	−7	12.49	16	−3.2	14.65	22	9.4%	−3.80 [−12.46, 4.86]
Total (95% CI)			**140**			**172**	**100.0%**	**−1.05 [−3.71, 1.61]**

Heterogeneity: Tau² = 0.00; Chi² = 0.72, df = 3 (P = 0.87); I² = 0%
Test for overall effect: Z = 0.78 (P = 0.44)

Figure 5. The pooled result of the difference of changes in systolic blood pressure between two groups [35–38].

On the other hand, aerobic plus resistance training significantly decreased HbA1c of patients with T2DM (MD −0.55%, 95% CI [−0.88, −0.22], $p = 0.001$, three studies included [34,36,37]). The heterogeneity was insignificant ($I^2 = 0\%$, $p = 0.72$) (Figure 6). This outcome was in consistent with the records of Maiorana et al. [39] that, at the final follow-up, the level of HbA1c was 7.9 ± 0.3% in patients with exercise, significantly lower than those without exercise (8.5 ± 0.4%).

Study or Subgroup	Exercise Mean	SD	Total	Control Mean	SD	Total	Weight	Mean Difference IV, Random, 95% CI
Baron 2012	−0.2	1.2	49	0.3	1.1	63	58.2%	−0.50 [−0.93, −0.07]
Dobrosielski 2012	−0.2	1.67	51	0.3	1.67	63	28.6%	−0.50 [−1.12, 0.12]
Loimaala 2003	−0.6	1.85	25	0.3	1.35	24	13.3%	−0.90 [−1.80, 0.00]
Total (95% CI)			**125**			**150**	**100.0%**	**−0.55 [−0.88, −0.22]**

Heterogeneity: Tau² = 0.00; Chi² = 0.65, df = 2 (P = 0.72); I² = 0%
Test for overall effect: Z = 3.29 (P = 0.001)

Figure 6. The pooled result of the difference of changes in hemoglobin A1c between two groups [35–37].

4. Discussion

Numerous meta-analyses have discussed the benefit of various types of exercise training on T2DM in glycemic control, psychosocial performance, the level of inflammatory cytokines, et al. [40–42]. In the current study, we primarily focused on the effect of aerobic plus machine-assisted resistance training on vascular function in patients with T2DM. Based on the data available, we failed to detect a statistical significance of this combined training method for vascular condition, as indicated by PWV or SBP. On the other hand, TSA suggested that this insignificant difference might be attributed to a relatively small sample size. Moreover, aerobic plus machine-assisted resistance training significantly reduced the level of HbA1c, which is associated with cardiovascular risk. Therefore, it is currently not appropriate to negate the benefit of this training method on vascular health in T2DM population.

Resistance training can be either machine-assisted [38,39], elastic band-assisted [43], or even free weight [44]. Some studies used elastic bands in resistance training section, but did not notice an improvement in flow-mediated dilation or endothelium-independent vasodilation in T2DM population [43,45]. On the other hand, aerobic plus free weight-based resistance training could significantly decrease carotid intima-media thickness and arterial stiffness [44,46]. Considering that the uncertainty in body weight or the elasticity of bands may act as confounders, we focused specifically on machine-assisted resistance training.

As the widely used structural and functional index for measuring arterial stiffness [47], PWV is usually faster in T2DM population [48], indicating vascular stiffening and high cardiovascular risk [49]. Surprisingly, the present data did not support the application of this exercise protocol for improving vascular condition in T2DM population. This may be explained by two factors. First, as aforementioned, those receiving free weight exercise have improved vascular condition, so one can speculate that different resistance training protocol may yield different outcomes. Second, by conducting TSA, we noted that the required sample size was not reached, therefore more clinical trials are still needed.

Next, we compared the change in hemodynamic index, SBP. As an reflection of the plasticity in vasculature [16], SBP is always higher in stiffened vessel [50]. We found that the change of SBP following aerobic plus resistance training was comparable to that in control group, indicating that this training protocol may not be able to improve vascular function in T2DM population.

However, in agreement with a recent meta-analysis [42], we noticed a significant decrease of HbA1c in T2DM population with exercise, implying that aerobic plus machine-assisted resistance training could help control blood glucose. In hyperglycemia-induced complications of T2DM, especially vascular dysfunction, oxidative stress plays a pivotal role [51]. Oxidative damage caused by excessive reactive oxygen species can lead to endothelial damage via several signaling pathways, aggravating vascular stiffness and impairing vasorelaxation [52,53]. To prevent or retard the progression of complications, long-term control of blood glucose is of vital importance [54], the benefit of aerobic plus machine-assisted resistance training on blood glucose control was an indirect evidence that this exercise protocol could be meaningful for controlling vascular complications. This was in accordance with previous researches that high HbA1c was associated vascular risk and could be predictive of vascular events [55,56].

Previously, several systematic reviews and meta-analyses studied the influence of exercise on vascular function in T2DM. By measuring brachial artery flow-mediated dilation, Lee found that exercise as a whole, regardless of the pattern, significantly improved vascular endothelial function [57]. Dos et al. noticed that aerobic plus resistance training could improve vascular function in T2DM [14]. However, some of the included studies were not RCTs, which may act as the origin of divergence compared with ours.

The current findings should be interpreted with caution. First, some data we input were based on estimation, which might introduce impreciseness. The sample size was also not statistically sufficient, as indicated by TSA. In addition, the relatively short follow-up duration may contribute to the insignificant difference of PWV or SBP. Contrarily, we found that HbA1c was improved by training. Since HbA1c is related to better glucose metabolism, which indicates greater redox balance, one can expect a better vascular system [58]. Next, the evaluation of vascular condition should be multi-dimensional. A comprehensive understanding of vascular status in T2DM patients with exercise can be conducted in the future. Thirdly, albeit an exact protocol of exercise in each study, confounders were unavoidable. The age ranges from 40 to over 60, the follow-up duration ranges from 16 to 52 weeks, and even one study only recruited male patients. To reveal the effect of aerobic plus resistance training on vascular health, a longer follow-up period in a group of patients with closer age range is necessary. Finally, HbA1c does not indicate the variation of the glycemic profile, which is also a risk factor for cardiovascular events in T2DM population [59]. The effect of exercise on glycemic variability can be detected in further trials.

In conclusion, the outcome of the current meta-analysis was not supportive of the benefit of aerobic plus machine-assisted resistance training on vascular condition in T2DM population. However, this finding could be a result of small sample size. Considering that there was a significant improvement of HbA1c after training, this method may still have the potential of maintaining vascular health. More studies with longer follow-up duration are required to verify this potential.

Author Contributions: Conceptualization, Z.L.; methodology, H.Z.; software, writing-original draft preparation: X.G.; software: S.G.; investigation, X.G. and S.G. All authors have read and agreed to the published version of the manuscript.

Funding: Chenguang Plan of Yangpu Hospital, Tongji University (2020-14). Fund for psychosomatic medicine, key discipline of district level of Shanghai Yangpu District mental health center ([2019] No. 108).

Institutional Review Board Statement: Not applicable.

Conflicts of Interest: The authors declare no conflict of interest.

References

1. Cho, N.H.; Shaw, J.E.; Karuranga, S.; Huang, Y.; da Rocha Fernandes, J.D.; Ohlrogge, A.W.; Malanda, B. IDF Diabetes Atlas: Global estimates of diabetes prevalence for 2017 and projections for 2045. *Diabetes Res. Clin. Pract.* **2018**, *138*, 271–281. [CrossRef]
2. Solomon, S.D.; Chew, E.; Duh, E.J.; Sobrin, L.; Sun, J.K.; VanderBeek, B.L.; Wykoff, C.C.; Gardner, T.W. Diabetic Retinopathy: A Position Statement by the American Diabetes Association. *Diabetes Care* **2017**, *40*, 412–418, Erratum in *Diabetes Care* **2017**, *40*, 1285. [CrossRef] [PubMed]
3. Ismail-Beigi, F.; Craven, T.; Banerji, M.A.; Basile, J.; Calles, J.; Cohen, R.M.; Cuddihy, R.; Cushman, W.C.; Genuth, S.; Grimm, R.H., Jr.; et al. Effect of intensive treatment of hyperglycaemia on microvascular outcomes in type 2 diabetes: An analysis of the ACCORD randomised trial. *Lancet* **2010**, *376*, 419–430. [CrossRef]
4. Yun, J.S.; Ko, S.H. Current trends in epidemiology of cardiovascular disease and cardiovascular risk management in type 2 diabetes. *Metabolism* **2021**, *123*, 154838. [CrossRef] [PubMed]
5. Monteiro-Alfredo, T.; Oliveira, S.; Amaro, A.; Rosendo-Silva, D.; Antunes, K.; Pires, A.S.; Teixo, R.; Abrantes, A.M.; Botelho, M.F.; Castelo-Branco, M.; et al. Hypoglycaemic and Antioxidant Properties of Acrocomia aculeata (Jacq.) Lodd Ex Mart. Extract Are Associated with Better Vascular Function of Type 2 Diabetic Rats. *Nutrients* **2021**, *13*, 2856. [CrossRef]
6. Choi, J.H.; Cho, Y.J.; Kim, H.J.; Ko, S.H.; Chon, S.; Kang, J.H.; Kim, K.K.; Kim, E.M.; Kim, H.J.; Song, K.H.; et al. Effect of carbohydrate-restricted diets and intermittent fasting on obesity, type 2 diabetes mellitus, and hypertension management: Consensus statement of the Korean Society for the Study of obesity, Korean Diabetes Association, and Korean Society of Hypertension. *Clin. Hypertens.* **2022**, *28*, 26. [CrossRef]
7. Salzberg, L. Risk Factors and Lifestyle Interventions. *Prim. Care.* **2022**, *49*, 201–212. [CrossRef]
8. Delevatti, R.S.; Bracht, C.G.; Lisboa, S.D.C.; Costa, R.R.; Marson, E.C.; Netto, N.; Kruel, L.F.M. The Role of Aerobic Training Variables Progression on Glycemic Control of Patients with Type 2 Diabetes: A Systematic Review with Meta-analysis. *Sports Med. Open* **2019**, *5*, 22. [CrossRef]
9. Way, K.L.; Keating, S.E.; Baker, M.K.; Chuter, V.H.; Johnson, N.A. The Effect of Exercise on Vascular Function and Stiffness in Type 2 Diabetes: A Systematic Review and Meta-analysis. *Curr. Diabetes Rev.* **2016**, *12*, 369–383. [CrossRef]
10. Sinacore, D.R.; Gulve, E.A. The role of skeletal muscle in glucose transport, glucose homeostasis, and insulin resistance: Implications for physical therapy. *Phys. Ther.* **1993**, *73*, 878–891. [CrossRef]
11. Okamoto, T.; Masuhara, M.; Ikuta, K. Combined aerobic and resistance training and vascular function: Effect of aerobic exercise before and after resistance training. *J. Appl. Physiol.* **2007**, *103*, 1655–1661. [CrossRef] [PubMed]
12. Li, Y.; Hanssen, H.; Cordes, M.; Rossmeissl, A.; Endes, S.; Schmidt-Trucksass, A. Aerobic, resistance and combined exercise training on arterial stiffness in normotensive and hypertensive adults: A review. *Eur. J. Sport Sci.* **2015**, *15*, 443–457. [CrossRef] [PubMed]

13. Liberati, A.; Altman, D.G.; Tetzlaff, J.; Mulrow, C.; Gotzsche, P.C.; Ioannidis, J.P.; Clarke, M.; Devereaux, P.J.; Kleijnen, J.; Moher, D. The PRISMA statement for reporting systematic reviews and meta-analyses of studies that evaluate healthcare interventions: Explanation and elaboration. *BMJ* **2009**, *339*, b2700. [CrossRef]
14. Dos Santos Araujo, J.E.; Nunes Macedo, F.; Sales Barreto, A.; Viana Dos Santos, M.R.; Antoniolli, A.R.; Quintans-Junior, L.J. Effects of Resistance and Combined training on Vascular Function in Type 2 Diabetes: A Systematic Review of Randomized Controlled Trials. *Rev. Diabet. Stud.* **2019**, *15*, 16–25. [CrossRef] [PubMed]
15. Sacks, D.; Baxter, B.; Campbell, B.C.V.; Carpenter, J.S.; Cognard, C.; Dippel, D.; Eesa, M.; Fischer, U.; Hausegger, K.; Hirsch, J.A.; et al. Multisociety Consensus Quality Improvement Revised Consensus Statement for Endovascular Therapy of Acute Ischemic Stroke. *Int. J. Stroke* **2018**, *13*, 612–632. [CrossRef] [PubMed]
16. Chen, H.; Chen, Y.; Wu, W.; Cai, Z.; Chen, Z.; Yan, X.; Wu, S. Total cholesterol, arterial stiffness, and systolic blood pressure: A mediation analysis. *Sci. Rep.* **2021**, *11*, 1330. [CrossRef]
17. Kwon, T.H.; Kim, K.D. Machine-Learning-Based Noninvasive In Vivo Estimation of HbA1c Using Photoplethysmography Signals. *Sensors* **2022**, *22*, 2963. [CrossRef]
18. Sun, Y.; Chen, J.; Li, H.; Jiang, J.; Chen, S. Steroid Injection and Nonsteroidal Anti-inflammatory Agents for Shoulder Pain: A PRISMA Systematic Review and Meta-Analysis of Randomized Controlled Trials. *Medicine* **2015**, *94*, e2216. [CrossRef]
19. Higgins, J.P.T.; Green, S. *Cochrane Handbook for Systematic Reviews of Interventions Version 5.1.0 [Updated March 2011]*; The Cochrane Collaboration: London, UK, 2011.
20. Higgins, J.P.; Thompson, S.G.; Deeks, J.J.; Altman, D.G. Measuring inconsistency in meta-analyses. *BMJ* **2003**, *327*, 557–560. [CrossRef]
21. Song, F.; Eastwood, A.J.; Gilbody, S.; Duley, L.; Sutton, A.J. Publication and related biases. *Health Technol. Assess.* **2000**, *4*, 1–115. [CrossRef]
22. Higgins, J.P.; Altman, D.G.; Gotzsche, P.C.; Juni, P.; Moher, D.; Oxman, A.D.; Savovic, J.; Schulz, K.F.; Weeks, L.; Sterne, J.A.; et al. The Cochrane Collaboration's tool for assessing risk of bias in randomised trials. *BMJ* **2011**, *343*, d5928. [CrossRef] [PubMed]
23. Guyatt, G.H.; Oxman, A.D.; Kunz, R.; Brozek, J.; Alonso-Coello, P.; Rind, D.; Devereaux, P.J.; Montori, V.M.; Freyschuss, B.; Vist, G.; et al. GRADE guidelines 6. Rating the quality of evidence—Imprecision. *J. Clin. Epidemiol.* **2011**, *64*, 1283–1293. [CrossRef] [PubMed]
24. Guyatt, G.H.; Oxman, A.D.; Kunz, R.; Woodcock, J.; Brozek, J.; Helfand, M.; Alonso-Coello, P.; Falck-Ytter, Y.; Jaeschke, R.; Vist, G.; et al. GRADE guidelines: 8. Rating the quality of evidence—Indirectness. *J. Clin. Epidemiol.* **2011**, *64*, 1303–1310. [CrossRef] [PubMed]
25. Guyatt, G.H.; Oxman, A.D.; Kunz, R.; Woodcock, J.; Brozek, J.; Helfand, M.; Alonso-Coello, P.; Glasziou, P.; Jaeschke, R.; Akl, E.A.; et al. GRADE guidelines: 7. Rating the quality of evidence—Inconsistency. *J. Clin. Epidemiol.* **2011**, *64*, 1294–1302. [CrossRef] [PubMed]
26. Guyatt, G.H.; Oxman, A.D.; Montori, V.; Vist, G.; Kunz, R.; Brozek, J.; Alonso-Coello, P.; Djulbegovic, B.; Atkins, D.; Falck-Ytter, Y.; et al. GRADE guidelines: 5. Rating the quality of evidence—Publication bias. *J. Clin. Epidemiol.* **2011**, *64*, 1277–1282. [CrossRef] [PubMed]
27. Guyatt, G.H.; Oxman, A.D.; Vist, G.; Kunz, R.; Brozek, J.; Alonso-Coello, P.; Montori, V.; Akl, E.A.; Djulbegovic, B.; Falck-Ytter, Y.; et al. GRADE guidelines: 4. Rating the quality of evidence—Study limitations (risk of bias). *J. Clin. Epidemiol.* **2011**, *64*, 407–415. [CrossRef]
28. Brok, J.; Thorlund, K.; Gluud, C.; Wetterslev, J. Trial sequential analysis reveals insufficient information size and potentially false positive results in many meta-analyses. *J. Clin. Epidemiol.* **2008**, *61*, 763–769. [CrossRef]
29. Thorlund, K.; Devereaux, P.J.; Wetterslev, J.; Guyatt, G.; Ioannidis, J.P.; Thabane, L.; Gluud, L.L.; Als-Nielsen, B.; Gluud, C. Can trial sequential monitoring boundaries reduce spurious inferences from meta-analyses? *Int. J. Epidemiol.* **2009**, *38*, 276–286. [CrossRef]
30. Sun, Y.; Zhang, P.; Liu, S.; Li, H.; Jiang, J.; Chen, S.; Chen, J. Intra-articular Steroid Injection for Frozen Shoulder: A Systematic Review and Meta-analysis of Randomized Controlled Trials With Trial Sequential Analysis. *Am. J. Sports Med.* **2017**, *45*, 2171–2179. [CrossRef]
31. Guo, S.; Guo, X.; Zhang, H.; Zhang, X.; Li, Z. The Effect of Diacerein on Type 2 Diabetic Mellitus: A Systematic Review and Meta-Analysis of Randomized Controlled Trials with Trial Sequential Analysis. *J. Diabetes Res.* **2020**, *2020*, 2593792. [CrossRef]
32. Wetterslev, J.; Thorlund, K.; Brok, J.; Gluud, C. Estimating required information size by quantifying diversity in random-effects model meta-analyses. *BMC Med. Res. Methodol.* **2009**, *9*, 86. [CrossRef] [PubMed]
33. Okada, S.; Hiuge, A.; Makino, H.; Nagumo, A.; Takaki, H.; Goto, H.K.; Yoshimasa, Y.; Miyamoto, Y. Effect of exercise intervention on endothelial function and incidence of cardiovascular disease in patients with type 2 diabetes. *J. Atheroscler. Thromb.* **2010**, *17*, 828–833. [CrossRef] [PubMed]
34. Loimaala, A.; Groundstroem, K.; Rinne, M.; Nenonen, A.; Huhtala, H.; Parkkari, J.; Vuori, I. Effect of long-term endurance and strength training on metabolic control and arterial elasticity in patients with type 2 diabetes mellitus. *Am. J. Cardiol.* **2009**, *103*, 972–977. [CrossRef] [PubMed]
35. Loimaala, A.; Huikuri, H.V.; Kööbi, T.; Rinne, M.; Nenonen, A.; Vuori, I. Exercise training improves baroreflex sensitivity in type 2 diabetes. *Diabetes* **2003**, *52*, 1837–1842. [CrossRef]

36. Barone, G.B.; Dobrosielski, D.; Bonekamp, S.; Stewart, K.; Clark, J. A randomized trial of exercise for blood pressure reduction in type 2 diabetes: Effect on flow-mediated dilation and circulating biomarkers of endothelial function. *Atherosclerosis* **2012**, *224*, 446–453. [CrossRef]
37. Dobrosielski, D.; Gibbs, B.; Ouyang, P.; Bonekamp, S.; Clark, J.; Wang, N.; Silber, H.; Shapiro, E.; Stewart, K. Effect of exercise on blood pressure in type 2 diabetes: A randomized controlled trial. *J. Gen. Intern. Med.* **2012**, *27*, 1453–1459. [CrossRef]
38. Magalhães, J.; Melo, X.; Correia, I.; Ribeiro, R.; Raposo, J.; Dores, H.; Bicho, M.; Sardinha, L. Effects of combined training with different intensities on vascular health in patients with type 2 diabetes: A 1-year randomized controlled trial. *Cardiovasc. Diabetol.* **2019**, *18*, 34. [CrossRef]
39. Maiorana, A.; O'Driscoll, G.; Cheetham, C.; Dembo, L.; Stanton, K.; Goodman, C.; Taylor, R.; Green, D. The effect of combined aerobic and resistance exercise training on vascular function in type 2 diabetes. *J. Am. Coll. Cardiol.* **2001**, *38*, 860–866. [CrossRef]
40. Jayedi, A.; Emadi, A.; Shab-Bidar, S. Dose-Dependent Effect of Supervised Aerobic Exercise on HbA(1c) in Patients with Type 2 Diabetes: A Meta-analysis of Randomized Controlled Trials. *Sports Med.* **2022**. online ahead of print. [CrossRef]
41. Jiahao, L.; Jiajin, L.; Yifan, L. Effects of resistance training on insulin sensitivity in the elderly: A meta-analysis of randomized controlled trials. *J. Exerc. Sci. Fit.* **2021**, *19*, 241–251. [CrossRef]
42. Mannucci, E.; Bonifazi, A.; Monami, M. Comparison between different types of exercise training in patients with type 2 diabetes mellitus: A systematic review and network metanalysis of randomized controlled trials. *Nutr. Metab. Cardiovasc. Dis.* **2021**, *31*, 1985–1992. [CrossRef] [PubMed]
43. Miche, E.; Herrmann, G.; Nowak, M.; Wirtz, U.; Tietz, M.; Hürst, M.; Zoller, B.; Radzewitz, A. Effect of an exercise training program on endothelial dysfunction in diabetic and non-diabetic patients with severe chronic heart failure. *Clin. Res. Cardiol.* **2006**, *95* (Suppl. S1), i117–i124. [CrossRef] [PubMed]
44. Brozic, A.P.; Marzolini, S.; Goodman, J.M. Effects of an adapted cardiac rehabilitation programme on arterial stiffness in patients with type 2 diabetes without cardiac disease diagnosis. *Diab. Vasc. Dis. Res.* **2017**, *14*, 104–112. [CrossRef] [PubMed]
45. Kwon, H.R.; Min, K.W.; Ahn, H.J.; Seok, H.G.; Lee, J.H.; Park, G.S.; Han, K.A. Effects of Aerobic Exercise vs. Resistance Training on Endothelial Function in Women with Type 2 Diabetes Mellitus. *Diabetes Metab. J.* **2011**, *35*, 364–373. [CrossRef] [PubMed]
46. Byrkjeland, R.; Stensæth, K.H.; Anderssen, S.; Njerve, I.U.; Arnesen, H.; Seljeflot, I.; Solheim, S. Effects of exercise training on carotid intima-media thickness in patients with type 2 diabetes and coronary artery disease. Influence of carotid plaques. *Cardiovasc. Diabetol.* **2016**, *15*, 13. [CrossRef]
47. Miyamoto, M.; Kotani, K.; Okada, K.; Ando, A.; Hasegawa, H.; Kanai, H.; Ishibashi, S.; Yamada, T.; Taniguchi, N. Arterial wall elasticity measured using the phased tracking method and atherosclerotic risk factors in patients with type 2 diabetes. *J. Atheroscler. Thromb.* **2013**, *20*, 678–687. [CrossRef]
48. Kotb, N.A.; Gaber, R.; Salama, M.; Nagy, H.M.; Elhendy, A. Clinical and biochemical predictors of increased carotid intima-media thickness in overweight and obese adolescents with type 2 diabetes. *Diab. Vasc. Dis. Res.* **2012**, *9*, 35–41. [CrossRef]
49. Lorenz, M.W.; Markus, H.S.; Bots, M.L.; Rosvall, M.; Sitzer, M. Prediction of clinical cardiovascular events with carotid intima-media thickness: A systematic review and meta-analysis. *Circulation* **2007**, *115*, 459–467. [CrossRef]
50. Beckman, J.A.; Creager, M.A.; Libby, P. Diabetes and Atherosclerosis: Epidemiology, Pathophysiology, and Management. *JAMA J. Am. Med. Assoc.* **2002**, *287*, 2570. [CrossRef]
51. Pulakazhi Venu, V.K.; El-Daly, M.; Saifeddine, M.; Hirota, S.A.; Ding, H.; Triggle, C.R.; Hollenberg, M.D. Minimizing Hyperglycemia-Induced Vascular Endothelial Dysfunction by Inhibiting Endothelial Sodium-Glucose Cotransporter 2 and Attenuating Oxidative Stress: Implications for Treating Individuals With Type 2 Diabetes. *Can. J. Diabetes* **2019**, *43*, 510–514. [CrossRef]
52. Srinivasan, S.; Hatley, M.E.; Bolick, D.T.; Palmer, L.A.; Edelstein, D.; Brownlee, M.; Hedrick, C.C. Hyperglycaemia-induced superoxide production decreases eNOS expression via AP-1 activation in aortic endothelial cells. *Diabetologia* **2004**, *47*, 1727–1734. [CrossRef] [PubMed]
53. Lai, T.C.; Chen, Y.C.; Cheng, H.H.; Lee, T.L.; Tsai, J.S.; Lee, I.T.; Peng, K.T.; Lee, C.W.; Hsu, L.F.; Chen, Y.L. Combined exposure to fine particulate matter and high glucose aggravates endothelial damage by increasing inflammation and mitophagy: The involvement of vitamin D. *Part. Fibre Toxicol.* **2022**, *19*, 25. [CrossRef] [PubMed]
54. Kohnert, K.D.; Heinke, P.; Zander, E.; Vogt, L.; Salzsieder, E. Glycemic Key Metrics and the Risk of Diabetes-Associated Complications. *Rom. J. Diabetes Nutr. Metab. Dis.* **2016**, *23*, 403–413. [CrossRef]
55. D'Souza, J.M.; D'Souza, R.P.; Vijin, V.F.; Shetty, A.; Arunachalam, C.; Pai, V.R.; Shetty, R.; Faarisa, A. High predictive ability of glycated hemoglobin on comparison with oxidative stress markers in assessment of chronic vascular complications in type 2 diabetes mellitus. *Scand. J. Clin. Lab. Investig.* **2016**, *76*, 51–57. [CrossRef]
56. Kostov, K.; Blazhev, A. Use of Glycated Hemoglobin (A1c) as a Biomarker for Vascular Risk in Type 2 Diabetes: Its Relationship with Matrix Metalloproteinases-2, -9 and the Metabolism of Collagen IV and Elastin. *Medicina* **2020**, *56*, 231. [CrossRef]
57. Lee, J.H.; Lee, R.; Hwang, M.H.; Hamilton, M.T.; Park, Y. The effects of exercise on vascular endothelial function in type 2 diabetes: A systematic review and meta-analysis. *Diabetol. Metab. Syndr.* **2018**, *10*, 15. [CrossRef]
58. Dhawan, P.; Vasishta, S.; Balakrishnan, A.; Joshi, M.B. Mechanistic insights into glucose induced vascular epigenetic reprogramming in type 2 diabetes. *Life Sci.* **2022**, *298*, 120490. [CrossRef]
59. Martinez, M.; Santamarina, J.; Pavesi, A.; Musso, C.; Umpierrez, G.E. Glycemic variability and cardiovascular disease in patients with type 2 diabetes. *BMJ Open Diabetes Res. Care* **2021**, *9*, e002032. [CrossRef]

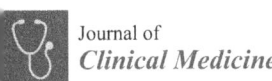

Article

Knee Cartilage Change within 5 Years after Aclr Using Hamstring Tendons with Preserved Tibial-Insertion: A Prospective Randomized Controlled Study Based on Magnetic Resonance Imaging

Yuhan Zhang [1], Shaohua Liu [2], Yaying Sun [2], Yuxue Xie [3] and Jiwu Chen [4,*]

1. Department of Orthopaedics, Beijing Chaoyang Hospital, Capital Medical University, Beijing 100020, China
2. Department of Sports Medicine, Huashan Hospital, Fudan University, Shanghai 200040, China
3. Department of Radiology & Institute of Medical Functional and Molecular Imaging, Huashan Hospital, Fudan University, Shanghai 200040, China
4. Department of Sports Medicine, Shanghai General Hospital, Shanghai Jiaotong University, Shanghai 200080, China
* Correspondence: jeevechen@gmail.com

Abstract: Background: Comparing to anterior cruciate ligament reconstructions (ACLR) with free hamstring tendon (FHT), ACLR with preserved tibial-insertion hamstring tendon (HT-PTI) could ensure the blood supply of the graft and avoid graft necrosis. Yet, whether HT-PTI could protect the cartilage and clinical outcomes in mid-long period after ACLR was still unclear. **Purpose:** To compare the cartilage change and clinical results between the HT-PTI and FHT in 5 years after ACLR. **Study design:** Randomized controlled trial; Level of evidence, 2. **Methods:** A total of 45 patients who underwent isolated ACLR with the autograft of hamstring tendons were enrolled and randomized into 2 groups. The study group undertook ACLR with HT-PTI, whereas the control group had FHT. At pre-operation, and 6, 12, 24, and 60 months post-operation, all cases underwent evaluation with Knee Injury and Osteoarthritis Outcome Score (KOOS), and MR examination. The knee cartilage was divided into 8 sub-regions of which the T2 value and cartilage volume on MRI were measured and documented. The data of two groups were compared and their correlations were analyzed. **Results:** A total of 18 patients in the HT-PTI group and 19 patients in the FHT group completed the follow-up. The KOOS scores were improved at each follow-up time point ($p < 0.001$), reached the most superior at 12 months and maintained until 60 months but had no significant difference between the two groups. At 60 months, the cartilage in most subregions in FHT group had higher T2 values than those of pre-operation ($p < 0.05$) and also higher than HT-PTI group; The cartilage volume changes (CV%) are positive at 6 months and negative from 12 to 60 months in the FHT group, while being negative at all time points in the HT-PTI group. The values of absolute CV% in most subregions in FHT group were significantly higher than those in the HT-PTI group at 6 and 60 months ($p < 0.05$). **Conclusion:** The improvement of KOOS score peaked at 12 months in all cases and had no difference between the two groups. The cartilage in the FHT group had more volume loss, earlier and wider damage than that in the HT-PTI group within 5 years. No significant correlation was found among KOOS score, CV%, and T2 value.

Keywords: ACLR; hamstring tendon with preserved tibial insertion; MRI; T2; cartilage volume

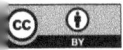

1. Introduction

The instability of the knee joint after the injury of the anterior cruciate ligament (ACL) will lead to the wear of articular cartilage. At present, relevant research shows that ACL reconstruction (ACLR) can effectively correct the instability of the knee joint, thereby reducing the wear of articular cartilage [1]. However, various studies showed that the damage of articular cartilage was still progressing after ACLR had corrected joint instability [2–6]. It was proved that various inflammatory factors including IL-1β, IL-6, IL-10 and TNF-α were released into the joint during the graft necrosis and proliferation stages after ACLR, activated matrix metalloproteinases to digest collagen and proteoglycan in cartilage matrix, and resulted in cartilage degeneration [7,8]. Therefore, the potential biochemical and metabolic factors could lead to the occurrence of knee OA after ACLR [1,9].

In the early stage of cartilage degeneration, the cartilage would have increased water content, decreased proteoglycan content [10] and reduced volume [11,12]. MRI is the most commonly used to evaluate cartilage injury [12–14] because its sensitivity in detecting the water change in cartilage [15]. As the T2 relaxation time of cartilage is directly proportional to the water distribution in cartilage and inversely proportional to the specific distribution of proteoglycan [12,16,17], MRI quantitative T2 value is used for detecting early cartilage lesions through the changes of cartilage matrix and water content [18].

The growing activity in the field of cartilage damage creates a need for validated clinical outcome scores whose special emphasis was given to patients with cartilage injuries [19]. Different from the Lysholm, Tegner, and international knee documentation committee (IKDC) scores, the Western Ontario and McMaster Universities Index (WOMAC) is commonly used to measure the patients with osteoarthritis (OA) [20]. However, the population presenting with focal cartilage lesions after ACLR is generally younger and more active as compared to patients with OA [21]. The Knee Injury and Osteoarthritis Outcome Score (KOOS) was developed as an extension of the WOMAC and designed to assess symptoms and function in younger or more active patients with ACL injuries and cartilage damage [19]. Therefore, the KOOS would fit this population better. In addition, the KOOS have been proved to be a measure of sufficient reliability, validity, and responsiveness for surgery and physical therapy after ACLR [19,22].

Given the hamstring tendon with intact tibial insertion (HT-PTI) had much less necrosis than the free hamstring tendon (FHT) after ACLR [7,23], and could avoid necrosis and reduced the level of intra-articular inflammation [7,23,24], we hypothesized that the knee after ACLR using HT-PTI might have less cartilage degeneration than those using FHT.

The purpose of this study was to investigate and compare the KOOS score and cartilage degeneration measured on MRI after ACLR in 5 years with HT-PTI and FHT, then to analyze which operation could help to slow down the cartilage degeneration after surgery and analyze the potential correlations between knee function and cartilage degeneration.

2. Methods

2.1. Participants

This study was approved by the local ethical committee and all patients signed informed consent before enrollment. This single-center, prospective, randomized trial was conducted in our hospital. The patients with ACL injury were consecutively enrolled from January to December 2014, and the indication, inclusion criteria, and other detail information were described in the methods of our previous study [24]. The inclusion criteria for participants were (1) unilateral ACL injury, (2) no history of surgery in the injured knee, and (3) age between 18 and 45 years. The participants were excluded if they had any of the following: (1) osteoarthritis; (2) combined ligament injuries; (3) multisystem trauma, nerve injuries, or fractures; or (4) cartilage injury more severe than grade 2 using the Outerbridge grading system [25] (determined during diagnostic arthroscopy) [7]. Differences of demographic data between the 2 groups were not statistically significant (all p values < 0.05) [7]. In all, 45 patients who qualified for inclusion were recruited and randomly distributed into 2 groups, including 21 patients underwent ACLR with HT-PTI and 24 with FHT, were performed follow-up during the periodic follow-up (Figure 1). 17.8% of the patients were lost to the follow-up.

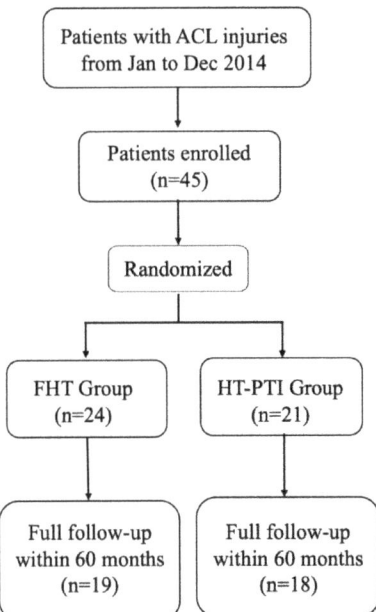

Figure 1. Flowchart of the randomized clinical trial. Full follow-up within 60 months included patients who had follow-up at pre-operation and 6, 12, 24, and 60 months postoperatively. The HT-PTI group had ACLR with an insertion preserved hamstring tendon autograft, and the FHT group had ACLR with a free hamstring tendon autograft. HT-PTI, hamstring tendon with intact tibial insertion; FHT, free hamstring tendon; ACL, anterior cruciate ligament; ACLR, ACL reconstruction.

2.2. Surgical Technique and Postoperative Rehabilitation

The surgical techniques had been published previously. All operations were performed by the same senior surgeon using the same instrumentation and the same arthroscopic single-bundle ACLR techniques. All patients received the same protocol of postoperative rehabilitation [1].

2.3. Clinical Evaluation

Considering the assessment of the outcomes during inflammatory processes and stable-state condition postoperatively [7], the evaluations were performed and documented before surgery and at 6, 12, 24, and 60 months after surgery. As our previous study summarized and published the clinical outcomes based on objective scores within 60 months postoperatively [1], the KOOS score was evaluated at pre-operation and 6, 12, 24 and 60 months post-operatively in this study. The score includes five subscales: symptoms, pain, activities of daily living (ADL), sport and recreation function (Sports/rec), and quality of life (QoL). The higher the total score, the better the outcome of knee joint after ACLR.

2.4. MRI Scan and Image Analysis

MRI examinations were conducted by 3.0-T MRI scanner (MAGNETOM Verio, A Tim System; Siemens, Shanghai, China) and performed at 6, 12, 24 and 60 months after ACLR. Three-dimensional double echo steady states (3D-DESS) in sagittal plane was used to quantify cartilage. The repetition time was 14.45 ms, the echo time was 5.17 ms, and the turn angle was 25°, The thickness was 1.5 mm. In sagittal T2 mapping sequence, the repetition time was 2820 ms, echo time was 13.8/27.6/41.4/55.2/69.0 ms, and turn angle was 180°, The voxel size was $0.4 \times 0.4 \times 3.0$ mm; The visual field was 160 mm; The imaging time was 5 min 48 s. All image data were collected by Siemens software package (numaris/7, syngomr B17; Siemens) measurement and processing.

The MRI data of 3D-DESS sequence were imported into Siemens knee cap (version 1.5) workstation for automatic recognition of knee cartilage. The software could automatically divide articular cartilage into eight sub-regions [26,27]: patella (P), femoral trochlea (TrF), anterior area of lateral femoral condyle (aLFC), posterior area of lateral femoral condyle (pLFC), and anterior area of medial femoral condyle, (aMFC), posterior area of medial femoral condyle (pMFC), lateral tibia plateau (LT), medial tibia plateau (MT). The volume of cartilage in each subregion was obtained by manual fine-tuning. The aLFC and pLFC were divided by the posterior horn of the lateral meniscus, and the aMFC and pMFC were divided by the posterior horn of the medial meniscus. The specific operation interface of the software was shown in Figure 2, and the 3D model established by the software according to the preoperative knee cartilage of the patient is shown in Figure 3.

After all the MRI images being input into PACS Image processing software, two experienced radiologists independently measured the T2 value and cartilage value (CV) of each sub-region of cartilage after operation without knowing the specific grouping of FHT and HT-PTI. The repeated measurements were made on 2 days at 1–2 weeks apart [1].

The T2 values of cartilage were measured on three consecutive sagittal planes of the medial, lateral tibiofemoral and patellofemoral joints respectively (Figure 4). When manually sketching the cartilage contour for measurement, tried to avoid the subchondral bone plate and joint fluid and remove the extreme value. The average T2 value of all 3 consecutive layers was the T2 value corresponding to the measured cartilage subregion. All data of T2 mapping sequence were imported into Siemens workstation (syngi mrb17 software) for reconstruction to obtain T2 mapping.

The percent of cartilage volume changing (CV%) [17] of 8 sub-regions were measured and compared between HT-PTI and FHT groups preoperatively and at 6, 12, 24, and 60 months after ACLR. The volume change rate CV% of cartilage was calculated according to the following formula:

$$CV\% = \frac{\text{postoperative CV} - \text{preoperative CV}}{\text{preoperative CV}} \times 100\%$$

The negative value of CV% indicated that the cartilage volume decreased at this follow-up time point comparing to the preoperative CV, while the positive value indicated increased cartilage volume. The larger the absolute value of CV%, the greater the change of cartilage volume.

2.5. Statistical Analysis

Stata software (v13.0; Stata Corp., College Station, TX, USA). Continuous variables are represented by means ± standard deviation. The differences of T2 value, CV% and KOOS score between HT-PTI group and FHT group were compared. If the data obeyed normal distribution and the variance was homogeneous, the independent sample t-test was used; otherwise, the nonparametric Mann Whitney rank sum test was used. When comparing within groups, paired t-test was used if the data obeyed normal distribution and the variance was homogeneous, otherwise nonparametric Wilcoxon signed ranks test was used. Spearman correlation analysis was used to calculate and analyze the correlation between knee cartilage KOOS score, T2 and CV%. Intra correlation coefficient (ICC) was used to evaluate the consistency between the two measurements and scores (ICC < 0.4 was defined as poor; $0.4 \leq ICC \leq 0.75$ was defined as medium; ICC > 0.75 was defined as good). The significance level was set at 0.05. Using G*Power software (version 3.1) to calculate the sample size, according to the previous relevant research to determine the corresponding research index threshold [15], set the test level α = 0.5, test efficiency $(1 - \beta)$. Additionally, post hoc power analysis found that each group needs at least 16 patients to achieve significant difference. Therefore, the number of patients included in this study meets the minimum sample size requirements.

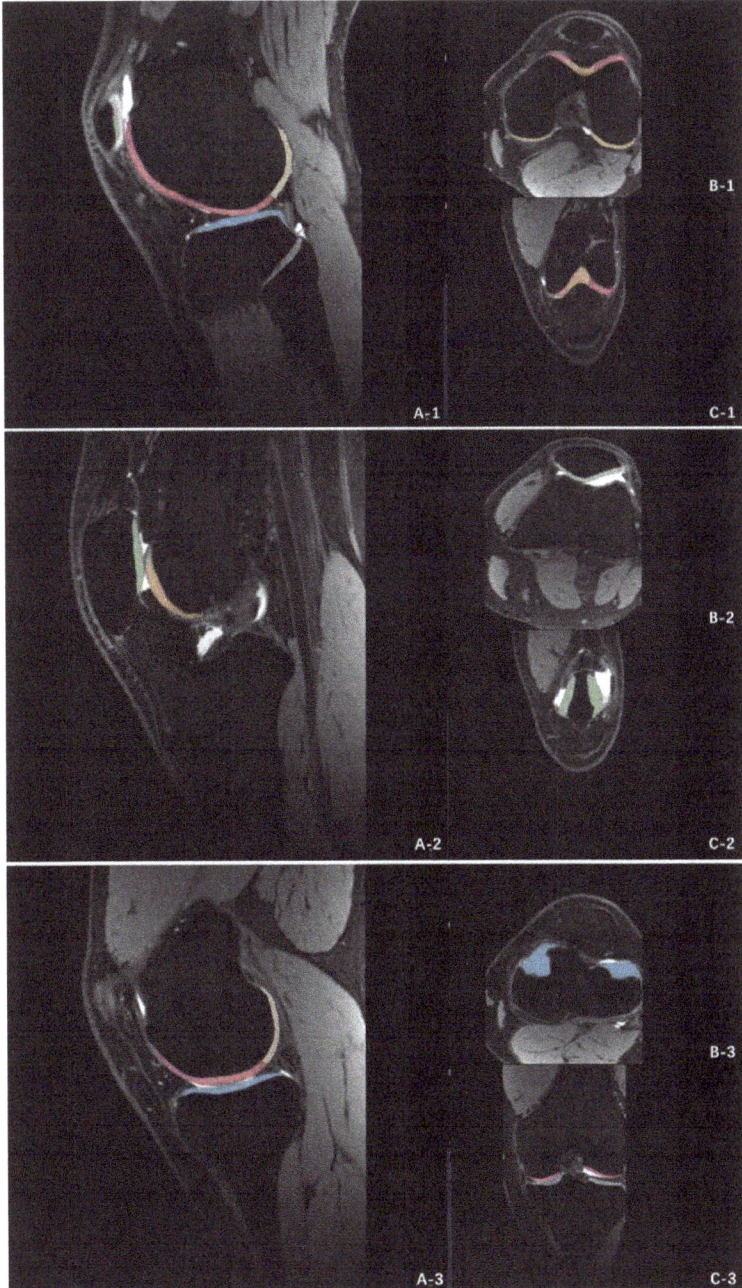

Figure 2. Siemens knee cap (version 1.5) software 3D-DESS image workstation operation interface. The software can automatically recognize and calculate the volume of each cartilage subregion of the knee joint. (**A-1**), Sagittal position of lateral knee joint; (**B-1**), Horizontal position of lateral knee joint; (**C-1**), Coronal position of lateral knee joint; (**A-2**), Sagittal position of middle knee joint; (**B-2**), Horizontal position of middle knee joint; (**C-2**), Coronal position of middle knee joint; (**A-3**), Sagittal position of medial knee joint; (**B-3**), Horizontal position of medial knee joint; (**C-3**), Coronal position of medial knee joint.

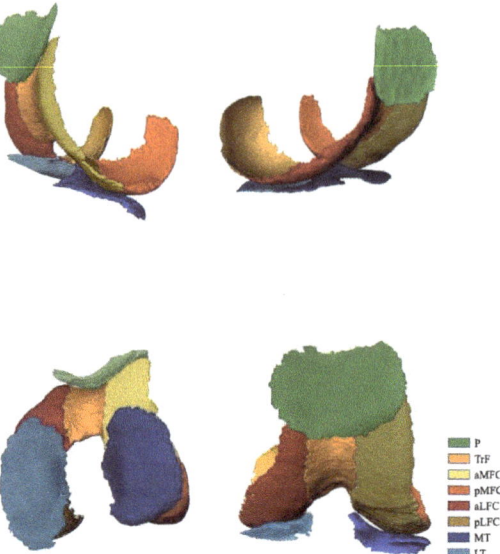

Figure 3. 3D model of knee joint cartilage. The 3D reconstruction model of complete knee cartilage was automatically divided into 8 subregions: P, TrF, aMFC, pMFC, aLFC, pLFC, MT and LT by Siemens knee cap (version 1.5). Different cartilage subareas are marked with different colors. The corresponding cartilage subareas of each color are shown in the far right of this figure. P, patella. TrF, femoral trochlea. aLFC, anterior area of lateral femoral condyle. pLFC, posterior area of lateral femoral condyle. aMFC, anterior area of medial femoral condyle. pMFC, posterior area of medial femoral condyle. LT, lateral tibia plateau. MT, medial tibia plateau.

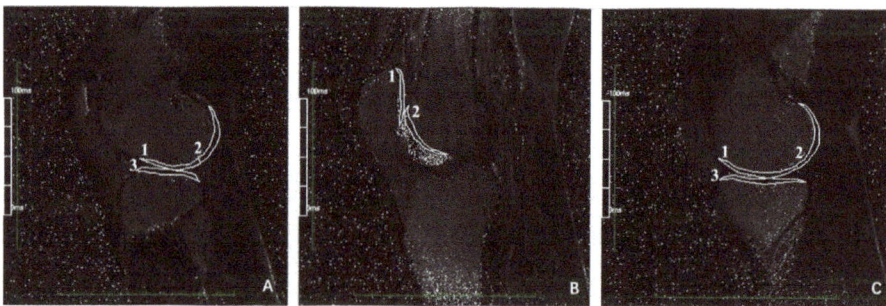

Figure 4. Measurements of T2 value of cartilage in each sub region of knee joint. (**A**) the lateral tibiofemoral joint of the knee: the measurement sub zone 1 is the aLFC, the measurement sub zone 2 is the pLFC, and the measurement sub zone 3 is the LT; (**B**) patellofemoral joint of knee joint: the measurement sub zone 1 is P, and the measurement sub zone 2 is TrF; (**C**) medial tibiofemoral joint of knee joint: the measurement subzone 1 is aMFC, the measurement subzone 2 is pMFC, and the measurement subzone 3 is MT.

3. Results

Finally, 5 patients in the control group and 3 patients in the study group were lost to full follow-up. 37 participants (82.2%) undergone complete follow-ups in this study: 18 patients in the study group and 19 patients in the control group, and relevant demographic data has been published in our previous study [24]. Differences of demographic data between the two groups were not statistically significant (all p values > 0.05) [1].

3.1. Clinical Outcomes

In our previous study [24], the clinical outcomes including the International Knee Documentation Committee (IKDC), Tegner scores, Lysholm activity score, and KT-1000 arthrometer measurements were improved compared with before surgery ($p < 0.001$) and were similar in both groups.

As shown in Table 1, the scores of KOOS in the two groups showed the same trend with time, which significantly improved at 6 months ($p < 0.001$), further significantly improved at 12 months ($p < 0.05$), and then maintained at a relatively stable level from 12 months to 60 months after ACLR. The differences were statistically significant ($p < 0.001$). There was no significant difference between HT-PTI group and FHT group in the symptoms, pain, activities of daily living, sport and recreation function, and quality of life scores of KOOS at pre-operation, 6, 12, 24 and 60 months after ACLR ($p > 0.05$).

Table 1. KOOS Outcomes in the Study and Control Groups [a].

	Symptoms	Pain	ADL	Sports/Rec	QoL
Control Group					
Pre-operative	67.1 ± 22.3	75.2 ± 23.8	80.8 ± 21.7	51.3 ± 18.9	47.3 ± 24.9
6-month	82.5 ± 15.3 *	84.9 ± 13.8 *	89.9 ± 11.3 *	63.3 ± 21.2 *	81.6 ± 17.3 *
12-month	90.2 ± 11.7 *#	91.0 ± 9.9 *#	95.6 ± 5.5 *#	80.4 ± 8.7 *#	92.4 ± 7.2 *#
24-month	92.1 ± 13.9 *#	93.7 ± 7.4 *#	97.1 ± 4.2 *#	86.9 ± 10.6 *#	93.8 ± 6.1 *#
60-month	92.3 ± 10.6 *#	93.3 ± 6.3 *#	96.7 ± 4.4 *#	86.3 ± 11.1 *#	92.1 ± 5.8 *#
Study group					
Pre-operative	68.9 ± 23.7	73.7 ± 21.1	79.8 ± 22.5	53.7 ± 19.6	50.1 ± 22.8
6-month	83.1 ± 15.9 *	86.3 ± 12.6 *	88.5 ± 10.9 *	65.1 ± 19.7 *	80.8 ± 15.9 *
12-month	89.9 ± 10.8 *#	92.2 ± 13.3 *#	96.8 ± 5.3 *#	81.2 ± 10.4 *#	91.7 ± 9.9 *#
24-month	91.9 ± 12.5 *#	94.5 ± 7.1 *#	98.1 ± 4.7 *#	87.5 ± 12.0 *#	93.2 ± 7.7 *#
60-month	92.7 ± 11.2 *#	93.6 ± 7.7 *#	97.3 ± 4.5 *#	85.6 ± 11.5 *#	92.5 ± 6.2 *#

[a] Clinical-outcomes in the study and control groups at pre-operation, 6, 12, 24 and 60 months after ACLR. KOOS: Knee Injury and Osteoarthritis Outcome Score, ADL: activities of daily living, Sports/Rec: sport and recreation function, QoL: quality of life. Comparing with the pre-operative clinical outcome, * $p < 0.001$. Comparing with the 6-month clinical outcome, # $p < 0.05$. Values were shown as mean ± SD.

3.2. MRI Findings

On the MR images, no ligament re-tear or obvious cartilage defects were observed. The ICC index of inter-observer reliability was 0.786, and the ICC index of intra-observer reliability was 0.803.

3.3. T2 Value

The T2 mapping color scale of articular cartilage in HT-PTI group and FHT group at 6, 12, 24 and 60 months after operation is shown in Figures 5 and 6. If the false color of cartilage is close to red, the cartilage had higher T2 value and more damage. Meanwhile, if the color is closer to dark blue, the cartilage had lower T2 value and less damage.

As shown in Figure 7, the preoperative cartilage T2 values had no significant difference in each sub-region of knee joint between groups ($p > 0.05$). Compared with HT-PTI group, the FHT group had higher T2 values in P, TrF, pMFC, MT and LT at 6th month, in aLFC, aMFC, MT and LT at 12 months, in TrF, aLFC, aMFC, LT and MT at 24 months, and in TrF, aLFC, aMFC, LT and MT at 60 months (all $p < 0.05$).

As shown in Table 2, in the FHT group, except from pMFC, the T2 value increased within 60 months after operation in all measured areas. In HT-PTI group, the T2 value did not change in P, TrF, pMFC and pLFC, and increased in aMFC, aLFC, MT and LT.

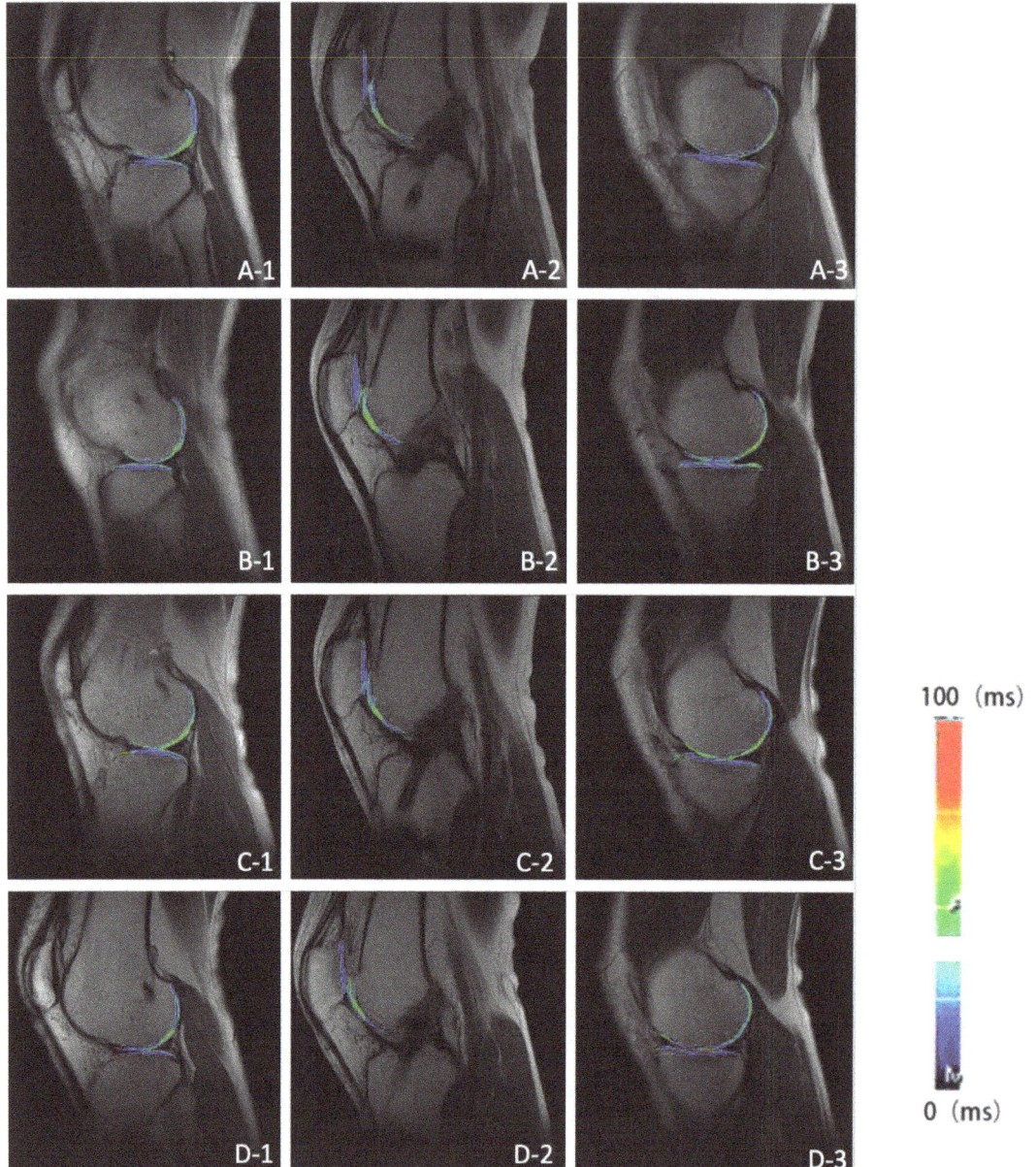

Figure 5. Sagittal T2 mapping of knee joint in HT-PTI group. (**A-1–A-3**) show the lateral tibiofemoral joint, patellofemoral joint and medial tibiofemoral joint in HT-PTI group at 6 months after operation; (**B-1–B-3**) show the lateral tibiofemoral joint, patellofemoral joint and medial tibiofemoral joint in HT-PTI group 12 months after operation; (**C-1–C-3**) show the lateral tibiofemoral joint, patellofemoral joint and medial tibiofemoral joint in HT-PTI group 24 months after operation; (**D-1–D-3**) show the lateral tibiofemoral joint, patellofemoral joint and medial tibiofemoral joint in HT-PTI group 60 months after operation.

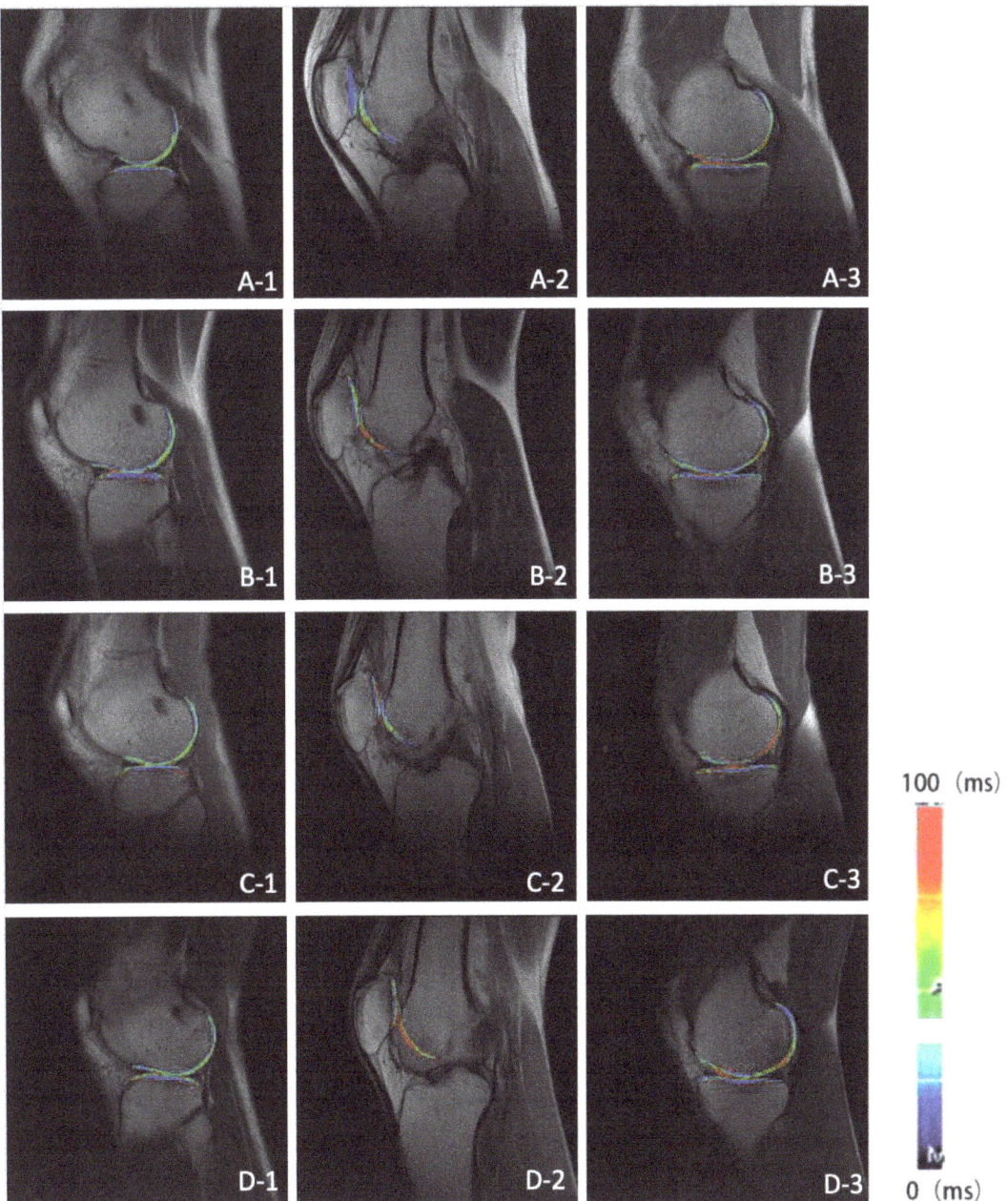

Figure 6. T2 mapping of knee joint sagittal plane in FHT group. (**A-1–A-3**) show the lateral tibiofemoral joint, patellofemoral joint and medial tibiofemoral joint at 6 months after operation in FHT group; (**B-1–B-3**) show the lateral tibiofemoral joint, patellofemoral joint and medial tibiofemoral joint 12 months after operation in FHT group; (**C-1–C-3**) show the lateral tibiofemoral joint, patellofemoral joint and medial tibiofemoral joint 24 months after operation in FHT group; (**D-1–D-3**) show the lateral tibiofemoral joint, patellofemoral joint and medial tibiofemoral joint in FHT group 60 months after operation.

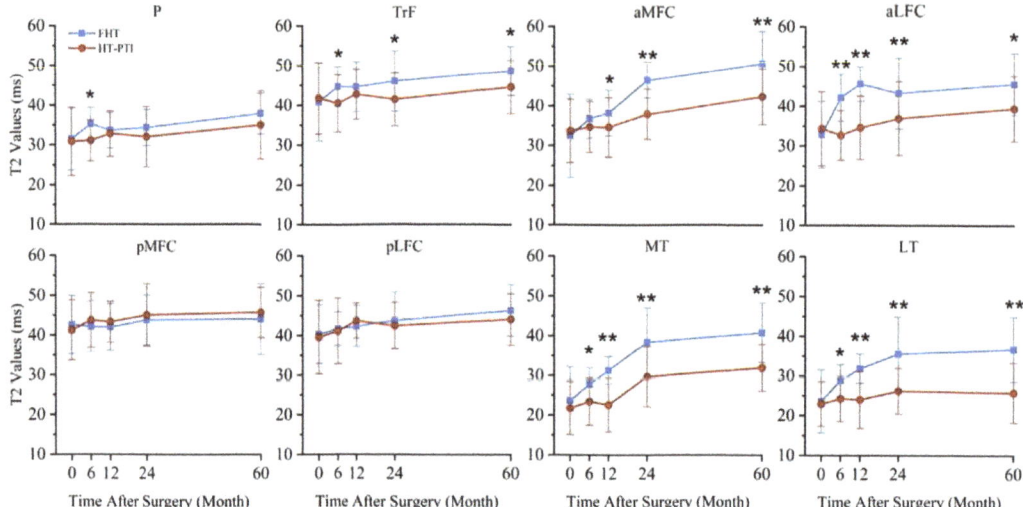

Figure 7. The T2 values of cartilage in each subregion were compared between FHT group and HT-PTI group. There was no significant difference in T2 value between the two groups before operation; The difference of P T2 value between two groups was significant at 6 months after operation; The differences of TrF T2 values between two groups were significant at 6, 24 and 60 months after operation; The differences of aMFC T2 values between two groups were significant at 12, 24 and 60 months after operation; The T2 values of aLFC, MT and LT between two groups were significantly different within 60 months after operation. * $p < 0.05$; ** $p < 0.001$. FHT, free hamstring tendon; HT-PTI, hamstring tendon with intact tibial insertion; P, patella; TrF, femoral trochlea; aLFC, anterior area of lateral femoral condyle; pLFC, posterior area of lateral femoral condyle; aMFC, anterior area of medial femoral condyle; pMFC, posterior area of medial femoral condyle; LT, lateral tibia plateau; MT; medial tibia plateau.

3.4. Cartilage Volume Change

In comparison with the FHT group, the HT-PTI group had similar CV% at 12 and 24 months after operation ($p > 0.05$), but significantly lower |CV%| all subregions at 6 month (all $p < 0.05$) and significantly lower |CV%| P, TrF, aMFC, aLFC, MT and LT at 60 months (all $p < 0.05$) (Figure 8).

In FHT group, the cartilage CV in all 8 sub-regions showed a transient increase at 6 months after operation, and reduced from 12 to 60th month with the increased |CV%| ($p < 0.05$). In HT-PTI group, the cartilage CV decrease with the increased |CV%| in aLFC, pMFC, pLFC, MT and LT at 24 and 60 months, and in P, TrF and aMFC at 60 months ($p < 0.05$) (Table 3).

3.5. Correlation Analysis

Possible associations among KOOS, T2 values and CV% are shown in Appendix A Tables A1–A3. However, no correlation was found between T2 value and KOOS scores, between CV% of each cartilage sub-region and KOOS scores, or between T2 value and CV% of each cartilage sub-region in FHT group and HT-PTI group at all timepoints (all $p > 0.05$).

Table 2. T2 values at Different Subregions and Timepoints in Two Groups [α].

	P	TrF	aMFC	aLFC	pMFC	pLFC	MT	LT
FHT group								
Pre-operative	31.52 ± 7.84	40.85 ± 9.77	32.46 ± 10.46	32.89 ± 8.35	42.63 ± 7.32	40.28 ± 7.39	23.63 ± 8.57	23.58 ± 7.92
6 m	35.28 ± 4.16	44.83 ± 5.04	36.73 ± 4.88	42.19 ± 5.89 [a]	42.18 ± 6.37	41.73 ± 4.22	27.78 ± 4.20	28.82 ± 4.01 [a]
12 m	33.72 ± 4.49	44.79 ± 6.27	38.18 ± 5.75 [a]	45.64 ± 4.28 [a]	42.04 ± 5.86	42.35 ± 5.14	31.32 ± 3.48 [a]	31.83 ± 3.69 [a]
24 m	34.38 ± 4.56	46.21 ± 7.61 [a]	46.51 ± 4.52 [abc]	43.33 ± 8.87 [a]	43.81 ± 6.27	43.77 ± 7.14	38.42 ± 8.59 [abc]	35.53 ± 9.31 [ab]
60 m	37.93 ± 5.12 [a]	48.73 ± 6.16 [a]	50.62 ± 8.18 [abcd]	45.61 ± 7.79 [a]	44.11 ± 8.92	46.29 ± 6.51 [ab]	40.78 ± 7.47 [abc]	36.67 ± 8.15 [ab]
HT-PTI group								
Pre-operative	30.86 ± 8.56	41.75 ± 8.97	33.72 ± 7.93	34.38 ± 9.28	41.24 ± 7.53	39.56 ± 9.31	21.74 ± 6.62	22.94 ± 5.61
6 m	31.16 ± 5.18	40.63 ± 7.21	34.63 ± 6.39	32.74 ± 6.23	43.81 ± 6.89	41.13 ± 8.35	23.42 ± 5.96	24.27 ± 5.75
12 m	32.84 ± 5.73	42.94 ± 6.33	34.56 ± 7.49	34.62 ± 7.97	43.38 ± 5.12	43.74 ± 4.42	22.56 ± 6.77	24.01 ± 7.20
24 m	32.06 ± 7.58	41.60 ± 6.73	37.92 ± 6.32	36.96 ± 9.27	45.06 ± 7.85	42.42 ± 5.84	29.74 ± 7.62 [abc]	26.19 ± 5.75
60 m	35.05 ± 8.53	44.65 ± 6.69	42.34 ± 7.05 [abcd]	39.43 ± 8.21 [b]	45.79 ± 6.29	44.02 ± 6.47	31.94 ± 5.87 [abc]	27.75 ± 7.53 [a]

[α] Values were shown as mean ± SD. [a] Comparing with the pre-operative T2-values, $p < 0.05$. [b] Comparing with the 6-month-T2-values, $p < 0.05$. [c] Comparing with the 12-month-T2-values, $p < 0.05$. [d] Comparing with the 24-month-T2-values, $p < 0.05$. FHT, free hamstring tendon; HT-PTI, hamstring tendon with intact tibial insertion; P, patella; TrF, femoral trochlea; aLFC, anterior area of lateral femoral condyle; pLFC, posterior area of lateral femoral condyle; aMFC, anterior area of medial femoral condyle; pMFC, posterior area of medial femoral condyle; LT, lateral tibia plateau; MT, medial tibia plateau.

Table 3. CV% at Different Subregions and Timepoints in Two Groups [α].

	P	TrF	aMFC	aLFC	pMFC	pLFC	MT	Lt
FHT group								
6 m	6.1 ± 13.4	6.8 ± 12.7	4.3 ± 9.2	5.4 ± 9.4	2.9 ± 8.3	2.8 ± 8.1	4.5 ± 10.6	4.2 ± 11.3
12 m	−0.9 ± 3.0 *	0.2 ± 4.8 *	−1.7 ± 5.3 *	−2.1 ± 5.4 *	−0.8 ± 4.9 *	−1.1 ± 5.2 *	−3.8 ± 6.6 *	−4.5 ± 5.9 *
24 m	−3.8 ± 6.3 *#	−2.6 ± 7.2 *#	−4.9 ± 7.1 *#	−5.6 ± 9.3 *#	−3.4 ± 7.1 *#	−4.0 ± 7.3 *#	−6.7 ± 10.5 *#	−6.3 ± 11.2 *#
60 m	−9.8 ± 16.8 *#	−9.5 ± 12.6 *#	−12.3 ± 16.9 *#	−12.8 ± 15.7 *#	−7.7 ± 13.2 *#	−8.1 ± 13.5 *#	−13.3 ± 18.6 *#	−14.9 ± 19.3 *#
HT-PTI group								
6 m	0.3 ± 4.8	0.7 ± 2.4	−0.7 ± 3.1	−0.5 ± 3.8	−0.3 ± 4.2	−0.6 ± 3.9	−0.8 ± 4.9	−0.9 ± 4.7
12 m	−0.7 ± 5.9	−0.3 ± 4.1	−1.8 ± 6.1	−1.6 ± 7.8	−0.9 ± 6.3	−1.0 ± 6.1	−3.1 ± 7.4	−3.3 ± 6.9
24 m	−2.1 ± 2.5	−1.9 ± 6.5	−3.1 ± 7.1	−3.8 ± 8.2 *	−3.5 ± 8.2 *	−4.4 ± 8.5 *	−5.8 ± 9.9 *	−5.3 ± 12.7 *
60 m	−5.2 ± 13.3 *#	−4.1 ± 6.9 *#	−6.8 ± 7.2 *#	−7.1 ± 9.3 *#	−5.4 ± 12.9 *#	−5.7 ± 13.4 *#	−7.2 ± 10.3 *#	−6.9 ± 9.7 *#

[α] Values were presented as mean ± SD. * Comparing with the 6 m-CV%, $p < 0.05$. # Comparing with the 12 m-CV%, $p < 0.05$. [+] Comparing with the 24 m-CV%, $p < 0.05$. CV%, the percent of cartilage volume changing; FHT, free hamstring tendon; HT-PTI, hamstring tendon with intact tibial insertion; P, patella; TrF, femoral trochlea; aLFC, anterior area of lateral femoral condyle; pLFC, posterior area of lateral femoral condyle; aMFC, anterior area of medial femoral condyle; pMFC, posterior area of medial femoral condyle; LT, lateral tibia plateau; MT, medial tibia plateau.

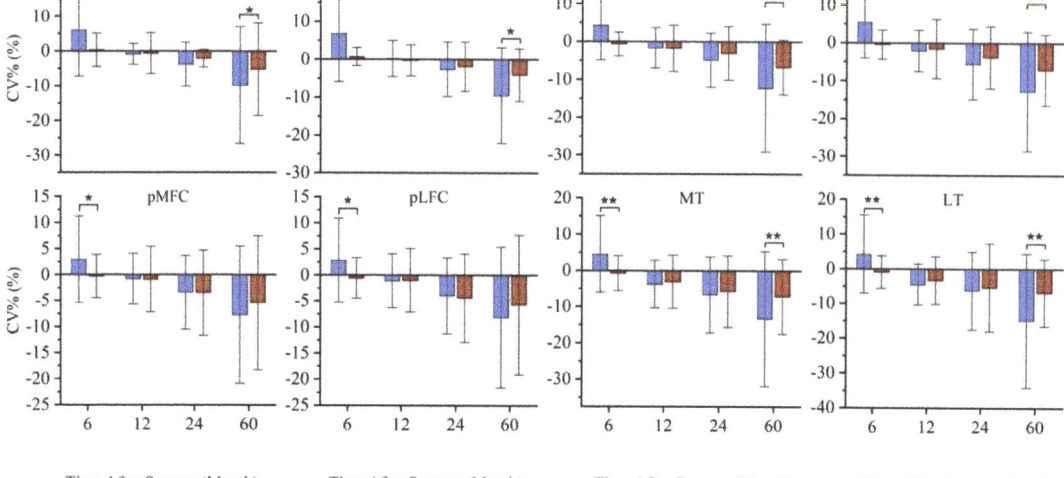

Figure 8. The CV% of cartilage between FHT group and HT-PTI group were compared. At 6 months after operation, significant differences were observed in all subgroups; Significant differences were observed in P, TrF, aMFC, aLFC, MT and LT at 60 months between two groups after operation. * $p < 0.05$; ** $p < 0.001$. CV%, the percent of cartilage volume changing; FHT, free hamstring tendon; HT-PTI, hamstring tendon with intact tibial insertion; P, patella; TrF, femoral trochlea; aLFC, anterior area of lateral femoral condyle; pLFC, posterior area of lateral femoral condyle; aMFC, anterior area of medial femoral condyle; pMFC, posterior area of medial femoral condyle; LT, lateral tibia plateau; MT; medial tibia plateau.

4. Discussion

In this study, we compared the clinical KOOS score, T2 value and CV of cartilage in 5 years after ACLR with HT-PTI and FHT. The results showed that the clinical KOOS scores of all cases were significantly improved comparing to pre-operation, and there was no significant difference between the two groups. Within the 5 years after ACLR, knee cartilage injury was found in all patients, and mainly in the aMFC, aLFC, MT and LT areas. Compared to the FHT group, the cartilage damage in the HT-PTI group occurred later with the smaller area. No correlation among KOOS score, CV% and T2 values were found in all cases.

The KOOS scores of HT-PTI group and FHT group had no significant difference within 60 months after ACLR, and it had a significant improvement compared with pre-operation from the 6-month, reached the peak at the 12-month, and maintained until the 60-month after ACLR. In our previous study [24], the clinical outcomes including the IKDC, Tegner, Lysholm activity score, and KT-1000 arthrometer measurements were improved compared with before surgery ($p < 0.001$) and were similar in both groups. Different with IKDC, Tegner and Lysholm activity score, KOOS was created as a need for clinical or researching outcomes tool given to patients with cartilage injuries [19] and was designed to assess symptoms and function in younger or more active patients with ACL injuries, cartilage damage [19]. Furthermore, the KOOS has adequate internal consistency, test-retest reliability and construct validity for surgery and physical therapy after reconstruction of the ACL [19,22]. Cristiani et al. evaluated the preoperative KOOS of 73 patients undergoing ACLR with FHT for the first time, and found that the average score of the preoperative KOOS subscales were consistent with the preoperative KOOS scores of the two groups in this study. In addition, consistent with the results of this study, Macri et al. evaluated ACLR with FHT at 5 years and found that the average score of KOOS subscales were significantly improved after ACLR.

Based on T2 value on MRI, the cartilage damage in FHT group was found earlier and in more sub-regions than that in HT-PTI group in this study. Compared to pre-operation, the higher T2 values were found in aLFC and LT at 6 months in FHT group, in aMFC and MT at 12 months in FHT group, and in MT at 24 months in HT-PTI group. The similar findings were also reported in other studies of ACLR with FHT. Related studies have found that ACL injury is easy to cause contusion to the lateral tibiofemoral joint cartilage. Histologically, the proteoglycan content of the cartilage matrix in the above subregions is significantly reduced, while imageology shows that the T2 value of the cartilage in the above subregions is significantly increased [28]. It can be inferred that the cartilage degeneration in the aLFC and LT subregions occurred 6 months after the operation in this study may be due to the further aggravation of the cartilage damage in the lateral femur of the patient before the operation. Based on T2 value evaluation within one year after ACLR using FHT, Poter et al. [29] reported the risk of cartilage damage in LT sub-region was doubled, which further supported the conclusion that the cartilage of LT subregion in FHT group would degenerate in the early stage after ACLR in our study. In addition, many other related studies also found similar conclusions to this study, that the T2 value of cartilage in the medial area of tibiofemoral joint was significantly higher in the follow-up of 6-36 months than that before operation [28,30].

Regarding the CV change evaluated on MRI, the CV decreased significantly in both groups. The absolute value of CV% at 5 years in HT-PTI group was smaller than that in FHT group, which means the cartilage degenerate less in HT-PTI group. Although ACLR was to maintain knee stability and avoid cartilage damage, it had been proved that the incidence of cartilage degeneration would still high after ACLR [1]. In addition to the possible mechanical factors leading to cartilage injury after ACLR, the changes of biochemical environment in the articular cavity after reconstruction had also been proved to play a role in cartilage injury [7,8]. Among them, most of the research was the inflammation after ACL reconstruction [31–34]. Our previous studies had confirmed that ACLR with HT-PTI had less graft necrosis and less inflammation than FHT [7,23]. Therefore, HT-PTI might reduce the effect of postoperative articular cartilage by reducing necrosis and inflammation.

Interestingly, the CV% was positive at 6 months in FHT group. Relevant studies also found that compared with pre-operation, the cartilage volume increased in 3–24 months and then decreased using traditional FHT [12,13,35,36]. Wang et al. [37] conducted relevant studies and concluded that the volume increase might be caused by cartilage edema and swelling after ACLR with FHT, and they also found that there was a certain correlation between the late cartilage defect after ACLR with FHT and the early cartilage volume increase after ACLR.

Although the knee cartilage degeneration was different between two groups, both the HT-PTI and FHT groups had similar KOOS scores at all time points. The postoperative KOOS scores were significantly higher than pre-operation from the 6th month after the operation, reached the best at the 12 months and maintained until the 60 months. The correlation analysis of each group showed that there was no correlation among the KOOS score, CV% and T2 value. This might be due to the fact that the clinical score used to evaluate the prognosis was mainly based on the subjective feelings of patients [7].

5. Limitation

There were still some limitations in this study. Firstly, this study was limited to the quantitative monitoring of the changes of knee cartilage by MRI, but lacked of relevant clinicopathological and histological verification. However, considering the related problems of clinical ethics, it was difficult to obtain the cartilage tissue of patients after ACLR for related pathological and histological research. In addition, the current measurement of T2 value was mainly based on the measurement of cartilage T2 at multiple levels, and the average value was taken, although the measurement bias was reduced to a certain extent.

However, it was also limited to the selected cartilage MRI layers, which was not the actual T2 value of the complete cartilage in some regions.

6. Conclusions

No matter whether FHT or HT-PTI was used for ACLR, the KOOS scores of all patients were significantly improved after their operations, and there was no significant change within 5 years after operations for both groups. The clinical outcomes of T2 and CV based on MRI confirmed that there was a certain degree of articular cartilage degeneration in both groups, and FHT group was more severe. However, there was no correlation among KOOS score, CV%, and T2 in all patients.

Author Contributions: Data curation, Y.X.; Investigation, S.L.; Methodology, Y.S.; Writing—original draft, Y.Z.; Writing—review & editing, J.C. All authors have read and agreed to the published version of the manuscript.

Funding: This research received no external funding.

Institutional Review Board Statement: The study was conducted in accordance with the Declaration of Helsinki, and approved by the Institutional Review Board of Huashan Hospital of Fudan University (protocol code 2011 (256) and date of approval 16 November 2011).

Informed Consent Statement: Informed consent was obtained from all subjects involved in the study. Written informed consent has been obtained from the patients to publish this paper.

Conflicts of Interest: The authors declare no conflict of interest.

Appendix A

Table A1. Correlation between T2 value and KOOS of each cartilage sub-region before and after operation (r value).

	KOOS-Symptoms			KOOS-Pain			KOOS-ADL			KOOS-Sports/Rec			KOOS-QoL		
	Total (n = 37)	FHT (n = 19)	HT-PTI (n = 18)	Total (n = 37)	FHT (n = 19)	HT-PTI (n = 18)	Total (n = 37)	FHT (n = 19)	HT-PTI (n = 18)	Total (n = 37)	FHT (n = 19)	HT-PTI (n = 18)	Total (n = 37)	FHT (n = 19)	HT-PTI (n = 18)
Pre-operation															
P	−0.034	−0.170	−0.054	−0.062	−0.077	−0.153	−0.046	−0.043	−0.072	−0.062	−0.033	−0.183	−0.254	−0.057	−0.032
TrF	−0.072	−0.031	−0.284	−0.029	−0.072	−0.085	−0.027	−0.017	−0.026	−0.036	−0.173	−0.047	−0.039	−0.063	−0.028
aMFC	−0.063	−0.163	−0.294	−0.035	−0.026	−0.082	−0.053	−0.063	−0.084	−0.168	−0.229	−0.062	−0.052	−0.149	−0.062
aLFC	−0.140	−0.062	−0.072	−0.048	−0.082	−0.027	−0.081	−0.229	−0.118	−0.053	−0.085	−0.072	−0.044	−0.084	−0.084
pMFC	−0.194	−0.285	−0.063	−0.027	−0.019	−0.007	−0.083	−0.044	−0.247	−0.002	−0.062	−0.068	−0.082	−0.183	−0.225
pLFC	−0.009	−0.072	−0.074	−0.007	−0.173	−0.294	−0.273	−0.057	−0.074	−0.042	−0.063	−0.027	−0.018	−0.092	−0.005
MT	−0.057	−0.073	−0.173	−0.239	−0.052	−0.074	−0.052	−0.226	−0.062	−0.095	−0.167	−0.073	−0.075	−0.086	−0.003
LT	−0.007	−0.036	−0.073	−0.086	−0.081	−0.172	−0.297	−0.016	−0.091	−0.007	−0.032	−0.082	−0.109	−0.101	−0.098
6-month															
P	−0.263	−0.285	−0.274	−0.073	−0.052	−0.071	−0.011	−0.078	−0.035	−0.273	−0.227	−0.074	−0.045	−0.025	−0.193
TrF	−0.082	−0.073	−0.133	−0.047	−0.082	−0.175	−0.227	−0.246	−0.062	−0.084	−0.082	−0.036	−0.075	−0.052	−0.074
aMFC	−0.077	−0.094	−0.019	−0.005	−0.291	−0.063	−0.259	−0.081	−0.071	−0.082	−0.219	−0.006	−0.078	−0.062	−0.198
aLFC	−0.033	−0.199	−0.242	−0.026	−0.089	−0.037	−0.073	−0.005	−0.018	−0.266	−0.061	−0.088	−0.206	−0.019	−0.054
pMFC	−0.041	−0.207	−0.019	−0.268	−0.211	−0.106	−0.142	−0.215	−0.042	−0.121	−0.271	−0.104	−0.218	−0.204	−0.133
pLFC	−0.150	−0.240	−0.130	−0.073	−0.191	−0.126	−0.130	−0.273	−0.062	−0.299	−0.051	−0.272	−0.236	−0.114	−0.293
MT	−0.058	−0.176	−0.265	−0.084	−0.282	−0.062	−0.110	−0.109	−0.253	−0.082	−0.042	−0.072	−0.005	−0.271	−0.054
LT	−0.091	−0.230	−0.279	−0.148	−0.201	−0.238	−0.059	−0.022	−0.174	−0.174	−0.190	−0.191	−0.012	−0.284	−0.003
12-month															
P	−0.185	−0.042	−0.287	−0.266	−0.152	−0.040	−0.020	−0.129	−0.102	−0.197	−0.258	−0.138	−0.169	−0.081	−0.008
TrF	−0.113	−0.275	−0.270	−0.029	−0.154	−0.222	−0.183	−0.159	−0.158	−0.044	−0.146	−0.222	−0.013	−0.175	−0.120
aMFC	−0.067	−0.274	−0.230	−0.214	−0.120	−0.155	−0.158	−0.143	−0.238	−0.211	−0.034	−0.075	−0.182	−0.095	−0.184
aLFC	−0.080	−0.126	−0.052	−0.167	−0.299	−0.068	−0.275	−0.169	−0.092	−0.268	−0.136	−0.009	−0.004	−0.230	−0.059
pMFC	−0.227	−0.036	−0.044	−0.187	−0.285	−0.130	−0.012	−0.178	−0.255	−0.121	−0.049	−0.172	−0.116	−0.051	−0.184
pLFC	−0.189	−0.224	−0.237	−0.007	−0.209	−0.154	−0.128	−0.235	−0.297	−0.223	−0.174	−0.127	−0.142	−0.085	−0.145
MT	−0.074	−0.171	−0.158	−0.084	−0.181	−0.279	−0.094	−0.045	−0.043	−0.167	−0.122	−0.146	−0.151	−0.187	−0.091
LT	−0.214	−0.098	−0.092	−0.282	−0.166	−0.113	−0.219	−0.156	−0.171	−0.206	−0.299	−0.019	−0.266	−0.171	−0.129
24-month															
P	−0.241	−0.039	−0.058	−0.184	−0.204	−0.004	−0.135	−0.169	−0.259	−0.047	−0.198	−0.226	−0.211	−0.226	−0.284

Table A1. Cont.

	KOOS-Symptoms			KOOS-Pain			KOOS-ADL			KOOS-Sports/Rec			KOOS-QoL		
	Total (n = 37)	FHT (n = 19)	HT-PTI (n = 18)	Total (n = 37)	FHT (n = 19)	HT-PTI (n = 18)	Total (n = 37)	FHT (n = 19)	HT-PTI (n = 18)	Total (n = 37)	FHT (n = 19)	HT-PTI (n = 18)	Total (n = 37)	FHT (n = 19)	HT-PTI (n = 18)
TrF	−0.202	−0.094	−0.020	−0.033	−0.117	−0.175	−0.163	−0.128	−0.235	−0.124	−0.075	−0.138	−0.145	−0.129	−0.015
aMFC	−0.125	−0.190	−0.102	−0.030	−0.172	−0.181	−0.078	−0.112	−0.127	−0.052	−0.029	−0.089	−0.041	−0.158	−0.257
aLFC	−0.072	−0.088	−0.070	−0.185	−0.217	−0.102	−0.065	−0.015	−0.232	−0.014	−0.104	−0.054	−0.256	−0.099	−0.054
pMFC	−0.045	−0.295	−0.130	−0.170	−0.190	−0.176	−0.083	−0.291	−0.250	−0.280	−0.093	−0.073	−0.085	−0.179	−0.064
pLFC	−0.132	−0.216	−0.274	−0.021	−0.191	−0.203	−0.218	−0.170	−0.163	−0.087	−0.296	−0.255	−0.177	−0.007	−0.012
MT	−0.096	−0.132	−0.144	−0.287	−0.185	−0.062	−0.258	−0.199	−0.287	−0.180	−0.009	−0.262	−0.116	−0.172	−0.233
LT	−0.254	−0.064	−0.280	−0.157	−0.023	−0.091	−0.004	−0.232	−0.182	−0.218	−0.007	−0.173	−0.133	−0.277	−0.135

60-month

	Total (n = 37)	FHT (n = 19)	HT-PTI (n = 18)	Total (n = 37)	FHT (n = 19)	HT-PTI (n = 18)	Total (n = 37)	FHT (n = 19)	HT-PTI (n = 18)	Total (n = 37)	FHT (n = 19)	HT-PTI (n = 18)	Total (n = 37)	FHT (n = 19)	HT-PTI (n = 18)
P	−0.175	−0.018	−0.102	−0.240	−0.169	−0.089	−0.172	−0.020	−0.256	−0.196	−0.264	−0.248	−0.017	−0.098	−0.012
TrF	−0.043	−0.149	−0.202	−0.246	−0.125	−0.147	−0.069	−0.142	−0.240	−0.272	−0.101	−0.175	−0.294	−0.240	−0.174
aMFC	−0.027	−0.185	−0.130	−0.118	−0.187	−0.261	−0.240	−0.034	−0.218	−0.222	−0.015	−0.015	−0.246	−0.117	−0.166
aLFC	−0.295	−0.043	−0.135	−0.271	−0.115	−0.206	−0.240	−0.152	−0.180	−0.078	−0.162	−0.061	−0.155	−0.136	−0.036
pMFC	−0.015	−0.197	−0.213	−0.260	−0.224	−0.055	−0.083	−0.291	−0.126	−0.185	−0.216	−0.039	−0.264	−0.038	−0.293
pLFC	−0.065	−0.123	−0.284	−0.263	−0.109	−0.093	−0.084	−0.115	−0.112	−0.016	−0.237	−0.247	−0.106	−0.063	−0.220
MT	−0.175	−0.172	−0.081	−0.234	−0.062	−0.087	−0.053	−0.019	−0.244	−0.176	−0.054	−0.294	−0.238	−0.001	−0.272
LT	−0.139	−0.156	−0.123	−0.022	−0.135	−0.218	−0.086	−0.058	−0.254	−0.150	−0.238	−0.240	−0.059	−0.123	−0.093

FHT: free hamstring tendon, HT-PTI: preserved tibial-insertion hamstring tendon, KOOS: Knee Injury and Osteoarthritis Outcome Score, ADL: activities of daily living, Sports/rec: sport and recreation function, QoL: quality of life.

Table A2. Correlation between value CV% and KOOS of each cartilage sub-region after operation (r value).

	KOOS-Symptoms			KOOS-Pain			KOOS-ADL			KOOS-Sports/Rec			KOOS-QoL		
	Total (n = 37)	FHT (n = 19)	HT-PTI (n = 18)	Total (n = 37)	FHT (n = 19)	HT-PTI (n = 18)	Total (n = 37)	FHT (n = 19)	HT-PTI (n = 18)	Total (n = 37)	FHT (n = 19)	HT-PTI (n = 18)	Total (n = 37)	FHT (n = 19)	HT-PTI (n = 18)

6-month

	Total (n = 37)	FHT (n = 19)	HT-PTI (n = 18)	Total (n = 37)	FHT (n = 19)	HT-PTI (n = 18)	Total (n = 37)	FHT (n = 19)	HT-PTI (n = 18)	Total (n = 37)	FHT (n = 19)	HT-PTI (n = 18)	Total (n = 37)	FHT (n = 19)	HT-PTI (n = 18)
P	0.288	0.001	0.128	0.020	0.212	0.012	0.101	0.267	0.069	0.169	0.269	0.275	0.213	0.207	0.185
TrF	0.178	0.073	0.135	0.269	0.187	0.191	0.262	0.300	0.181	0.057	0.176	0.189	0.022	0.113	0.167
aMFC	0.258	0.245	0.052	0.087	0.082	0.146	0.035	0.153	0.028	0.018	0.137	0.173	0.247	0.257	0.249
aLFC	0.183	0.238	0.273	0.222	0.190	0.239	0.183	0.225	0.074	0.067	0.052	0.275	0.210	0.076	0.071
pMFC	0.181	0.092	0.265	0.226	0.011	0.021	0.076	0.152	0.044	0.164	0.051	0.010	0.241	0.290	0.156
pLFC	0.139	0.085	0.227	0.122	0.010	0.052	0.296	0.279	0.160	0.273	0.251	0.033	0.148	0.221	0.043

Table A2. Cont.

	KOOS-Symptoms			KOOS-Pain				KOOS-ADL				KOOS-Sports/Rec				KOOS-QoL		
	Total (n = 37)	FHT (n = 19)	HT-PTI (n = 18)	Total (n = 37)	FHT (n = 19)	HT-PTI (n = 18)	Total (n = 37)	FHT (n = 19)	HT-PTI (n = 18)		Total (n = 37)	FHT (n = 19)	HT-PTI (n = 18)		Total (n = 37)	FHT (n = 19)	HT-PTI (n = 18)
MT	0.190	0.177	0.121	0.004	0.144	0.273	0.119	0.102	0.068		0.037	0.108	0.069		0.261	0.270	0.079
LT	0.101	0.169	0.171	0.083	0.033	0.200	0.099	0.119	0.178		0.120	0.144	0.259		0.087	0.128	0.295
12-month																	
P	0.018	0.298	0.051	0.061	0.239	0.275	0.100	0.138	0.029		0.093	0.294	0.172		0.106	0.248	0.118
TrF	0.027	0.061	0.242	0.122	0.183	0.135	0.283	0.171	0.064		0.142	0.113	0.085		0.152	0.123	0.062
aMFC	0.230	0.104	0.189	0.295	0.116	0.217	0.173	0.155	0.149		0.021	0.016	0.210		0.228	0.224	0.133
aLFC	0.087	0.179	0.091	0.232	0.265	0.254	0.138	0.064	0.105		0.231	0.170	0.161		0.199	0.053	0.064
pMFC	0.079	0.169	0.297	0.153	0.239	0.114	0.086	0.143	0.119		0.061	0.289	0.059		0.166	0.264	0.262
pLFC	0.111	0.107	0.235	0.293	0.247	0.114	0.053	0.003	0.154		0.058	0.068	0.191		0.288	0.097	0.099
MT	0.052	0.057	0.253	0.226	0.249	0.294	0.251	0.269	0.245		0.120	0.049	0.050		0.209	0.081	0.291
LT	0.289	0.067	0.020	0.184	0.285	0.032	0.117	0.092	0.037		0.178	0.093	0.131		0.278	0.110	0.005
24-month																	
P	0.045	0.233	0.208	0.095	0.002	0.091	0.145	0.070	0.150		0.279	0.025	0.233		0.032	0.130	0.100
TrF	0.025	0.208	0.089	0.083	0.289	0.188	0.178	0.258	0.012		0.289	0.249	0.093		0.102	0.295	0.033
aMFC	0.074	0.221	0.010	0.036	0.246	0.115	0.118	0.097	0.089		0.291	0.194	0.258		0.045	0.114	0.024
aLFC	0.038	0.107	0.107	0.239	0.184	0.155	0.227	0.275	0.118		0.162	0.253	0.239		0.252	0.021	0.204
pMFC	0.062	0.015	0.009	0.151	0.122	0.295	0.210	0.275	0.213		0.044	0.094	0.100		0.058	0.018	0.032
pLFC	0.199	0.253	0.159	0.048	0.148	0.190	0.254	0.012	0.164		0.050	0.292	0.276		0.162	0.030	0.021
MT	0.087	0.165	0.072	0.117	0.242	0.129	0.049	0.067	0.125		0.062	0.140	0.003		0.167	0.239	0.269
LT	0.224	0.187	0.240	0.171	0.088	0.014	0.138	0.146	0.017		0.281	0.212	0.287		0.224	0.109	0.257
60-month																	
P	0.076	0.182	0.044	0.269	0.203	0.116	0.225	0.221	0.094		0.291	0.239	0.102		0.030	0.095	0.059
TrF	0.057	0.181	0.056	0.269	0.160	0.145	0.067	0.031	0.077		0.185	0.261	0.280		0.172	0.255	0.269
aMFC	0.028	0.176	0.042	0.051	0.162	0.209	0.100	0.130	0.051		0.187	0.259	0.005		0.210	0.095	0.107
aLFC	0.024	0.210	0.239	0.107	0.130	0.097	0.101	0.264	0.245		0.243	0.143	0.199		0.074	0.277	0.037
pMFC	0.102	0.272	0.123	0.165	0.092	0.093	0.083	0.177	0.084		0.188	0.281	0.015		0.275	0.098	0.182
pLFC	0.014	0.234	0.274	0.253	0.294	0.247	0.113	0.068	0.212		0.220	0.096	0.261		0.171	0.099	0.296
MT	0.282	0.107	0.089	0.163	0.054	0.204	0.239	0.215	0.123		0.110	0.070	0.057		0.174	0.258	0.091
LT	0.000	0.115	0.257	0.049	0.091	0.024	0.258	0.170	0.239		0.084	0.096	0.016		0.208	0.046	0.266

FHT: free hamstring tendon, HT-PTI: preserved tibial-insertion hamstring tendon, CV%: The percent of cartilage volume changing, KOOS: Knee Injury and Osteoarthritis Outcome Score, ADL: activities of daily living, Sports/rec: sport and recreation function, QoL: quality of life.

Table A3. Correlation between value CV% and T2 value of each cartilage sub-region after operation (r value).

	6-Month			12-Month			24-Month			60-Month		
	Total (n = 37)	FHT (n = 19)	HT-PTI (n = 18)	Total (n = 37)	FHT (n = 19)	HT-PTI (n = 18)	Total (n = 37)	FHT (n = 19)	HT-PTI (n = 18)	Total (n = 37)	FHT (n = 19)	HT-PTI (n = 18)
P	−0.048	−0.371	−0.223	−0.106	−0.140	−0.159	−0.266	−0.362	−0.143	−0.421	−0.392	−0.012
TrF	−0.458	−0.267	−0.305	−0.501	−0.420	−0.048	−0.142	−0.332	−0.325	−0.179	−0.366	−0.561
aMFC	−0.230	−0.207	−0.240	−0.541	−0.099	−0.207	−0.190	−0.436	−0.560	−0.569	−0.532	−0.523
aLFC	−0.545	−0.111	−0.496	−0.288	−0.024	−0.063	−0.075	−0.141	−0.322	−0.578	−0.102	−0.339
pMFC	−0.304	−0.151	−0.046	−0.156	−0.555	−0.586	−0.319	−0.049	−0.453	−0.029	−0.355	−0.169
pLFC	−0.495	−0.590	−0.177	−0.105	−0.352	−0.085	−0.564	−0.380	−0.043	−0.227	−0.588	−0.448
MT	−0.489	−0.357	−0.302	−0.366	−0.544	−0.364	−0.287	−0.497	−0.065	−0.094	−0.544	−0.334
LT	−0.281	−0.358	−0.429	−0.493	−0.493	−0.331	−0.532	−0.456	−0.431	−0.277	−0.537	−0.567

FHT: free hamstring tendon, HT-PTI: preserved tibial-insertion hamstring tendon, CV%: The percent of cartilage volume changing.

References

1. Ajuied, A.; Wong, F.; Smith, C.; Norris, M.; Earnshaw, P.; Back, D.; Davies, A. Anterior cruciate ligament injury and radiologic progression of knee osteoarthritis: A systematic review and meta-analysis. *Am. J. Sports Med.* **2014**, *42*, 2242–2252. [CrossRef] [PubMed]
2. Belk, J.W.; Kraeutler, M.J.; Carver, T.J.; McCarty, E.C. Knee Osteoarthritis After Anterior Cruciate Ligament Reconstruction With Bone–Patellar Tendon–Bone Versus Hamstring Tendon Autograft: A Systematic Review of Randomized Controlled Trials. *Arthrosc. J. Arthrosc. Relat. Surg.* **2018**, *34*, 1358–1365. [CrossRef] [PubMed]
3. Belk, J.W.; Kraeutler, M.J.; Houck, D.A.; McCarty, E.C. Knee Osteoarthritis After Single-Bundle Versus Double-Bundle Anterior Cruciate Ligament Reconstruction: A Systematic Review of Randomized Controlled Trials. *Arthroscopy* **2019**, *35*, 996–1003. [CrossRef]
4. Bellamy, N.; Buchanan, W.W.; Goldsmith, C.H.; Campbell, J.; Stitt, L.W. Validation study of WOMAC: A health status instrument for measuring clinically important patient relevant outcomes to antirheumatic drug therapy in patients with osteoarthritis of the hip or knee. *J. Rheumatol.* **1988**, *15*, 1833–1840. [PubMed]
5. Collins, N.J.; Prinsen, C.A.; Christensen, R.; Bartels, E.M.; Terwee, C.B.; Roos, E.M. Knee Injury and Osteoarthritis Outcome Score (KOOS): Systematic review and meta-analysis of measurement properties. *Osteoarthr. Cartil.* **2016**, *24*, 1317–1329. [CrossRef] [PubMed]
6. Corona, K.; Cerciello, S.; Vasso, M.; Toro, G.; D'Ambrosi, R.; Pola, E.; Ciolli, G.; Mercurio, M.; Panni, A.S. Age over 50 does not predict results in anterior cruciate ligament reconstruction. *Orthop. Rev.* **2022**, *14*, 37310. [CrossRef]
7. Cristiani, R.; Viheriävaara, S.; Janarv, P.-M.; Edman, G.; Janarv, P.-M.; Forssblad, M.; Stålman, A. Knee laxity and functional knee outcome after contralateral ACLR are comparable to those after primary ACLR. *Knee Surg. Sports Traumatol. Arthrosc.* **2021**, *29*, 3864–3870. [CrossRef]
8. Del Torto, M.; Enea, D.; Panfoli, N.; Filardo, G.; Pace, N.; Chiusaroli, M. Hamstrings anterior cruciate ligament reconstruction with and without platelet rich fibrin matrix. *Knee Surg. Sports Traumatol. Arthrosc.* **2015**, *23*, 3614–3622. [CrossRef]
9. Eckstein, F.; Wirth, W.; Lohmander, L.S.; Hudelmaier, M.I.; Frobell, R.B. Five-Year Followup of Knee Joint Cartilage Thickness Changes After Acute Rupture of the Anterior Cruciate Ligament. *Arthritis Rheumatol.* **2015**, *67*, 152–161. [CrossRef]
10. Figueroa, D.; Figueroa, F.; Calvo, R.; Vaisman, A.; Ahumada, X.; Arellano, S. Platelet-rich plasma use in anterior cruciate ligament surgery: Systematic review of the literature. *Arthroscopy* **2015**, *31*, 981–988. [CrossRef]
11. Frobell, R.B. Change in cartilage thickness, posttraumatic bone marrow lesions, and joint fluid volumes after acute ACL disruption: A two-year prospective MRI study of sixty-one subjects. *J. Bone Joint Surg. Am.* **2011**, *93*, 1096–1103. [CrossRef] [PubMed]
12. Frobell, R.; Le Graverand, M.-P.; Buck, R.; Roos, E.; Roos, H.; Tamez-Pena, J.; Totterman, S.; Lohmander, L. The acutely ACL injured knee assessed by MRI: Changes in joint fluid, bone marrow lesions, and cartilage during the first year. *Osteoarthr. Cartil.* **2009**, *17*, 161–167. [CrossRef] [PubMed]
13. Gong, X.; Jiang, D.; Wang, Y.-J.; Wang, J.; Ao, Y.-F.; Yu, J.-K. Second-Look Arthroscopic Evaluation of Chondral Lesions After Isolated Anterior Cruciate Ligament Reconstruction: Single-Versus Double-Bundle Reconstruction. *Am. J. Sports Med.* **2013**, *41*, 2362–2367. [CrossRef]
14. Kumar, D.; Su, F.; Wu, D.; Pedoia, V.; Heitkamp, L.; Ma, C.B.; Souza, R.B.; Li, X. Frontal Plane Knee Mechanics and Early Cartilage Degeneration in People With Anterior Cruciate Ligament Reconstruction: A Longitudinal Study. *Am. J. Sports Med.* **2018**, *46*, 378–387. [CrossRef] [PubMed]
15. Li, X.; Kuo, D.; Theologis, A.; Carballido-Gamio, J.; Stehling, C.; Link, T.M.; Ma, C.B.; Majumdar, S. Cartilage in Anterior Cruciate Ligament–Reconstructed Knees: MR imaging T1{rho} and T2—Initial Experience with 1-year Follow-up. *Radiology* **2011**, *258*, 505–514. [CrossRef] [PubMed]
16. Liu, S.; Li, H.; Tao, H.; Sun, Y.; Chen, S.; Chen, J. A Randomized Clinical Trial to Evaluate Attached Hamstring Anterior Cruciate Ligament Graft Maturity With Magnetic Resonance Imaging. *Am. J. Sports Med.* **2018**, *46*, 1143–1149. [CrossRef]
17. Liu, S.; Sun, Y.; Wan, F.; Ding, Z.; Chen, S.; Chen, J. Advantages of an Attached Semitendinosus Tendon Graft in Anterior Cruciate Ligament Reconstruction in a Rabbit Model. *Am. J. Sports Med.* **2018**, *46*, 3227–3236. [CrossRef] [PubMed]
18. Maerz, T.; Sherman, E.; Newton, M.; Yilmaz, A.; Kumar, P.; Graham, S.F.; Baker, K.C. Metabolomic serum profiling after ACL injury in rats: A pilot study implicating inflammation and immune dysregulation in post-traumatic osteoarthritis. *J. Orthop. Res.* **2018**, *36*, 1969–1979. [CrossRef] [PubMed]
19. McAlindon, T.E.; LaValley, M.P.; Harvey, W.F.; Price, L.L.; Driban, J.; Zhang, M.; Ward, R.J. Effect of Intra-articular Triamcinolone vs Saline on Knee Cartilage Volume and Pain in Patients With Knee Osteoarthritis: A Randomized Clinical Trial. *JAMA* **2017**, *317*, 1967–1975. [CrossRef]
20. McAlindon, T.E.; Nuite, M.; Krishnan, N.; Ruthazer, R.; Price, L.; Burstein, D.; Griffith, J.; Flechsenhar, K. Change in knee osteoarthritis cartilage detected by delayed gadolinium enhanced magnetic resonance imaging following treatment with collagen hydrolysate: A pilot randomized controlled trial. *Osteoarthr. Cartil.* **2011**, *19*, 399–405. [CrossRef]
21. Mendias, C.L.; Enselman, E.R.S.; Olszewski, A.M.; Gumucio, J.P.; Edon, D.L.; Konnaris, M.A.; Carpenter, J.E.; Awan, T.M.; Jacobson, J.A.; Gagnier, J.J.; et al. The Use of Recombinant Human Growth Hormone to Protect Against Muscle Weakness in Patients Undergoing Anterior Cruciate Ligament Reconstruction: A Pilot, Randomized Placebo—Controlled Trial. *Am. J. Sports Med.* **2020**, *48*, 1916–1928. [CrossRef] [PubMed]

22. Nishioka, H.; Hirose, J.; Nakamura, E.; Okamoto, N.; Karasugi, T.; Taniwaki, T.; Okada, T.; Yamashita, Y.; Mizuta, H. Detecting ICRS grade 1 cartilage lesions in anterior cruciate ligament injury using T1ρ and T2 mapping. *Eur. J. Radiol.* **2013**, *82*, 1499–1505. [CrossRef]
23. Nugzar, O.; Zandman-Goddard, G.; Oz, H.; Lakstein, D.; Feldbrin, Z.; Shargorodsky, M. The role of ferritin and adiponectin as predictors of cartilage damage assessed by arthroscopy in patients with symptomatic knee osteoarthritis. *Best Pract. Res. Clin. Rheumatol.* **2018**, *32*, 662–668. [CrossRef] [PubMed]
24. Papalia, R.; Franceschi, F.; Vasta, S.; Di Martino, A.; Maffulli, N.; Denaro, V. Sparing the anterior cruciate ligament remnant: Is it worth the hassle? *Br. Med. Bull.* **2012**, *104*, 91–111. [CrossRef]
25. Potter, H.G.; Jain, S.K.; Ma, Y.; Black, B.R.; Fung, S.; Lyman, S. Cartilage Injury After Acute, Isolated Anterior Cruciate Ligament Tear: Immediate and Longitudinal Effect with Clinical/MRI Follow-up. *Am. J. Sports Med.* **2012**, *40*, 276–285. [CrossRef]
26. Roos, E.M.; Roos, H.P.; Lohmander, L.S.; Ekdahl, C.; Beynnon, B.D. Knee Injury and Osteoarthritis Outcome Score (KOOS)—Development of a self-administered outcome measure. *J. Orthop. Sports Phys. Ther.* **1998**, *28*, 88–96. [CrossRef]
27. Song, E.-K.; Seon, J.-K.; Yim, J.-H.; Woo, S.-H.; Seo, H.-Y.; Lee, K.-B. Progression of Osteoarthritis After Double- and Single-Bundle Anterior Cruciate Ligament Reconstruction. *Am. J. Sports Med.* **2013**, *41*, 2340–2346. [CrossRef]
28. Song, G.-Y.; Zhang, H.; Zhang, J.; Li, X.; Chen, X.-Z.; Li, Y.; Feng, H. The Anterior Cruciate Ligament Remnant: To Leave It or Not? *Arthrosc. J. Arthrosc. Relat. Surg.* **2013**, *29*, 1253–1262. [CrossRef] [PubMed]
29. Su, F.; Hilton, J.F.; Nardo, L.; Wu, S.; Liang, F.; Link, T.; Ma, C.; Li, X. Cartilage morphology and T1ρ and T2 quantification in ACL-reconstructed knees: A 2-year follow-up. *Osteoarthr. Cartil.* **2013**, *21*, 1058–1067. [CrossRef]
30. Subburaj, K.; Kumar, D.; Souza, R.B.; Alizai, H.; Li, X.; Link, T.M.; Majumdar, S. The Acute Effect of Running on Knee Articular Cartilage and Meniscus Magnetic Resonance Relaxation Times in Young Healthy Adults. *Am. J. Sports Med.* **2012**, *40*, 2134–2141. [CrossRef]
31. Theologis, A.A.; Haughom, B.; Liang, F.; Zhang, Y.; Majumdar, S.; Link, T.M.; Ma, C.B.; Li, X. Comparison of T1rho relaxation times between ACL-reconstructed knees and contralateral uninjured knees. *Knee Surg. Sports Traumatol. Arthrosc.* **2014**, *22*, 298–307. [CrossRef]
32. Van Ginckel, A.; Verdonk, P.; Victor, J.; Witvrouw, E. Cartilage Status in Relation to Return to Sports After Anterior Cruciate Ligament Reconstruction. *Am. J. Sports Med.* **2013**, *41*, 550–559. [CrossRef] [PubMed]
33. Wang, H.-J.; Ao, Y.-F.; Jiang, D.; Gong, X.; Wang, Y.-J.; Wang, J.; Yu, J.-K. Relationship Between Quadriceps Strength and Patellofemoral Joint Chondral Lesions After Anterior Cruciate Ligament Reconstruction. *Am. J. Sports Med.* **2015**, *43*, 2286–2292. [CrossRef]
34. Wang, X.; Bennell, K.L.; Wang, Y.; Wrigley, T.V.; Van Ginckel, A.; Fortin, K.; Saxby, D.J.; Cicuttini, F.; Lloyd, D.; Vertullo, C.J.; et al. Tibiofemoral joint structural change from 2.5 to 4.5 years following ACL reconstruction with and without combined meniscal pathology. *BMC Musculoskelet. Disord.* **2019**, *20*, 312. [CrossRef] [PubMed]
35. Wang, X.; Wrigley, T.V.; Bennell, K.L.; Wang, Y.; Fortin, K.; Cicuttini, F.M.; Lloyd, D.G.; Bryant, A.L. Cartilage quantitative T2 relaxation time 2–4 years following isolated anterior cruciate ligament reconstruction. *J. Orthop. Res.* **2018**, *36*, 2022–2029. [CrossRef] [PubMed]
36. Woollard, J.D.; Gil, A.B.; Sparto, P.; Kwoh, C.K.; Piva, S.R.; Farrokhi, S.; Powers, C.M.; Fitzgerald, G.K. Change in Knee Cartilage Volume in Individuals Completing a Therapeutic Exercise Program for Knee Osteoarthritis. *J. Orthop. Sports Phys. Ther.* **2011**, *41*, 708–722. [CrossRef]
37. Zhang, Y.; Liu, S.; Chen, Q.; Hu, Y.; Sun, Y.; Chen, J. Maturity Progression of the Entire Anterior Cruciate Ligament Graft of Insertion—Preserved Hamstring Tendons by 5 Years: A Prospective Randomized Controlled Study Based on Magnetic Resonance Imaging Evaluation. *Am. J. Sports Med.* **2020**, *48*, 2970–2977. [CrossRef]

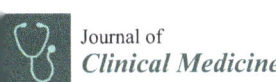

Article

Adaptive Posture-Balance Cardiac Rehabilitation Exercise Significantly Improved Physical Tolerance in Patients with Cardiovascular Diseases

Mei Ma [2,†], Bowen Zhang [1,†], Xinxin Yan [3], Xiang Ji [1], Deyu Qin [2], Chaodong Pu [2], Jingxiang Zhao [2], Qian Zhang [2], Heinz Lowis [4] and Ting Li [1,*]

1. Institute of Biomedical Engineering, Chinese Academy of Medical Sciences and Peking Union Medical College, Tianjin 300192, China
2. Department of Rehabilitation Medicine, Tianjin Chest Hospital, Tianjin 300192, China
3. Department of Cardiology, Key Laboratory of Pulmonary Vascular Medicine, Fuwai Hospital, Chinese Academy of Medical Sciences and Peking Union Medical College, Beijing 100037, China
4. Drei-Burgen-Klinik of German Pension Insurance of Rhineland-Palatinate, 55583 Bad Kreuznach, Germany
* Correspondence: liting@bme.cams.cn; Tel.: +86-180-0212-7296
† These authors contributed equally to this work.

Abstract: Cardiac rehabilitation (CR) requires more professional exercise modalities to improve the efficiency of treatment. Adaptive posture-balance cardiac rehabilitation exercise (APBCRE) is an emerging, balance-based therapy from clinical experience, but lacks evidence of validity. Our study aimed to observe and assess the rehabilitation effect of APBCRE on patients with cardiovascular diseases (CVDs). All participants received one-month APBCRE therapy evenly three times per week and two assessments before and after APBCRE. Each assessment included cardiopulmonary exercise testing (CPET), resting metabolic rate (RMR) detection, and three questionnaires about general health. The differences between two assessments were analyzed to evaluate the therapeutic effects of APBCRE. A total of 93 participants (80.65% male, 53.03 ± 12.02 years) were included in the analysis. After one-month APBCRE, oxygen uptake (VO_2, 11.16 ± 2.91 to 12.85 ± 3.17 mL/min/kg, $p < 0.01$) at anaerobic threshold (AT), ventilation (VE, 28.87 ± 7.26 to 32.42 ± 8.50 mL/min/kg, $p < 0.01$) at AT, respiratory exchange ratio (RER, 0.93 ± 0.06 to 0.95 ± 0.05, $p < 0.01$) at AT and oxygen uptake efficiency slope (OUES, 1426.75 ± 346.30 to 1547.19 ± 403.49, $p < 0.01$) significantly improved in CVD patients. The ≤55-year group had more positive improvements (VO_2 at AT, 23% vs. 16%; OUES, 13% vs. 6%) compared with the >55-year group. Quality of life was also increased after APBCRE (47.78 ± 16.74 to 59.27 ± 17.77, $p < 0.001$). This study proved that APBCRE was a potentially available exercise rehabilitation modality for patients with CVDs, which performed significant increases in physical tolerance and quality of life, especially for ≤55-year patients.

Keywords: cardiac rehabilitation; exercise therapy; balance exercises; cardiovascular diseases

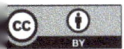

1. Introduction

Cardiovascular diseases (CVDs) are a group of disorders of heart and blood vessel disorders, such as coronary heart disease [1] and heart failure [2]. CVDs are the leading cause of death and disability in the world [3]. Approximately 330 million people in China suffer from CVDs, and the prevalence continues to increase [4]. With the progression of CVDs, physical tolerance in patients gradually declines until complete loss, along with increasing dyspnea. It seriously affects the quality of life of patients and causes a huge social burden [5]. Therefore, it is critical to improve the physical tolerance of CVDs patients.

The American College of Cardiology guidelines emphasize [6] that cardiac rehabilitation (CR) is an important and effective approach to preventing and treating CVDs and is strongly recommended for clinical practice. Moreover, numerous studies confirm [7,8]

that CR improves physical tolerance [9] and quality of life in patients with CVDs [10,11], reduces the incidence risk of CVDs [12], and decreases the rate of hospital readmission.

At present, the main modality of CR is physical exercise [13], occasionally supplemented with health education and psychological counseling [7]. Patients could choose to finish CR at home or in center depending on their condition. Although there are no significant differences in rehabilitation effects between home-based CR and center-based CR, home-based CR provides better satisfaction and comfort for patients [14,15]. The general exercise methods of CR [16] include walking, jogging, cycling and other aerobic exercises, combined with resistance training. Emerging techniques and traditional exercises have been explored and are found to be effective, such as high-intensity interval training (HIIT) [17,18], yoga [19,20] and Tai Chi [21]. In most studies, the exercise intensity is controlled at 40% to 80% of the maximum heart rate (HR) [22,23], and the exercise frequency ranges from 3 to 6 times per week [24,25]. However, the above sports methods and rehabilitation modalities are mainly based on existing general exercise models [6,17], rather than exclusively focusing on CVDs. Universal models usually do not achieve the expected effect due to lack of pertinence, although they are intensively adopted.

Based on balance exercise, a new rehabilitation approach was designed and named as adaptive posture-balance cardiac rehabilitation exercise (APBCRE). The approach was inspired by clinical practice about CVDs, specifically designed to reduce the risk of falls. To better understand the clinical effectiveness of APBCRE on CVDs patients, the current study aimed to assess whether APBCRE could enhance physical tolerance and improve the quality of life in patients with CVDs.

2. Materials and Methods

2.1. Study Design

This experiment was performed among CVDs patients from December 2020 to March 2021 in Tianjin Chest Hospital. This study protocol was approved by the local ethics committee (IRB-SOP-016(F)-001-02, 9 August 2021). All subjects have signed informed consent forms before being enrolled. The whole experiment included one month of APBCRE and two clinical assessments before and after APBCRE interventions. The one-month APBCRE consisted of twelve exercise sessions, evenly three times per week. Each assessment included cardiopulmonary exercise testing (CPET), resting metabolism rate (RMR) detection, and questionnaires about quality of life (QoL), depression levels and anxiety levels. The primary outcome was physical tolerance assessed by oxygen uptake (VO_2) at anaerobic threshold (AT). The secondary endpoints were the resting metabolism level and QoL measured by RMR and 12-item Short Form Survey (SF-12), respectively. A flowchart of this study is provided in Figure 1.

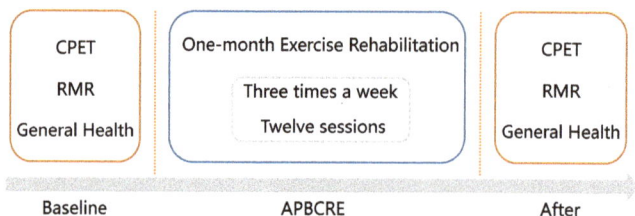

Figure 1. Flowchart of this study. CPET cardiopulmonary exercise testing, RMR resting metabolism rate, APBCRE adaptive posture-balance cardiac rehabilitation exercise.

2.2. Patient Selection

Subjects were recruited from patients with CVDs. The inclusion criteria were (1) age over 18 years old; (2) diagnosed as CVDs, including coronary heart disease (CHD), old myocardial infarction (MI), arrhythmias and heart valve disease; (3) without percutaneous coronary intervention (PCI) or one week after PCI; (4) without coronary artery bypass graft

(CABG) or one month after CABG. Patients were excluded if having abnormal blood pressure response, acute heart failure, unstable angina, acute myocardial infarction, congenital heart disease, and severe musculoskeletal diseases limiting [23].

2.3. Rehabilitation Protocol

Depending on personal physical conditions, participants were assigned to three danger levels: low-level, medium-level, and high-level. The standards of danger level are shown in Table A1 in Appendix A. The different danger-level patients underwent individualized APBCRE with matched different exercise thresholds and accepted comprehensive guidance from professional nurses.

The fundamental process of APBCRE consisted of four parts: breathing training and warm-up, aerobic exercise, resistance exercise, and flexibility exercise. The first part generally lasted 5–15 min for any danger level. For better effects of sport rehabilitation, our study designed a new warm-up method based on balance exercise, which was the essence of APBCRE. Figure 2a outlined the specific steps of the new warm-up method, including stretching of upper limbs, legs, waist, and other parts. The first part mainly contributed to improving body coordination and balance. The second part was moderate-intensity endurance exercise. The intensity was controlled at 40–60% AT, 60–70% of peak HR and Borg grade 12–13. The exercise duration of aerobic exercise was usually 30 min. Moreover, a body-building vehicle was used for resistance exercise in the third part for 10–15 min. The resistance power of the bicycle was adjusted depending on danger level and VO_2 at AT. The last part was the continuation of low-intensity aerobic training for 5–10 min. It was designed to slow flow of blood from the skeletal muscles back to the heart, which could effectively prevent a significant increase in cardiac stress. In summary, the total exercise time for one session was generally 50–70 min, varying with physical function of patients. Although there is no specific date for each training, patients were required to complete 12 sessions within one month.

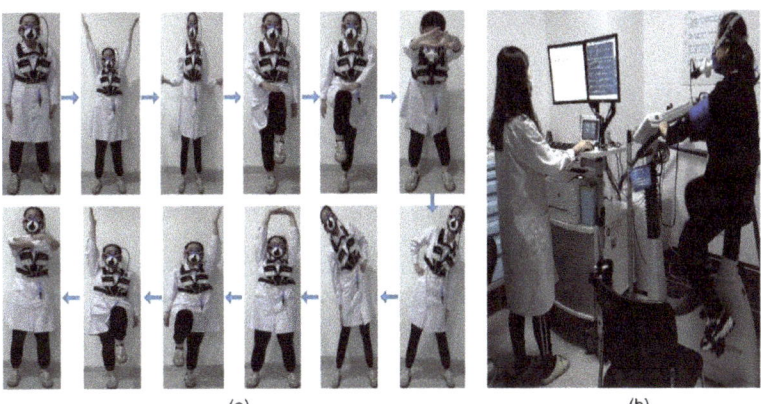

Figure 2. (**a**) Critical steps of balance exercise in APBCRE; (**b**) operation diagram of CPX. APBCRE adaptive posture-balance cardiac rehabilitation exercise. CPX exercise cardiopulmonary function measurement system.

2.4. Outcome Measure

- Cardiopulmonary Exercise Testing (CPET)

CPET was performed on the exercise cardiopulmonary function measurement system (Oxycon Mobile, JAEGER-CareFusion, Hoechberg, Germany) (CPX, Figure 2b). Individualized ramp protocol was used for CPET. HR, VO_2, respiratory exchange ratio (RER) and ventilation (VE) were collected at resting state and AT, respectively. AT was defined by the V-slope method. VE-VCO_2 slope (VE/VCO_2) and oxygen uptake efficiency slope

(OUES) was calculated based on VO_2, VE and carbon dioxide output (VCO_2). The power of the bicycle at AT (WAT) in CPET was also collected to evaluate sports performance in participants. Maximum effort was reached when RER was above 1.05.

- Resting Metabolic Rate (RMR)

Resting metabolic rate was also measured by CPX. The energy expenditure (ee) of RMR was calculated by detecting VO_2 and VCO_2 in the resting state. The equation was 'ee = $1.59 \times VCO_2 + 5.68 \times VO_2 + 2.17 \times \alpha^2$', in which α was a fixed variable depending on patients. RMR consisted of three parts: fat energy (fat), carbohydrate energy (cho) and protein energy. Protein energy was set as a constant (405 Kcal/d), and the others were computed as ee.

- General health assessment of quality of life, anxiety and depression

Three validated questionnaires were used to assess general health of participants. It included quality of life assessed by SF-12, level of anxiety assessed by Generalized Anxiety Disorder 7-item (GAD-7), level of depression assessed by Patient Health Questionnaire-9 (PHQ-9). The score of SF-12 was a continuous variable, ranging from 0 to 100. Closer to 0 meant lower quality of life, and closer to 100 was opposite. GAD-7 and PHQ-9 were grade variables, which were respectively divided into 4 groups and 5 groups. Higher score presented higher severity of anxiety or depression.

2.5. Sample Size

Sample size calculation was performed for primary outcome physical tolerance measured by VO_2 at AT. Michitaka K. et al. [16] found that VO_2 at AT notably increased around 11.7% (11.1 ± 1.1 to 12.4 ± 2.4 mL/min/kg) after rehabilitation. We hypothesized that significance level was 0.05, power was 0.90 and the improvement of before and after intervention was 15%. The sample size was calculated as at least 21 participants per group. Since our study was a self-controlled experiment, at least 21 patients were needed in total. The sample size was calculated using online free tool from Harvard University (http://hedwig.mgh.harvard.edu/sample_size/js/js_parallel_quant.html, accessed on 7 October 2020).

2.6. Statistical Analysis

Continuous variables were described by mean and standard deviation (SD), and categorical variables were described by absolute count and relative frequency. K-NearestNeighbor (KNN) algorithm was used to fill in the missing values. The differences of continuous variables between before and after APBCRE were compared by two-tailed paired Student's t test. Fisher's exact test was used for categorical variables. Moreover, all participants were divided into two subgroups (≤55-year group and >55-year group) by the mean age in order to analyze age differences in rehabilitation effect of APBCRE. The same analysis methods were applied to compare differences within subgroups between two time points. We also counted the rate of changes in outcomes for each patient after APBCRE, which aimed to compare the alteration degree of multiple indicators.

Two-tailed $p < 0.05$ was regarded as the significant level for all tests. Data analyses and visualization were conducted with R (version 3.6.2, created by Robert Clifford Gentleman and George Ross Ihaka, https://www.r-project.org/, accessed on 30 July 2022) and Python (version 3.7, created by Guido van Rossum, https://www.python.org/, accessed on 30 July 2022).

3. Results

3.1. Participants Characteristics

In our study, 93 enrolled patients were all eligible for analysis. Table 1 outlines the demographic characteristics and clinical profiles of patients. Overall, 80.65% of patients were male and the mean age was 53.03. Most of the participants (77.42%) were overweight (body mass index (BMI) > 24.0 kg/m^2), even 29.03% obesity (BMI ≥ 28.0 kg/m^2). In

CVDs composition, 72 (77.42%) patients had CHD, 47 (50.54%) had MI, 21 (22.58%) had arrhythmias and 7 (7.53%) had heart valve disease. Of these, 44 patients were complicated with hypertension, and 17 with diabetes. More than one-third of patients (44.09%) have accepted PCI, and 14 patients have undergone CABG.

Table 1. Characteristics of study participants.

Characteristics	Normal
Sex (Male)	75 (80.65%)
Mean age (years)	53.03 (12.02)
Mean body mass index (kg/m^2)	
<18.5	3 (3.22%)
18.5~24.0	18 (19.35%)
24.0~28.0	45 (48.39%)
≥28.0	27 (29.03%)
Coronary Heart Disease (%)	72 (77.42%)
Old Myocardial Infarction (%)	47 (50.54%)
Arrhythmias (%)	21 (22.58%)
Heart Valve disease (%)	7 (7.53%)
Hypertension (%)	44 (47.31%)
Diabetes (%)	17 (18.28%)
Percutaneous Coronary Intervention (%)	41 (44.09%)
Coronary Artery Bypass Graft (%)	14 (15.05%)

3.2. Physical Tolerance

VO$_2$ at AT increased significantly after one-month APBCRE (11.16 ± 2.91 to 12.85 ± 3.17 mL/min/kg, $p < 0.01$) (Table 2). VE at AT, RER at AT were also significantly different (respectively, 28.87 ± 7.26 to 32.42 ± 8.50 mL/min/kg, $p < 0.001$; 0.93 ± 0.06 to 0.95 ± 0.05, $p < 0.01$). Moreover, the variation of VE was higher than VO$_2$ (3.55 vs. 1.69 mL/min/kg). VE at AT and VO$_2$ at AT had higher changing proportions (more than 15%) compared with other notably different variables. There were no significant differences between before and after APBCRE in resting state (all $p > 0.05$).

To explore the specific efficiency of APBCRE in different age groups, participants were divided into ≤55-year group and >55-year group by the average age. The ≤55-year group contained 54 patients (49 male, 44.67 ± 6.73 years), and the >55-year group contained 39 patients (26 male, 64.62 ± 7.04 years). VO$_2$ at AT increased significantly in both groups ($p < 0.01$) (Figure 3a), while the ≤55-year group had higher changing proportion (0.23 (95%CI, 0.1 to 0.35)) compared with >55-year group (0.16 (95%CI, 0.09 to 0.23)) (Figure 4). But the rate of change of VE at AT was similar in two subgroups (0.17 (95%CI, 0.06 to 0.28) vs. 0.17 (95%CI, 0.08 to 0.26)). OUES was significantly different (1531.19 ± 265.11 to 1706.60 ± 363.39, $p < 0.01$) in the ≤55-year group, but not different in the >55-year group ($p = 0.22$). More details about CPET results being significantly different were shown in Figure 3, including VE at AT, VO$_2$ at AT, RER at AT and OUES.

Table 2. CPET parameters at before and after rehabilitation in different groups.

	Overall					≤55 year					>55 year				
	Before		After		Before vs. After p (t Test)	Before		After		Before vs. After p (t Test)	Before		After		Before vs. After p (t Test)
	Mean	SD	Mean	SD		Mean	SD	Mean	SD		Mean	SD	Mean	SD	
Resting State (RS) [a]															
HR (cpm)	78.52	11.88	76.18	10.70	0.06	78.54	11.98	77.83	11.51	0.65	78.49	11.88	73.90	9.13	0.01 *
VO$_2$ (mL/min/kg)	4.33	1.18	4.25	1.28	0.57	4.20	0.95	4.12	1.10	0.63	4.52	1.43	4.42	1.50	0.73
VE (mL/min/kg)	13.22	4.44	13.11	4.53	0.84	13.43	4.71	13.50	4.86	0.91	12.92	4.06	12.56	4.02	0.68
RER	0.81	0.07	0.82	0.08	0.11	0.80	0.06	0.82	0.07	0.07	0.82	0.07	0.83	0.09	0.63
Anaerobic Threshold (AT) [b]															
HR (cpm)	104.03	15.55	105.81	14.04	0.21	105.19	14.76	108.19	14.38	0.10	102.44	16.65	102.51	13.03	0.97
VO$_2$ (mL/min/kg)	11.16	2.91	12.85	3.17	0.00 **	11.58	2.64	13.54	3.25	0.00 **	10.58	3.19	11.90	2.81	0.00 **
VE (mL/min/kg)	28.87	7.26	32.42	8.50	0.00 **	30.59	7.46	34.02	8.51	0.01 *	26.49	6.33	30.21	8.07	0.00 **
RER	0.93	0.06	0.95	0.05	0.00 **	0.94	0.05	0.95	0.04	0.02 *	0.92	0.06	0.94	0.05	0.00 **
Slope															
VE/VCO$_2$	29.94	5.18	29.69	5.42	0.58	28.36	3.33	28.17	3.69	0.61	32.12	6.40	31.80	6.65	0.56
OUES	1426.75	346.30	1547.19	403.49	0.00 **	1531.19	265.11	1706.60	363.39	0.00 **	1282.14	394.15	1326.47	351.94	0.22

* $p < 0.05$; ** $p < 0.01$; when comparing. [a] at the beginning of the whole test with rest state. [b] in the process of the whole test reaching the critical value of AT. SD standard deviation, cpm counts per minutes, HR heart rates, VO$_2$ oxygen uptake, RER respiratory exchange ratio, VE ventilation, VE/VCO$_2$ VE–VCO$_2$ slope, OUES oxygen uptake efficiency slope.

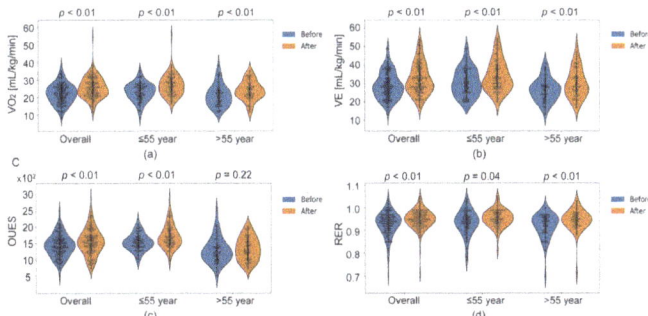

Figure 3. Distribution of significantly different variables in CPET between before and after APBCRE in all participants, the ≤55-year group and the >55-year group. (**a**) VO_2 at AT; (**b**) VE at AT; (**c**) OUES; (**d**) RER at AT. CPET cardiopulmonary exercise testing, APBCRE adaptive posture-balance cardiac rehabilitation exercise, VO_2 oxygen uptake, VE ventilation, OUES: oxygen uptake efficiency slope, RER respiratory exchange ratio, AT anaerobic threshold.

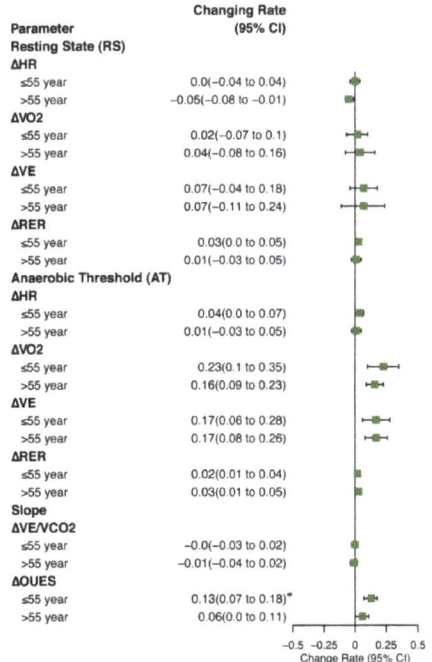

Figure 4. Changing rate of the ≤55-year group and >55-year group about CPET. * $p < 0.05$, comparing the increment between the ≤55-year group and >55-year group. Δ refers to the changing rate of variables. CPET cardiopulmonary exercise, HR heart rates, VO_2 oxygen uptake, RER respiratory exchange ratio, VE ventilation, VE/VCO_2 VE–VCO_2 slope, OUES, oxygen uptake efficiency slope, CI Confidence interval.

3.3. Secondary Endpoints

The resting metabolic rate was not significantly different between before and after APBCRE (Figure 5a), including total energy, fat energy, and carbohydrate energy. However, the score of SF-12 significantly increased after one-month APBCRE (47.78 ± 16.74 to 59.27 ± 17.77, $p < 0.001$) (Figure 5b). The level distribution of PHQ-9 also varied significantly ($p < 0.05$), but the GAD-7 had no difference ($p = 0.06$, data not shown). The number of

PHQ-9 scores below 10 changed from 26 (83.87%) to 29 (93.55%). WAT also increased significantly after APBCRE intervention (56.56 ± 23.55 to 68.85 ± 24.46 watt, $p < 0.001$) (Figure 5c).

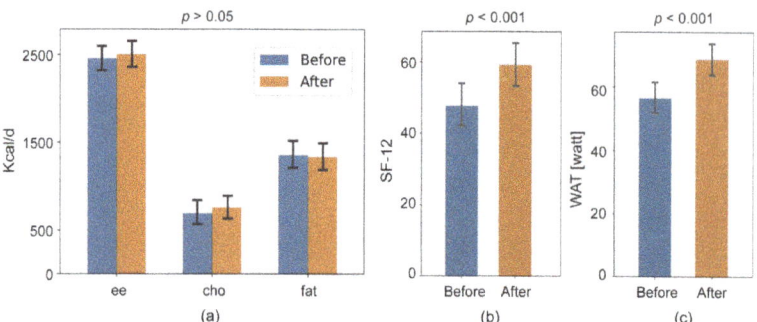

Figure 5. Secondary endpoint results before and after APBCRE: (**a**) resting metabolic rate, including energy expenditure, carbohydrate energy and fat energy; (**b**) the score of SF-12; (**c**) bicycle power at AT. APBCRE adaptive posture-balance cardiac rehabilitation exercise, AT anaerobic threshold.

4. Discussion

Our study demonstrated that APBCRE was a potentially safe and effective rehabilitation approach for patients with CVDs. Patients performed a significant increase in physical tolerance after undergoing one-month APBCRE. The ≤55-year group was more positive than the >55-year group. Quality of life and level of anxiety were also notably improved. APBCRE is the combination of existing exercise modalities and traditional medicine. It starts from respiratory regulation, and gradually extends the limb movement to the whole body through aerobic exercise, resistance exercise and flexibility training. APBCRE aims to improve neuroplasticity of the autonomic nerve through resetting the pattern of exercise.

European and American Heart Disease guidelines [26,27] recommend exercise rehabilitation as an adjuvant treatment for CVDs to compensate some shortcomings of pharmacological therapy. It is universally accepted that exercise rehabilitation is beneficial to improving physics tolerance [6], although there is controversial in specific exercise modalities and intensity [23]. In previous studies, physics tolerance is usually assessed by the peak oxygen uptake (VO_{2peak}) [8,10,28]. However, VO_{2peak} needs to be measured in the exhaustion state, which is easily interfered by subjective consciousness. Therefore, our study chose VO_2 at AT instead of VO_{2peak} to ensure the objectivity of measurements. We found that VO_2 at AT significantly improved by 19.79%, which was similar to other rehabilitation modalities (simple aerobic exercise [29] and HIIT [17]). Meanwhile, it confirmed the positive rehabilitation effect of APBCRE.

Moreover, we observed that VO_2, VE at AT in two age subgroups both significantly increased, while the ≤55-year group improved more. OUES only increased in the ≤55-year group ($p < 0.01$ vs. $p = 0.22$). OUES was an objective, reproducible measure of cardiopulmonary reserve, which integrated cardiovascular, musculoskeletal and respiratory function [30]. The differences between subgroups indicated that APBCRE had various modes of effect for different age levels. For lower-age patients, APBCRE improved both musculoskeletal, respiratory and cardiovascular function. However, for higher-age patients, APBCRE mainly enhanced ventilation when sporting rather than directly improving oxygen utilization of skeletal muscle. The improvement of ventilation was also relatively constrained. This result was consistent with the irreversible alterations in skeletal muscles and myocardium from aging. Thus, age is a nonnegligible factor when making exercise rehabilitation protocol for CVDs patients.

Furthermore, our study showed the positive therapeutic effect of exercise rehabilitation on elder patients with CVDs, which was similar to the results of Marchionni et al. [31] and Campo G et al. [32]. Lachman S et al. [33] found that moderate exercise training contributes to improving cardiovascular functions, even for elderly patients. These results confirmed that appropriate physical exercise played an important role in preventing and treating CVDs without age limitation.

The other important purpose of CR is to improve the quality of life [31], which is directly perceived by patients. Our study made individualized APBCRE programs and professional guidance for each participant to ensure more suitable exercise intensity and sports modality. The results showed that one-month APBCRE effectively improved quality of life, depression level and sports performance. However, the finding in previous studies was controversial. Snoek J.A. et al. [3] showed no differences in quality of life between the home-based mobile-guided cardiac rehabilitation group and controlled group. Yan-Wen Chen et al. [10] observes the opposite result in patients with chronic heart failure. It is indicated that the paradox possibly results from different types of CVDs and diverse sports modalities. Therefore, we will conduct additional experiments to verify the effectiveness of APBCRE on the quality of life of CVDs patients in the future.

In addition, cardiac function indicators or metabolic rate in resting state had no notable alterations after one-month APBCRE. The differences between AT and resting state indicated that short-term exercise rehabilitation mainly improved compensation capacity when sporting and had limited benefit for the whole organic function and basal metabolism. Eva Prescott et al. [5] showed that the rehabilitation efficacy was not well maintained at one year compared with the end of exercise. Therefore, we suggested that long-term regular rehabilitation was essential to improving overall function of the cardiovascular system.

There are some limitations in this study. Firstly, all patients in our study were recruited from a single center, and the sample distributions of gender and age were unbalanced. It limited the observation of the outcome of female and elderly patients, especially those over 75 years of age. Secondly, our study was a self-controlled experiment without the non-intervention control group. It led to a moderate decrease in the precision and explanation of experiments. Finally, the advantages of APBCRE were not fully explored due to a lack of comparing APBCRE with other exercise modalities. In the future, we plan to conduct a multi-center randomized controlled trial with more samples to cover the shortcomings of this study and further confirm our findings.

5. Conclusions

This study showed that the self-created rehabilitation method (adaptive posture-balance cardiac rehabilitation exercise, APBCRE) significantly improved the physical tolerance and quality of life of patients with CVDs. Moreover, compared with the >55-year group, the ≤55-year had more positive therapeutic efficiency.

Author Contributions: Conceptualization and methodology, M.M.; data curation, D.Q., C.P., J.Z. and Q.Z.; investigation, H.L.; formal analysis, and writing—original draft preparation, B.Z. and X.J.; writing—review and editing, X.Y. and T.L.; supervision, project administration and funding acquisition, T.L. All authors have read and agreed to the published version of the manuscript.

Funding: This research was funded by National Natural Science Foundation of China (no. 81971660), Medical & Health Innovation Project (2021-I2M-1-042, 2021-I2M-1-058), Sichuan Science and Technology Program (no. 2021YFH0004), Tianjin Outstanding Youth Fund Project (no. 20JCJQIC00230), Program of Chinese Institute for Brain Research in Beijing (2020-NKX-XM-14), and the Basic Research Program for Beijing–Tianjin–Hebei Coordination under grant no. 19JCZDJC65500(Z).

Institutional Review Board Statement: The study was conducted in accordance with the Declaration of Helsinki and was approved by the Ethics Committee of Tianjin Chest Hospital (IRB-SOP-016(F)-001-02, 9 August 2021) for studies involving humans.

Informed Consent Statement: Informed consent was obtained from all subjects involved in the study.

Data Availability Statement: The data used in this study are available from the corresponding author upon reasonable request.

Conflicts of Interest: The authors declare no conflict of interest.

Appendix A

Table A1. Detailed criteria for distinguishing danger levels.

Danger Level	Symptoms	Clinical Indicator	Standard
Low	<ul><li>No angina pectoris</li><li>No myocardial ischemia</li><li>No complex arrhythmias</li><li>No postoperative complications of PCI or CABG</li><li>No anxiety or depression</li></ul>	<ul><li>LVEF > 50%</li><li>METs > 7.0</li><li>cTn < 0.1 μg/L</li></ul>	Complies with all standards
Medium	<ul><li>Angina pectoris when medium-intensity exercise (5.0~6.9 METs)</li><li>Myocardial ischemia when low-intensity exercise (5.0~6.9 METs)</li><li>No complex ventricular arrhythmias when resting or sporting</li><li>No severe psychological disorders</li></ul>	<ul><li>LVEF: 40~49%</li><li>METs: 5.0~7.0</li><li>cTn < 0.1 μg/L</li></ul>	Does not comply with low-level and high-level
High	<ul><li>Angina pectoris when low-intensity exercise (<5.0 METs)</li><li>Myocardial ischemia when low-intensity exercise (<5.0 METs)</li><li>Complex ventricular arrhythmias when resting or sporting</li><li>Combined cardiogenic shock or heart failure after PCI or CABG</li><li>Severe psychological disorders</li></ul>	<ul><li>LVEF < 40%</li><li>METs ≤ 5.0</li><li>cTn > 0.1 μg/L</li></ul>	Complies with one standard

METs, metabolic equivalents; PCI, percutaneous coronary intervention; CABG, coronary artery bypass graft; LVEF, left ventricular ejection fraction; cTn, cardiac troponin.

References

1. Montalescot, G.; Sechtem, U.; Achenbach, S.; Andreotti, F.; Arden, C.; Budaj, A.; Bugiardini, R.; Crea, F.; Cuisset, T.; Di Mario, C.; et al. 2013 ESC Guidelines on the Management of Stable Coronary Artery Disease: The Task Force on the Management of Stable Coronary Artery Disease of the European Society of Cardiology. *Eur. Heart J.* **2013**, *34*, 2949–3003. [CrossRef] [PubMed]
2. Hao, G.; Wang, X.; Chen, Z.; Zhang, L.; Zhang, Y.; Wei, B.; Zheng, C.; Kang, Y.; Jiang, L.; Zhu, Z.; et al. Prevalence of Heart Failure and Left Ventricular Dysfunction in China: The China Hypertension Survey, 2012–2015. *Eur. J. Heart Fail.* **2019**, *21*, 1329–1337. [CrossRef] [PubMed]
3. Snoek, J.A.; Prescott, E.I.; van der Velde, A.E.; Eijsvogels, T.M.H.; Mikkelsen, N.; Prins, L.F.; Bruins, W.; Meindersma, E.; González-Juanatey, J.R.; Peña-Gil, C.; et al. Effectiveness of Home-Based Mobile Guided Cardiac Rehabilitation as Alternative Strategy for Nonparticipation in Clinic-Based Cardiac Rehabilitation Among Elderly Patients in Europe: A Randomized Clinical Trial. *JAMA Cardiol.* **2021**, *6*, 463–468. [CrossRef] [PubMed]
4. Ma, L.-Y.; Chen, W.-W.; Gao, R.-L.; Liu, L.-S.; Zhu, M.-L.; Wang, Y.-J.; Wu, Z.-S.; Li, H.-J.; Gu, D.-F.; Yang, Y.-J.; et al. China Cardiovascular Diseases Report 2018: An Updated Summary. *J. Geriatr. Cardiol.* **2020**, *17*, 1–8. [CrossRef] [PubMed]
5. Prescott, E.; Eser, P.; Mikkelsen, N.; Holdgaard, A.; Marcin, T.; Wilhelm, M.; Gil, C.P.; González-Juanatey, J.R.; Moatemri, F.; Iliou, M.C.; et al. Cardiac Rehabilitation of Elderly Patients in Eight Rehabilitation Units in Western Europe: Outcome Data from the EU-CaRE Multi-Centre Observational Study. *Eur. J. Prev. Cardiol.* **2020**, *27*, 1716–1729. [CrossRef]
6. Mampuya, W.M. Cardiac Rehabilitation Past, Present and Future: An Overview. *Cardiovasc. Diagn. Ther.* **2012**, *2*, 38–49.
7. Sibilitz, K.L.; Berg, S.K.; Rasmussen, T.B.; Risom, S.S.; Thygesen, L.C.; Tang, L.; Hansen, T.B.; Johansen, P.P.; Gluud, C.; Lindschou, J.; et al. Cardiac Rehabilitation Increases Physical Capacity but Not Mental Health after Heart Valve Surgery: A Randomised Clinical Trial. *Heart* **2016**, *102*, 1995–2003. [CrossRef]
8. Pratesi, A.; Baldasseroni, S.; Burgisser, C.; Orso, F.; Barucci, R.; Silverii, M.V.; Venturini, S.; Ungar, A.; Marchionni, N.; Fattirolli, F. Long-Term Functional Outcomes after Cardiac Rehabilitation in Older Patients. Data from the Cardiac Rehabilitation in Advanced AGE: EXercise TRaining and Active Follow-up (CR-AGE EXTRA) Randomised Study. *Eur. J. Prev. Cardiol.* **2019**, *26*, 1470–1478. [CrossRef]
9. Yang, X.; Li, Y.; Ren, X.; Xiong, X.; Wu, L.; Li, J.; Wang, J.; Gao, Y.; Shang, H.; Xing, Y. Effects of Exercise-Based Cardiac Rehabilitation in Patients after Percutaneous Coronary Intervention: A Meta-Analysis of Randomized Controlled Trials. *Sci. Rep.* **2017**, *7*, 44789. [CrossRef]

10. Chen, Y.-W.; Wang, C.-Y.; Lai, Y.-H.; Liao, Y.-C.; Wen, Y.-K.; Chang, S.-T.; Huang, J.-L.; Wu, T.-J. Home-Based Cardiac Rehabilitation Improves Quality of Life, Aerobic Capacity, and Readmission Rates in Patients with Chronic Heart Failure. *Medicine* **2018**, *97*, e9629. [CrossRef]
11. Campo, G.; Tonet, E.; Chiaranda, G.; Sella, G.; Maietti, E.; Bugani, G.; Vitali, F.; Serenelli, M.; Mazzoni, G.; Ruggiero, R.; et al. Exercise Intervention Improves Quality of Life in Older Adults after Myocardial Infarction: Randomised Clinical Trial. *Heart* **2020**, *106*, 1658–1664. [CrossRef] [PubMed]
12. Hammill, B.G.; Curtis, L.H.; Schulman, K.A.; Whellan, D.J. Relationship Between Cardiac Rehabilitation and Long-Term Risks of Death and Myocardial Infarction Among Elderly Medicare Beneficiaries. *Circulation* **2010**, *121*, 63–70. [CrossRef]
13. Clark, R.A.; Conway, A.; Poulsen, V.; Keech, W.; Tirimacco, R.; Tideman, P. Alternative Models of Cardiac Rehabilitation: A Systematic Review. *Eur. J. Prev. Cardiol.* **2015**, *22*, 35–74. [CrossRef] [PubMed]
14. Kraal, J.J.; Van den Akker-Van Marle, M.E.; Abu-Hanna, A.; Stut, W.; Peek, N.; Kemps, H.M. Clinical and Cost-Effectiveness of Home-Based Cardiac Rehabilitation Compared to Conventional, Centre-Based Cardiac Rehabilitation: Results of the FIT@Home Study. *Eur. J. Prev. Cardiol.* **2017**, *24*, 1260–1273. [CrossRef] [PubMed]
15. Bravo-Escobar, R.; González-Represas, A.; Gómez-González, A.M.; Montiel-Trujillo, A.; Aguilar-Jimenez, R.; Carrasco-Ruíz, R.; Salinas-Sánchez, P. Effectiveness and Safety of a Home-Based Cardiac Rehabilitation Programme of Mixed Surveillance in Patients with Ischemic Heart Disease at Moderate Cardiovascular Risk: A Randomised, Controlled Clinical Trial. *BMC Cardiovasc. Disord.* **2017**, *17*, 66. [CrossRef] [PubMed]
16. Kato, M.; Ogano, M.; Mori, Y.; Kochi, K.; Morimoto, D.; Kito, K.; Green, F.N.; Tsukamoto, T.; Kubo, A.; Takagi, H.; et al. Exercise-Based Cardiac Rehabilitation for Patients with Catheter Ablation for Persistent Atrial Fibrillation: A Randomized Controlled Clinical Trial. *Eur. J. Prev. Cardiol.* **2019**, *26*, 1931–1940. [CrossRef] [PubMed]
17. Villelabeitia-Jaureguizar, K.; Campos, D.V.; Senen, A.B.; Jiménez, V.H.; Bautista, L.R.; Garrido-Lestache, M.E.B.; Chicharro, J.L. Mechanical Efficiency of High versus Moderate Intensity Aerobic Exercise in Coronary Heart Disease Patients: A Randomized Clinical Trial. *Cardiol. J.* **2019**, *26*, 130–137. [CrossRef]
18. Taylor, J.L.; Holland, D.J.; Keating, S.E.; Leveritt, M.D.; Gomersall, S.R.; Rowlands, A.V.; Bailey, T.G.; Coombes, J.S. Short-Term and Long-Term Feasibility, Safety, and Efficacy of High-Intensity Interval Training in Cardiac Rehabilitation: The FITR Heart Study Randomized Clinical Trial. *JAMA Cardiol.* **2020**, *5*, 1382–1389. [CrossRef]
19. Prabhakaran, D.; Chandrasekaran, A.M.; Singh, K.; Mohan, B.; Chattopadhyay, K.; Chadha, D.S.; Negi, P.C.; Bhat, P.; Sadananda, K.S.; Ajay, V.S.; et al. Yoga-Based Cardiac Rehabilitation After Acute Myocardial Infarction. *J. Am. Coll. Cardiol.* **2020**, *75*, 1551–1561. [CrossRef]
20. Chandrasekaran, A.M.; Kinra, S.; Ajay, V.S.; Chattopadhyay, K.; Singh, K.; Singh, K.; Praveen, P.A.; Soni, D.; Devarajan, R.; Kondal, D.; et al. Effectiveness and Cost-Effectiveness of a Yoga-Based Cardiac Rehabilitation (Yoga-CaRe) Program Following Acute Myocardial Infarction: Study Rationale and Design of a Multi-Center Randomized Controlled Trial. *Int. J. Cardiol.* **2019**, *280*, 14–18. [CrossRef]
21. Salmoirago-Blotcher, E.; Wayne, P.M.; Dunsiger, S.; Krol, J.; Breault, C.; Bock, B.C.; Wu, W.; Yeh, G.Y. Tai Chi Is a Promising Exercise Option for Patients with Coronary Heart Disease Declining Cardiac Rehabilitation. *JAHA* **2017**, *6*, e006603. [CrossRef] [PubMed]
22. Piña, I.L.; Apstein, C.S.; Balady, G.J.; Belardinelli, R.; Chaitman, B.R.; Duscha, B.D.; Fletcher, B.J.; Fleg, J.L.; Myers, J.N.; Sullivan, M.J. Exercise and Heart Failure: A Statement from the American Heart Association Committee on Exercise, Rehabilitation, and Prevention. *Circulation* **2003**, *107*, 1210–1225. [CrossRef] [PubMed]
23. Donelli da Silveira, A.; Beust de Lima, J.; da Silva Piardi, D.; dos Santos Macedo, D.; Zanini, M.; Nery, R.; Laukkanen, J.A.; Stein, R. High-Intensity Interval Training Is Effective and Superior to Moderate Continuous Training in Patients with Heart Failure with Preserved Ejection Fraction: A Randomized Clinical Trial. *Eur. J. Prev. Cardiol.* **2020**, *27*, 1733–1743. [CrossRef] [PubMed]
24. Song, Y.; Ren, C.; Liu, P.; Tao, L.; Zhao, W.; Gao, W. Effect of Smartphone-Based Telemonitored Exercise Rehabilitation among Patients with Coronary Heart Disease. *J. Cardiovasc. Trans. Res.* **2020**, *13*, 659–667. [CrossRef]
25. Tang, L.H.; Kikkenborg Berg, S.; Christensen, J.; Lawaetz, J.; Doherty, P.; Taylor, R.S.; Langberg, H.; Zwisler, A.-D. Patients' Preference for Exercise Setting and Its Influence on the Health Benefits Gained from Exercise-Based Cardiac Rehabilitation. *Int. J. Cardiol.* **2017**, *232*, 33–39. [CrossRef]
26. Pelliccia, A.; Sharma, S.; Gati, S.; Bäck, M.; Börjesson, M.; Caselli, S.; Collet, J.-P.; Corrado, D.; Drezner, J.A.; Halle, M.; et al. 2020 ESC Guidelines on Sports Cardiology and Exercise in Patients with Cardiovascular Disease. *Eur. Heart J.* **2021**, *42*, 17–96. [CrossRef]
27. Price, K.J.; Gordon, B.A.; Bird, S.R.; Benson, A.C. A Review of Guidelines for Cardiac Rehabilitation Exercise Programmes: Is There an International Consensus? *Eur. J. Prev. Cardiol.* **2016**, *23*, 1715–1733. [CrossRef]
28. Reibis, R.; Salzwedel, A.; Buhlert, H.; Wegscheider, K.; Eichler, S.; Völler, H. Impact of Training Methods and Patient Characteristics on Exercise Capacity in Patients in Cardiovascular Rehabilitation. *Eur. J. Prev. Cardiol.* **2016**, *23*, 452–459. [CrossRef]
29. Boidin, M.; Trachsel, L.-D.; Nigam, A.; Juneau, M.; Tremblay, J.; Gayda, M. Non-Linear Is Not Superior to Linear Aerobic Training Periodization in Coronary Heart Disease Patients. *Eur. J. Prev. Cardiol.* **2020**, *27*, 1691–1698. [CrossRef]
30. Hollenberg, M.; Tager, I.B. Oxygen Uptake Efficiency Slope: An Index of Exercise Performance and Cardiopulmonary Reserve Requiring Only Submaximal Exercise. *J. Am. Coll. Cardiol.* **2000**, *36*, 194–201. [CrossRef]
31. Marchionni, N.; Fattirolli, F.; Fumagalli, S.; Oldridge, N.; Del Lungo, F.; Morosi, L.; Burgisser, C.; Masotti, G. Improved Exercise Tolerance and Quality of Life with Cardiac Rehabilitation of Older Patients After Myocardial Infarction: Results of a Randomized, Controlled Trial. *Circulation* **2003**, *107*, 2201–2206. [CrossRef] [PubMed]

32. Campo, G.; Tonet, E.; Chiaranda, G.; Sella, G.; Maietti, E.; Mazzoni, G.; Biscaglia, S.; Pavasini, R.; Myers, J.; Grazzi, G. Exercise Intervention to Improve Functional Capacity in Older Adults After Acute Coronary Syndrome. *J. Am. Coll. Cardiol.* **2019**, *74*, 2948–2950. [CrossRef] [PubMed]
33. Lachman, S.; Boekholdt, S.M.; Luben, R.N.; Sharp, S.J.; Brage, S.; Khaw, K.-T.; Peters, R.J.; Wareham, N.J. Impact of Physical Activity on the Risk of Cardiovascular Disease in Middle-Aged and Older Adults: EPIC Norfolk Prospective Population Study. *Eur. J. Prev. Cardiol.* **2018**, *25*, 200–208. [CrossRef] [PubMed]

Associations of Blood and Performance Parameters with Signs of Periodontal Inflammation in Young Elite Athletes—An Explorative Study

Cordula Leonie Merle [1,2,*], Lisa Richter [2], Nadia Challakh [2], Rainer Haak [2], Gerhard Schmalz [2], Ian Needleman [3,4], Peter Rüdrich [5], Bernd Wolfarth [5,6,7], Dirk Ziebolz [2,†] and Jan Wüstenfeld [5,6,†]

1. Department of Prosthetic Dentistry, UKR University Hospital Regensburg, 93053 Regensburg, Germany
2. Department of Cariology, Endodontology and Periodontology, University of Leipzig, 04103 Leipzig, Germany
3. Centre for Oral Health and Performance, UCL Eastman Dental Institute, London WC1E 6BT, UK
4. UK IOC Research Centre, London WC1E 6BT, UK
5. Department of Sports Medicine, Institute for Applied Scientific Training, 04109 Leipzig, Germany
6. Department of Sports Medicine, Charité University Medicine, 10115 Berlin, Germany
7. Institute of Sports Science, Humboldt University, 10099 Berlin, Germany
* Correspondence: cordula.merle@klinik.uni-regensburg.de
† These authors contributed equally to this work.

Abstract: This retrospective cross-sectional study aimed to explore interactions between signs of periodontal inflammation and systemic parameters in athletes. Members of German squads with available data on sports medical and oral examination were included. Groups were divided by gingival inflammation (median of papillary bleeding index, PBI ≥ median) and signs of periodontitis (Periodontal Screening Index, PSI ≥ 3). Age, gender, anthropometry, blood parameters, echocardiography, sports performance on ergometer, and maximal aerobic capacity (VO_{2max}) were evaluated. Eighty-five athletes (f = 51%, 20.6 ± 3.5 years) were included (PBI < 0.42: 45%; PSI ≥ 3: 38%). Most associations were not statistically significant. Significant group differences were found for body fat percentage and body mass index. All blood parameters were in reference ranges. Minor differences in hematocrit, hemoglobin, basophils, erythrocyte sedimentation rates, urea, and HDL cholesterol were found for PBI, in uric acid for PSI. Echocardiographic parameters (n = 40) did not show any associations. Athletes with PSI ≥ 3 had lower VO_{2max} values (55.9 ± 6.7 mL/min/kg vs. 59.3 ± 7.0 mL/min/kg; p = 0.03). In exercise tests (n = 30), athletes with PBI < 0.42 achieved higher relative maximal load on the cycling ergometer (5.0 ± 0.5 W/kg vs. 4.4 ± 0.3 W/kg; p = 0.03). Despite the limitations of this study, potential associations between signs of periodontal inflammation and body composition, blood parameters, and performance were identified. Further studies on the systemic impact of oral inflammation in athletes, especially regarding performance, are necessary.

Keywords: performance; systemic inflammation; physical endurance; physical fitness; maximal aerobic capacity; gingivitis

1. Introduction

The high-performance standards of elite athletes are built on foundations of physical fitness, health, and wellbeing. It may be a surprise, therefore, that oral ill health is common in elite athletes and results in an increased oral inflammatory burden [1]. The prevalence of both gingivitis and periodontitis can be high [1] and differs significantly from non-elite controls [2–4]. For instance, among footballers, a periodontitis prevalence of 41% was reported [5].

Oral infections, including periodontal diseases, cause increased systemic inflammation [6], which can resolve following treatment [7], although there are inconsistencies between studies [8]. The relationship between oral health and physical activity could be bidirectional. Some studies have reported an impairment from poor oral health on measures of physical activity and performance [9]. On the other hand, intensive physical activity leads to systemic changes: levels of (pro-)inflammatory cytokines [10,11] as well as stress hormones [12] increase. On the other side, immunoglobulin A levels decrease [13]. A transitional reduced cellular immune response [14,15] has been proposed to lead to an open window for infections [16]. However, the impact of these changes on oral inflammation is not clear.

The relationship between oral health and anaerobic capacity of athletes has received very little attention. A recent study in elite rowers did not find a relationship between dental caries and anaerobic capacity, although the study had few participants and differences in oral health status between comparison groups were small [17]. There has been no published research investigating the influence of oral inflammation on the performance of athletes or systemic biomarkers. Nevertheless, several studies have found negative impacts of poor oral health on self-reported measures of performance [18,19]. Consequently, this retrospective explorative study aimed to investigate associations between signs of periodontal inflammation and systemic parameters in elite athletes. Associations between gingival and periodontal inflammation to blood, echocardiographic, and performance parameters were investigated. It was hypothesized that these parameters would be affected in athletes with increased signs of periodontal inflammation.

2. Materials and Methods

2.1. Study Design and Participants

This pilot study was based on a retrospective data evaluation from a collaboration between the Department of Cariology, Endodontology and Periodontology and the Institute for Applied Scientific Training (IAT) Leipzig. Dental examinations were performed as a supplement to the annual sports medical and performance diagnostics.

Inclusion criteria were athletes of German national teams, perspective, or youth squads, aged between 18 and 30 years, male and female. The sports medical and standardized dental examination (performed on the same day) were conducted between May and December 2019. Participants with incomplete dental examination were excluded. A comprehensive description of the cohort and oral health status was already published elsewhere [4].

The study was reviewed and approved by the Ethics Committee of the medical faculty of Leipzig University, Germany (No. 091/20-ek). All participants were informed verbally and in writing about the scientific use of their clinical data and provided their informed consent for participation in research studies. The recommendations for strengthening the reporting of cross-sectional studies (STROBE) were considered [20].

2.2. Data Collection

Data on general characteristics, blood parameters, echocardiographic examination, and sports performance tests as part of the sports medical records were exported from the IAT database. Data on signs of periodontal inflammation were extracted from patients' dental records.

General characteristics. Recorded general characteristics were age, gender, training, and anthropometric data including body mass index (BMI), body fat percentage (BFP), lean body mass (LBM), and resting heart rate (RHR).

Blood parameters. The annual sports medical and performance diagnostics comprised extensive blood tests for all athletes. A complete blood count with the number of erythrocytes, leukocytes, thrombocytes, lymphocytes, neutrophils, basophils, eosinophils and monocytes, hematocrit, hemoglobin, mean corpuscular hemoglobin (MCH), mean corpuscular hemoglobin concentration (MCHC), mean corpuscular volume (MCV), immature reticulocyte fraction (IFR), high (HFR), medium (MFR), and low-fluorescence reticulocytes (LFR) was performed. Neutrophil–lymphocyte (NLR), monocyte–lymphocyte (MLR), and platelet–lymphocyte ratios (PLR) were calculated. Further determined blood parameters were erythrocyte sedimentation rates after 1 (ESR1h) and 2 h (ESR2h), iron, ferritin, natrium, calcium, potassium, magnesium, gamma-glutamyl transferase (GGT), glutamic-pyruvate-transaminase (GPT), urea, uric acid, creatine kinase, total protein, total cholesterol, low-density lipoprotein (LDL) and high-density lipoprotein (HDL) cholesterol, LDL/HDL ratio, glucose, and triglycerides.

Echocardiographic examination. Additionally, if available, sport-specific and performance-related measurements of transthoracic echocardiographic examination were exported: absolute heart volume (HV_abs), relative heart volume (HV_rel) (calculated by the equation of Dickhuth) [21], left atrial size (LA), left ventricular end-diastolic dimension (LVEDd), and tricuspid annular plane systolic excursion (TAPSE).

Sports performance. Maximal aerobic capacity (VO_{2max}) by spiroergometry was extracted if available. If not, it was estimated by the equation of Rexhepi and Brestoci [22]. Furthermore, data from sports performance tests with incremental exercise tests on running or cycle ergometer were considered: RHR, heart rates (HF), lactate, and power, respectively, and speed were extracted for analysis. Besides minimum, maximum, and differences, the speed/power output at individual anaerobic threshold (IAnT), lactate threshold 1 (LT1, initial rise after basal lactate), lactate threshold 2 (LT2, Dickhuth model: basal lactate + 1.5 mmol/L), without load ($p = 0$), and maximal load (P_{max}) at the ergometer were tested.

Signs of periodontal inflammation. Data for both gingival and periodontal inflammation were extracted from patients' dental records. A comprehensive (standardized) orofacial examination was performed using a headlight on an examination couch at the IAT. A single skilled dentist that was trained in these periodontal parameters examined all athletes (kappa > 80%). Gingival inflammation was assessed by the papillary bleeding index (PBI) [23] which discriminates five scores after probing (0: no bleeding; 1: single bleeding point; 2: several bleeding points or fine line; 3: interdental triangle filled with blood, 4: profuse bleeding). The PBI index was calculated per patient by division of the total sum by the total number of interdental papillae. Periodontal conditions (= sign of periodontitis/periodontal treatment need) were examined using the Periodontal Screening Index [24]: score 0 to 2 has probing depths less than 3.5 mm. Score 0 shows no bleeding, no calculus, score 1 bleeding on probing, and score 2 calculus. A score of 3 or 4 indicates increased probing depths (3: pocket depth 3.5–5.5 mm; 4: pocket depth > 5.5 mm) as a sign of periodontitis. Third molars were not included in this evaluation despite they took a more anterior position.

2.3. Statistical Analysis

Statistical analysis was performed with SPSS Statistics for Windows (version 23.0, IBM Corp., Armonk, NY, USA). Possible associations from signs of periodontal inflammation to anthropometric data, blood, echocardiographic, and exercise test parameters were examined. For analyzing associations to gingival inflammation, the athletes were divided into two groups by median of the PBI (PBI < median vs. PBI $\geq$ median). Regarding signs of periodontitis, group division was based on having increased probing depths ($\geq$3.5 mm) or not (PSI < 3 vs. PSI $\geq$ 3). Quantitative variables were presented by mean and standard deviation (SD). Independent, normal-distributed samples were analyzed with a t-test. For non-normal distributed samples, the Mann–Whitney U test was used. All tests were performed two sided, with a significance level at $p < 0.05$ and under exclusion of missing data. Normal distribution was verified by Kolmogorov–Smirnov test. For parameters with an association ($p < 0.1$) and plausible link to PBI or PSI, a multivariate analysis of variance (MANOVA) and, for significant models, linear regression were planned.

3. Results

3.1. Athletes

Records of 85 athletes from the German national elite, perspective, and youth squads (f = 51%, 20.6 ± 3.5 years) were included for retrospective evaluation. Table 1 shows their characteristics, training, and anthropometric data.

Table 1. Characteristics of the athletes (entire cohort).

	n	%
n—All disciplines	85	100.0
-Running	39	45.9
-Biathlon	24	28.2
-Cross-country skiing	10	11.8
-Rowing	8	9.4
-Triathlon	4	4.7
Female gender	43	50.6
	mean	SD
Age (years)	20.6	± 3.5
Training sessions per week	9.8	± 2.9
Training time (h) per week	17.3	± 4.8
Training history (years)	7.2	± 2.9
Body mass index (kg/m^2)	20.7	± 2.1
Body weight (kg)	65.9	± 10.5
Body height (cm)	177.8	± 9.6
Resting heart rate [a] (bpm)	49.0	± 8.2
Body fat percentage (by impedance) (%)	8.7	± 3.5
Body fat percentage (by skin folds) (%)	13.1	± 4.7
Lean body mass (%)	57.3	± 9.2
VO$_{2max}$ (mL/min/kg)	58.02	± 7.02

Abbreviations: n: number of participants; VO$_{2max}$: maximal aerobic capacity. [a] Missing data for eight participants (n = 77).

3.2. Signs of Periodontal Inflammation

Mean gingival inflammation (PBI) was 0.48 ± 0.29 and the median was 0.42 (IQR: 0.31; 0.69). The subgroup PBI < 0.42 contained 40 and the subgroup PBI ≥ 0.42 45 athletes. As such, 53 athletes had a PSI < 3 and 32 a PSI ≥ 3 with 11 having a PSI ≥ 3 in more than one sextant. No athlete showed a PSI score of 4. The associations between body composition and performance with periodontal health are shown in Table 2. Most associations were not statistically significant at $p < 0.05$. BFP was significantly lower in PBI ≥ 0.42 (PBI < 0.42: 14.4 ± 4.8 vs. PBI ≥ 0.42: 11.9 ± 4.3; $p = 0.02$) but significantly higher in PSI ≥ 3 (PSI < 3: 12.4 ± 4.9 vs. PSI ≥ 3: 14.3 ± 4.2; $p = 0.047$). Athletes with signs of periodontitis also had a higher BMI (PSI < 3: 20.3 ± 2.0 vs. PSI ≥ 3: 21.5 ± 2.0; $p = 0.01$).

3.3. Blood Parameters

Results of the complete blood count (Table 3) and further blood parameters (Table 4) are presented for the entire cohort and separately for the divided groups by PBI and PSI. Again, most associations were not statistically significant. However, statically significant differences between athletes with a lower and those with a higher PBI were found for hematocrit (PBI < 0.42: 41.5 ± 2.8% vs. PBI ≥ 0.42: 42.6 ± 2.4%; $p = 0.04$), hemoglobin (14.2 ± 1.2 g/dL vs. 14.7 ± 0.9 g/dL; $p = 0.04$), basophils (0.5 ± 0.2% vs. 0.4 ± 0.2%; $p = 0.03$), ESR1h (5.1 ± 3.3 mm vs. 3.8 ± 2.8 mm; $p = 0.01$), ESR2h (10.6 ± 7.2 mm vs. 8.0 ± 5.7 mm; $p = 0.04$), urea (6.3 ± 1.7 mmol/L vs. 5.5 ± 1.4 mmol/L; $p = 0.04$), and HDL cholesterol (1.9 ± 0.3 mmol/l vs. 1.7 ± 0.2 mmol/L; p = 0.02). In relation to periodontitis based on PSI ≥ 3, statistically significant differences were found only for uric acid (PSI < 3: 251.3 ± 74.1 μmol/L vs. PSI ≥ 3: 283.1 ± 60.8 μmol/L; p = 0.04). Multivariate linear regression was performed for urea, uric acid, HDL cholesterol, thrombocytes, and iron, whereby ANOVA revealed significance for two different models, including urea, uric acid, and thrombocytes, however, showing a small effect size (Supplementary Materials Table S1).

3.4. Echocardiographic Parameters

An echocardiographic examination was performed on a subgroup of 40 athletes. The results of the quantitative measurements are presented in Supplementary Materials Table S2. HV_rel was, on average, 12 mL/kg, LA 3.6 cm, and TAPSE 2.5 cm. There were no statistically significant associations with PBI or PSI.

3.5. Performance Parameters

Spiroergometric data were available for 41 athletes; 30 completed further performance diagnostics with incremental exercise tests (Table 5). Ergometer types were running (n = 20, biathletes) or cycling (n = 10, cross-country skiers). Overall, in athletes, those with signs of periodontitis had lower VO_{2max} values (55.9 ± 6.7 mL/min/kg vs. 59.3 ± 7.0 mL/min/kg; p = 0.03). Detailed data on power on the ergometer are presented in Table 6; the group with less gingival inflammation achieved a higher relative maximal load on the cycling ergometer (PBI < 0.42: 5.0 ± 0.5 W/kg vs. PBI ≥ 0.42: 4.4 ± 0.3 W/kg; p = 0.03).

Table 2. Characteristics of the athletes (entire cohort) and their associations with periodontal health (PBI and PSI).

	Association to PBI							Association to PSI						
	PBI < 0.42			PBI ≥ 0.42			p-Value	PSI < 3			PSI ≥ 3			p-Value
	n		%	n		%		n		%	n		%	
n	40		47.1	45		52.9	0.05	53		62.4	32		37.6	
Female gender	25		62.5	18		40.0		28			15			
	mean	±	SD	mean	±	SD	p-Value	mean	±	SD	mean	±	SD	p-Value
Age (years)	21.0	±	3.0	22.0	±	3.8	0.35	21.4	±	3.2	21.6	±	3.9	0.81
Training sessions per week	10.4	±	3.2	9.2	±	2.4	0.15	9.9	±	2.7	9.5	±	3.1	0.51
Training time (h) per week	16.8	±	4.0	17.7	±	5.4	0.58	17.4	±	5.1	17.1	±	4.3	0.99
Training history (years)	6.7	±	3.0	7.6	±	2.9	0.12	6.9	±	2.8	7.7	±	3.1	0.23
BMI (kg/m^2)	20.9	±	2.0	20.5	±	2.1	0.36	20.3	±	2.0	21.5	±	2.0	**0.01**
Body weight (kg)	65.9	±	10.5	66.0	±	10.5	0.99	64.5	±	10.2	68.3	±	10.6	0.11
Body height (cm)	176.8	±	9.4	178.6	±	9.9	0.35	177.8	±	9.7	177.6	±	9.6	0.96
RHR (bpm)	48.5	±	8.4	49.3	±	8.1	0.59	47.9	±	6.7	50.7	±	10.1	0.25
BFP (by impedance) (%)	9.5	±	3.7	7.9	±	3.1	0.07	8.1	±	3.7	9.6	±	2.8	**0.01**
BFP (by skin folds) (%)	14.4	±	4.8	11.9	±	4.3	**0.02**	12.4	±	4.9	14.3	±	4.2	0.05
LBM (%)	56.4	±	9.0	58.0	±	9.3	0.43	56.4	±	8.5	58.7	±	10.1	0.37
VO$_{2max}$ (mL/min/kg)	56.9	±	6.3	59.0	±	7.5	0.44	59.3	±	7.0	55.9	±	6.7	**0.03**

Abbreviations: BMI: body mass index, RHR: resting heart rate; BFP: body fat percentage; LBM: lean body mass; n: number of participants; PBI: Papillary Bleeding Index; PSI: Periodontal Screening Index with PSI ≥ 3 indicating increased probing depths as a sign of probable periodontitis; VO$_{2max}$: maximal aerobic capacity. Bold marks significant differences ($p < 0.05$).

Table 3. Complete blood count (BC) of the athletes (entire cohort) and their associations with periodontal health (PBI and PSI).

	Total n = 85	Reference Ranges	Association to PBI PBI < 0.42	Association to PBI PBI ≥ 0.42	Association to PBI p-Value	Association to PSI PSI < 3	Association to PSI PSI ≥ 3	Association to PSI p-Value
Erythrocytes ($\times 10^6/\mu L$)	4.8 ± 0.4	3.9–6.1	4.8 ± 0.4	4.9 ± 0.4	0.15	4.8 ± 0.4	4.8 ± 0.4	0.86
Hematocrit (%)	42.1 ± 2.6	34.1–44.9	41.5 ± 2.8	42.6 ± 2.4	**0.04**	42.0 ± 2.6	42.2 ± 2.7	0.71
Hemoglobin (g/dL)	14.5 ± 1.1	12–18	14.2 ± 1.2	14.7 ± 0.9	**0.04**	14.5 ± 1.1	14.5 ± 1.1	0.89
MCH (fmol)	1.9 ± 0.1	1.5–2.1	1.9 ± 0.1	1.9 ± 0.1	0.52	1.9 ± 0.1	1.9 ± 0.1	0.93
MCHC (mmol/L)	21.4 ± 0.5	20.0–22.7	21.3 ± 0.6	21.4 ± 0.5	0.30	21.4 ± 0.6	21.3 ± 0.5	0.71
MCV (fl)	87.3 ± 3.3	79.4–100	87.2 ± 3.5	87.5 ± 3.1	0.65	87.3 ± 3.8	87.4 ± 2.4	0.84
IRF (%)	3.7 ± 2.0	2.1–17.5	3.9 ± 2.3	3.4 ± 1.7	0.23	3.7 ± 2.3	3.6 ± 1.5	0.70
HFR (%)	0.2 ± 0.3	0–2.4	0.2 ± 0.4	0.2 ± 0.3	0.71	0.2 ± 0.4	0.2 ± 0.3	0.75
MFR (%)	3.4 ± 1.9	1.8–14.4	3.7 ± 2.2	3.2 ± 1.7	0.24	3.5 ± 2.2	3.4 ± 1.4	0.75
LFR (%)	96.3 ± 2.0	87.8–99.5	96.1 ± 2.3	96.6 ± 1.7	0.23	96.3 ± 2.3	96.4 ± 1.5	0.70
Leukocytes (/nl)	5.9 ± 1.3	3.6–9.8	5.7 ± 1.2	6.0 ± 1.4	0.19	5.8 ± 1.2	6.0 ± 1.5	0.35
Lymphocytes (%)	39.0 ± 7.3	19–53	40.5 ± 7.8	37.8 ± 6.5	0.08	39.1 ± 7.0	39.0 ± 7.7	0.96
Neutrophils (%)	46.7 ± 7.8	34–71	45.5 ± 8.7	47.8 ± 6.7	0.17	46.5 ± 7.3	47.1 ± 8.6	0.75
Basophils (%)	0.5 ± 0.2	0.1–1.2	0.5 ± 0.2	0.4 ± 0.2	**0.03**	0.5 ± 0.3	0.4 ± 0.2	0.62
Eosinophils (%)	3.3 ± 2.7	1–7	3.2 ± 2.0	3.3 ± 3.2	0.95	3.4 ± 3.1	3.1 ± 1.7	0.88
Monocytes (%)	10.5 ± 2.1	5.0–12.0	10.3 ± 1.8	10.7 ± 2.3	0.43	10.6 ± 2.2	10.4 ± 1.9	0.74
Thrombocytes (/nl)	236.7 ± 48.3	150–361	247.2 ± 49.2	227.4 ± 45.9	0.06	239.6 ± 47.1	232.1 ± 50.5	0.49
NLR	1.3 ± 0.5	0.1–3.2	1.22 ± 0.5	1.34 ± 0.5	0.09	1.27 ± 0.5	1.31 ± 0.6	0.84
MLR	0.3 ± 0.1	2.0–8.6	0.26 ± 0.1	0.30 ± 0.1	0.18	0.28 ± 0.1	0.28 ± 0.1	0.91
PLR	110.3 ± 32.3	46.8–218.0	113.8 ± 29.1	107.2 ± 35.0	0.14	112.8 ± 32.0	106.2 ± 33.0	0.33

Abbreviations: MCH: mean corpuscular hemoglobin (MCH); MCHC: mean corpuscular hemoglobin concentration; MCV: mean corpuscular volume (MCV); HFR: high fluorescence reticulocytes; IRF: immature reticulocyte fraction (IRF); LFR: low fluorescence reticulocytes; MFR: medium fluorescence reticulocytes; MLR: monocyte-lymphocyte ratio; n: number of participants; NLR: neutrophil-lymphocyte ratio; PBI: Papillary Bleeding Index; PLR: platelet-lymphocyte ratio; PSI: Periodontal Screening Index with PSI ≥ 3 indicating increased probing depths as a sign of probable periodontitis. Bold marks significant differences ($p < 0.05$).

Table 4. Further blood parameters of the athletes (entire cohort) and their associations to with periodontal health (PBI and PSI).

	Total n = 85	Reference Ranges	Association to PBI			Association to PSI		
			PBI < 0.42	PBI ≥ 0.42	p-Value	PSI < 3	PSI ≥ 3	p-Value
ESR1h (mm)	4.4 ± 3.1	<10	5.1 ± 3.3	3.8 ± 2.8	**0.01**	4.7 ± 3.3	4.0 ± 2.7	0.32
ESR2h (mm)	9.2 ± 6.5	<20	10.6 ± 7.2	8.0 ± 5.7	**0.04**	9.7 ± 7.0	8.5 ± 5.7	0.76
Iron (µmol/L)	16.8 ± 7.1	6.6–30.1	15.6 ± 6.6	17.9 ± 7.3	0.13	16.6 ± 7.3	17.1 ± 6.9	0.75
Ferritin (µg/L)	62.2 ± 39.0	15–280	56.4 ± 32.7	67.4 ± 43.6	0.32	62.1 ± 41.3	62.5 ± 35.6	0.73
Natrium [a] (mmol/L)	139.9 ± 2.3	15–280	140.0 ± 2.3	139.9 ± 2.3	0.64	140.0 ± 2.5	139.8 ± 2.1	0.78
Calcium (mmol/L)	2.4 ± 0.1	2.2–2.6	2.4 ± 0.1	2.4 ± 0.1	0.35	2.4 ± 0.1	2.4 ± 0.1	0.21
Potassium (mmol/L)	4.2 ± 0.3	3.6–5.5	4.2 ± 0.2	4.2 ± 0.3	0.95	4.2 ± 0.3	4.2 ± 0.3	0.75
Magnesium (mmol/L)	0.8 ± 0.1	15–280	0.8 ± 0.1	0.8 ± 0.1	0.95	0.8 ± 0.1	0.8 ± 0.1	0.30
GGT [b] (U/L)	22.3 ± 5.7	0–55	22.2 ± 4.4	22.4 ± 6.7	0.74	23.1 ± 6.6	21.3 ± 4.3	0.29
GPT [b] (U/L)	40.2 ± 41.5	10–50	36.1 ± 18.5	43.5 ± 53.4	0.58	36.5 ± 16.9	45.2 ± 61.3	0.80
Urea (mmol/L)	5.9 ± 1.6	2.6–8.9	6.3 ± 1.7	5.5 ± 1.4	**0.04**	5.8 ± 1.6	6.0 ± 1.6	0.62
Uric acid (µmol/L)	263.3 ± 70.7	120–416	247.6 ± 65.8	277.2 ± 72.7	0.05	251.3 ± 74.1	283.1 ± 60.8	**0.04**
Creatine kinase (U/L)	427.5 ± 799.6	24–350	360.2 ± 412.5	487.3 ± 1030.6	0.07	340.9 ± 317.8	571.0 ± 1236.5	0.64
Creatinine [b] (µmol/L)	79.5 ± 11.7	44–97	78.76 ± 11.3	80.1 ± 12.1	0.64	80.5 ± 11.7	78.1 ± 11.8	0.41
Total Protein (g/L)	70.6 ± 3.5	66–88	70.8 ± 3.5	70.5 ± 3.5	0.70	70.2 ± 3.4	71.4 ± 3.5	0.13
Total Cholesterol [b] (mmol/L)	4.5 ± 0.8	<5.2	4.7 ± 0.8	4.3 ± 0.7	0.30	4.5 ± 0.9	4.5 ± 0.6	0.79
LDL Cholesterol [b] (mmol/L)	2.3 ± 0.6	<4.1	2.3 ± 0.7	2.3 ± 0.6	0.74	2.3 ± 0.7	2.3 ± 0.5	0.91
HDL Cholesterol [b] (mmol/L)	1.8 ± 0.3	>0.9	1.9 ± 0.3	1.7 ± 0.2	**0.02**	1.8 ± 0.2	1.8 ± 0.3	0.51
LDL/HDL Ratio [b]	1.3 ± 0.4	<3.5	1.3 ± 0.4	1.4 ± 0.4	0.41	1.3 ± 0.4	1.4 ± 0.4	0.53
Glucose (mmol/L)	4.7 ± 0.6	3.4–5.6	4.8 ± 0.4	4.6 ± 0.7	0.29	4.7 ± 0.6	4.7 ± 0.5	0.78
Triglycerides [b] (mmol/L)	0.9 ± 0.4	<2.3	1.0 ± 0.5	0.8 ± 0.3	0.06	0.9 ± 0.5	0.9 ± 0.3	0.89

Abbreviations: ESR1h: erythrocyte sedimentation rate after 1 h; ESR2h: erythrocyte sedimentation rate after 2 h; GPT: glutamat-pyruvate-transaminase; HDL: high-density lipoprotein; LDL: low-density lipoprotein; n: number of participants; PBI: Papillary Bleeding Index; PSI: Periodontal Screening Index with PSI ≥ 3 indicating increased probing depths as a sign of probable periodontitis. Bold marks significant differences ($p < 0.05$); [a] Missing data for two participants (n = 83); [b] Missing data for 18 participants (n = 67).

Table 5. Performance test parameters, heart frequencies, and lactate values during incremental exercise test and their association with periodontal health (PBI and PSI).

	Total	Association to PBI			Association to PSI		
	n = 30	PBI < 0.46	PBI ≥ 0.46	p-Value	PSI < 3	PSI ≥ 3	p-Value
RHR (bpm)	52.0 ± 9.3	51.5 ± 9.3	52.5 ± 9.5	0.77	50.3 ± 7.3	53.8 ± 10.9	0.30
HF_LT (bpm)	143.9 ± 12.7	142.8 ± 14.1	144.8 ± 11.7	0.67	145.2 ± 12.20	142.5 ± 13.5	0.57
HF_IAnT (bpm)	174.4 ± 12.2	173.4 ± 13.4	175.2 ± 11.5	0.70	176.5 ± 11.1	172.3 ± 13.3	0.36
HF_Pmax (bpm)	194.6 ± 8.9	193.8 ± 7.3	195.4 ± 10.2	0.63	196.1 ± 7.4	193.2 ± 10.2	0.39
HF_max (bpm)	201.9 ± 1.3	202.1 ± 1.2	201.6 ± 1.4	0.39	201.7 ± 1.3	202.0 ± 1.4	0.51
Lactate_LT1 (mmol/L)	1.2 ± 0.3	1.2 ± 0.3	1.3 ± 0.3	0.31	1.2 ± 0.3	1.3 ± 0.4	0.52
Lactate_LT2 (mmol/L)	2.7 ± 0.3	2.7 ± 0.3	2.8 ± 0.3	0.31	2.7 ± 0.3	2.8 ± 0.4	0.52
Lactate_max (mmol/L)	9.5 ± 2.2	10.1 ± 1.9	8.9 ± 2.3	0.13	9.5 ± 2.1	9.4 ± 2.3	0.97

Abbreviations: IAnT: individual anaerobic threshold; HF: heart frequency LT1: lactate threshold 1, LT2: lactate threshold 2; max: maximal value; n: number of participants; PBI: Papillary Bleeding Index; PSI: Periodontal Screening Index with PSI ≥ 3 indicating increased probing depths as a sign of probable periodontitis; Pmax: maximal load; RHR: resting heart rate.

Table 6. Power on ergometer during incremental exercise tests and their association with periodontal health (PBI and PSI).

	Total	Association to PBI			Association to PSI		
		PBI < 0.46	PBI ≥ 0.46	p-Value	PSI < 3	PSI ≥ 3	p-Value
Power (Running) (n = 20)							
P_la = 2 mmol/L (km/h)	12.0 ± 1.5	11.6 ± 1.1	12.3 ± 1.7	0.30	12.3 ± 1.1	11.8 ± 1.8	0.49
P_LT2 (km/h)	13.3 ± 1.4	12.9 ± 1.0	13.6 ± 1.6	0.28	13.4 ± 1.2	13.3 ± 1.7	0.92
P_LT1 (km/h)	9.8 ± 1.1	9.4 ± 0.8	10.0 ± 1.2	0.22	9.7 ± 1.0	9.8 ± 1.3	0.85
P$_{max}$ (km/h)	16.4 ± 1.7	16.1 ± 1.3	16.5 ± 2.0	0.55	16.6 ± 1.6	16.1 ± 1.9	0.58
Power (Cycling) (n = 10)							
P_la = 2 mmol/L (W)	217.9 ± 62.8	244.5 ± 52.9	178.0 ± 60.3	0.10	220.2 ± 69.3	215.6 ± 63.8	0.92
P_LT2 (W)	238.4 ± 65.9	263.3 ± 60.5	201.0 ± 62.0	0.09	245.8 ± 68.6	231.0 ± 70.3	0.92
P_LT1 (W)	150.3 ± 47.4	165.0 ± 46.5	128.3 ± 45.5	0.29	157.8 ± 47.6	142.8 ± 51.6	0.53
P$_{max}$ (W)	326.5 ± 77.1	360.5 ± 65.3	275.5 ± 70.4	0.09	332.8 ± 74.1	320.2 ± 88.3	0.81
P$_{max\_rel}$ (W/kg)	4.8 ± 0.5	5.0 ± 0.5	4.4 ± 0.3	**0.03**	4.9 ± 0.7	4.6 ± 0.4	0.25

Abbreviations: P_la = 2 mmol/l: power on ergometer when having lactate value of 2 mmol/L; P_LT1: power at lactate threshold 1; P_LT2: power at lactate threshold 2; PBI: Papillary Bleeding Index; PSI: Periodontal Screening Index with PSI ≥ 3 indicating increased probing depths as a sign of probable periodontitis; P$_{max}$: maximum power on ergometer; P$_{max\_rel}$: relative maximum power. Bold marks significant differences (p < 0.05).

4. Discussion

Overall, young athletes showed low mean gingival inflammation (PBI = 0.48 ± 0.29) but, importantly, signs of periodontitis (PSI ≥ 3) were present in 38% of the athletes. Group differences between athletes with lower or higher gingival inflammation were found for several blood parameters (hematocrit, hemoglobin, basophils, ESR1h, ESR2h, and urea), maximal aerobic capacity (VO_{2max}), and maximum load on the cycling ergometer. Athletes with signs of periodontitis differed in body composition (BMI, BFP), uric acid, and VO_{2max}.

One explanation for the differences between groups of different oral health status is that increased oral inflammation affects systemic parameters. Despite controversial discussion [8], various changes in blood values have been observed in periodontitis patients, including inflammation markers, cytokines, and changes in both white and red blood cell counts [25–29]. Furthermore, periodontal treatment that reduces local inflammation also reduces these systemic effects [7,30,31]. In the presented cohort of young athletes, the prevalence of signs of periodontitis was quite high (38%) in comparison to the overall population (1.7%) at this young age [32]. Moreover, this cohort of elite athletes showed a higher prevalence for signs of periodontitis than amateur athletes, despite similar oral health behavior [4]. Moderately elevated periodontal pockets (PSI score 3: none above 5.5 mm) were assessed. This low severity is in line with a previous study on periodontitis in footballers that reported overall mild periodontitis and a similar prevalence of periodontitis [5]. Even though the extent of systemic changes depends on the severity of periodontitis [28], increased CRP values have also been stated due to experimental gingivitis caused by cessation of oral hygiene [33]. Consequently, a systemic impact is possible, even for mild periodontitis and gingivitis. Regarding the gingival inflammation status in the present study, the PBI per papilla was below one (median: 0.42, IQR: 0.31;0.69), indicating mild or localized gingivitis.

Interestingly, the current study also revealed differences in the anthropometric data depending on periodontal status: individuals with probable signs of periodontitis showed higher BMI and BFP (Table 2). In contrast, another study could not reveal such differences between athletes, with and without periodontitis [5]. The values of BMI and BFP of the athletes were generally at a low level. For low BMI (18 to 22), a negative correlation between BMI and generalized aggressive periodontitis was already described [34] as well as in athletes, between BFP and periodontal probing depths [5]. In athletes with lower BMI and BFP, the phenomena of 'Relative Energy Deficiency in Sport' must be considered [35]. However, the results of the current study are inconclusive between the groups of gingival and periodontal inflammation: athletes with higher gingival inflammation showed lower BFP measured by skin folds (Table 2).

Some blood parameters showed significant differences: basophils, hematocrit, hemoglobin, ESR1, ESR2, urea, HDL cholesterol (by PBI), and uric acid (by PSI). The detected extensions were not of clinical relevance, as all investigated blood markers were within the reference ranges and the differences were small. As the direction of the group differences was inconsistent between the groups of gingival and periodontal inflammation and partly even in the same comparison (ESR1 and ESR 2), the significance of these differences is questionable in general. Nevertheless, the direction and extent of the revealed differences for uric acid, hemoglobin, and hematocrit would be in line with the results of a study in blood donors with increased probing depths compared to periodontally "healthy" ones [36]. In contrast to the stated difference in HDL cholesterol in the present study, experimental gingivitis did not lead to differences in cholesterol fractions [33].

Regarding the results of the performance tests, on the cycling ergometer, athletes with a lower level of signs of periodontal inflammation consistently reached higher power. Despite the small subgroup size, several trends for gingival inflammation became apparent and athletes with less gingival inflammation reached a significantly higher relative maximum power (Table 6). The revealed differences are relevant, especially as the subgroup is a homogeneous elite group from one sport discipline. Furthermore, in general, athletes with signs of periodontitis achieved lower VO_{2max} values (Table 2). These results are in line with the stated negative influence of periodontitis on physical fitness in other population cohorts [9]. Athletes with higher oral inflammation could be compromised in their performance due to a systemic effect. In contrast, no impact of caries on the anaerobic capacity of athletes was found by another study [17]. However, this does not contradict a potential influence of oral inflammation as superficial caries generally have less systemic impact. The possibility of such systemic influence of oral health in athletes is underlined by potential associations between poor oral health and injuries [5,37,38].

Strengths and limitations: This explorative study was, to the best of the author's knowledge, the first published on possible associations between signs of periodontal inflammation and systemic parameters in competitive athletes. Including data from 85 athletes from the German national elite, perspective, or youth squads, allowed us to evaluate a considerable cohort. The limitation in athletes between 18 and 30 years indicates to include the typical age of elite athletes. With the resulting medium age of 21 years, this study presents the stage of young elite athletes. Moreover, a detailed description of the oral health status and oral health behavior of this cohort of elite athletes is available [4]. A major strength of the current study is the comprehensive number of available parameters, including blood parameters, echocardiographic parameters, as well as performance parameters. One limitation of the present study is the multiple statistical testing. Nevertheless, due to the explorative character, data were not adjusted [39]. Therefore, all statistical differences should be interpreted with caution. Overall, this applies to the performance and echocardiographic examinations, as only small subgroups could be analyzed. In addition, a potential selection bias must be considered, because it cannot be excluded that athletes with more severe signs of periodontal inflammation were more strongly affected and could not fulfill the squad levels for inclusion. In addition, the methods for the assessment of signs of periodontal inflammation must be discussed. The evaluated data originate from oral examinations that were part of the annual sports medical diagnostics and aimed to detect treatment need. Regarding the PSI, it must be considered that this screening index only indicates gingival inflammation and/or increased probing depths as a sign of probable periodontitis [23] and could also be caused by local swelling due to gingivitis. However, the stated prevalence of signs of periodontitis (38%) complies with the prevalence of a study with comprehensive periodontal examination, according to the current classification (41%, initial periodontitis, stage I, in all but two athletes) [5]. The current classification of periodontal disease (staging/grading matrix) [40] allows for the correct diagnosis with periodontitis. Nevertheless, these diagnoses are mainly based on attachment loss and may be in a stable status without inflammation [40]. The question of current periodontal inflammation and stability depends on periodontal probing depths and bleeding on probing (BOP) [40] but the BOP is not integrated in the basis diagnosis (stage/grade) of periodontitis. For the precise identification to periodontitis and/or periodontal inflammation, a complete periodontal chart (periodontal probing depths, clinical attachment loss for stage, and grade as well as BOP) would be necessary. The concept of the periodontal inflammation surface area (PISA) [41] could quantify the resulting inflammatory burden. These data were not available in the present study. This should be taken into account for interpretation of the presented data and for future studies. Nevertheless, despite not exactly identifying the diagnosis of periodontitis, the PSI identifies elevated periodontal probing depths in the case of full mouth and all-around-the-tooth examination [42]. Thus, it can detect current signs of periodontal inflammation (= inflammatory burden) and periodontal treatment need (PSI Score $\geq$ 3). Regarding the periodontal attachment loss, under- and, in young age groups, overestimation by the PSI have been discussed [43]. For gingival inflammation, such strict group definition (health vs. presence of inflammation) was not possible, as all athletes showed bleeding as a sign of gingivitis or periodontitis (no PSI score 0) [4]. The performed PBI is a gingivitis index that evaluates the gingival inflammation by the intensity of bleeding on probing at the interdental sites [23]. Generally, gingival inflammation as well as signs of periodontitis were only mild or localized. Due to the resulting small inflammation (PBI: median: 0.42, IQR: 0.31;0.69; PSI $\geq$ 3 in 38%, localized in 34% of them), the group size could still be too small for detecting these slight systemic effects. Further limitations must be addressed regarding the compared subgroups. The group differences of gingival inflammation (PBI < 0.42 vs. PBI ≥ 0.42) were small and might have limited the ability to assess the differences in the systemic effects. As, in addition to PSI score 1 to 2, score 3 could indicate the status of gingivitis due to localized swelling, the group division by PSI might not distinguish clearly enough between those athletes with and those without periodontal inflammation. A larger sample size as well as comprehensive periodontal examination might improve the identification of the small, but potentially important, systemic effects for both initial periodontitis and gingival inflammation. In addition, cohorts with more severe periodontal inflammation or experimental gingivitis are further interesting research possibilities. The blood parameters investigated in this study were those from routine medical tests due to the retrospective nature of the project. Thus, the available blood parameters are an unspecific part of the routine diagnostics. Even though, for periodontitis patients, some studies could reveal such differences [26,28,29], these parameters are probably not sensitive enough for such localized, mild inflammatory group differences. Furthermore, VO_{2max} was determined by spiroergometry in only less than half of the participants. The used formula for VO_{2max} in the others is based on age, body mass, and RHR. Nevertheless, it can be considered an appropriate estimation in case of missing exercise tests [22].

5. Conclusions

The present study supports the hypothesis for an influence of oral inflammation in athletes; body composition, blood, and performance test parameters differed slightly between athletes with different levels of signs of periodontal inflammation. A potential systemic impact of oral inflammation on athletic performance should be investigated.

This explorative study identifies some aspects for future research; prospective studies during a uniform exercise test with spiroergometry of all participants should be carried out. Blood analysis should include more sensitive inflammatory parameters, such as CRP and interleukins. As a marker for the oral status, the PISA and salivary biomarkers would be recommendable. A cohort with a higher level of inflammation burden could simplify the discrimination. Similarly, a larger sample size, based on an appropriate power calculation with consideration for the variability in outcome measures, will be important. Furthermore, an intervention study could prove the connection by showing the systemic effect of periodontal treatment in athletes.

Supplementary Materials: The following supporting information can be downloaded at: https://www.mdpi.com/article/10.3390/jcm11175161/s1, Table S1: Multivariate linear regression analysis of the influence of some blood parameters on gingival inflammation (PBI); Table S2: Echocardiographic parameters and their associations with periodontal health (PBI and PSI).

Author Contributions: Conceptualization, D.Z., J.W., G.S., R.H., B.W. and C.L.M.; methodology, G.S., D.Z., J.W. and C.L.M.; formal analysis, P.R. and C.L.M.; investigation, L.R. and J.W.; resources, R.H., B.W., D.Z. and J.W.; data curation, L.R. and C.L.M.; writing—original draft preparation, C.L.M.; writing—review and editing, G.S., D.Z., J.W., I.N., R.H. and N.C.; visualization, C.L.M.; supervision, D.Z. and J.W.; project administration, C.L.M. and D.Z. All authors have read and agreed to the published version of the manuscript.

Funding: This publication was supported by Open Access Publishing Fund of the University of Regensburg.

Institutional Review Board Statement: The study was conducted according to the guidelines of the Declaration of Helsinki and approved by the ethics committee of the medical faculty of Leipzig University, Germany (No. 091/20-ek, 26 May 2020).

Informed Consent Statement: Informed consent was obtained from all subjects involved in the study.

Data Availability Statement: The data supporting this study's findings are available from the corresponding author upon reasonable request.

Conflicts of Interest: The authors declare no conflict of interest.

References

1. Ashley, P.; Di Iorio, A.; Cole, E.; Tanday, A.; Needleman, I. Oral health of elite athletes and association with performance: A systematic review. *Br. J. Sports Med.* **2015**, *49*, 14–19. [CrossRef] [PubMed]
2. Merle, C.L.; Rott, T.; Challakh, N.; Schmalz, G.; Kottmann, T.; Kastner, T.; Blume, K.; Wolfarth, B.; Haak, R.; Ziebolz, D.; et al. Clinical findings and self-reported oral health status of biathletes and cross-country skiers in the preseason—A cohort study with a control group. *Res. Sports Med.* **2022**, 1–15. [CrossRef] [PubMed]
3. Minty, M.; Canceill, T.; Lê, S.; Dubois, P.; Amestoy, O.; Loubieres, P.; Christensen, J.E.; Champion, C.; Azalbert, V.; Grasset, E.; et al. Oral health and microbiota status in professional rugby players: A case-control study. *J. Dent.* **2018**, *79*, 53–60. [CrossRef]
4. Merle, C.L.; Richter, L.; Challakh, N.; Haak, R.; Schmalz, G.; Needleman, I.; Wolfarth, B.; Ziebolz, D.; Wüstenfeld, J. Orofacial conditions and oral health behavior of young athletes—A comparison of amateur and competitive sports. *Scand. Med. Sci. Sports* **2022**, *32*, 903–912. [CrossRef]
5. Botelho, J.; Vicente, F.; Dias, L.; Júdice, A.; Pereira, P.; Proença, L.; Machado, V.; Chambrone, L.; Mendes, J.J. Periodontal Health, Nutrition and Anthropometry in Professional Footballers: A Preliminary Study. *Nutrients* **2021**, *13*, 1792. [CrossRef]
6. Linden, G.J.; Lyons, A.; Scannapieco, F.A. Periodontal systemic associations: Review of the evidence. *J. Clin. Periodontol.* **2013**, *40* (Suppl. S14), S8–S19. [CrossRef] [PubMed]
7. Orlandi, M.; Muñoz Aguilera, E.; Marletta, D.; Petrie, A.; Suvan, J.; D'Aiuto, F. Impact of the treatment of periodontitis on systemic health and quality of life: A systematic review. *J. Clin. Periodontol.* **2021**, *49*, 314–327. [CrossRef] [PubMed]
8. Loos, B.G. Systemic Markers of Inflammation in Periodontitis. *J. Periodontol.* **2005**, *76*, 2106–2115. [CrossRef]
9. Bramantoro, T.; Hariyani, N.; Setyowati, D.; Purwanto, B.; Zulfiana, A.A.; Irmalia, W.R. The impact of oral health on physical fitness: A systematic review. *Heliyon* **2020**, *6*, e03774. [CrossRef]
10. Scherr, J.; Braun, S.; Schuster, T.; Hartmann, C.; Moehlenkamp, S.; Wolfarth, B.; Pressler, A.; Halle, M. 72-h kinetics of high-sensitive troponin T and inflammatory markers after marathon. *Med. Sci. Sports Exerc.* **2011**, *43*, 1819–1827. [CrossRef]
11. Pedersen, B.K.; Steensberg, A.; Fischer, C.; Keller, C.; Ostrowski, K.; Schjerling, P. Exercise and cytokines with particular focus on muscle-derived IL-6. *Exerc. Immunol. Rev.* **2001**, *7*, 18–31.
12. Nieman, D.C.; Ahle, J.C.; Henson, D.A.; Warren, B.J.; Suttles, J.; Davis, J.M.; Buckley, K.S.; Simandle, S.; Butterworth, D.E.; Fagoaga, O.R. Indomethacin does not alter natural killer cell response to 2.5 h of running. *J. Appl. Physiol.* **1995**, *79*, 748–755. [CrossRef]
13. Fahlman, M.M.; Engels, H.J.; Hall, H. SIgA and Upper Respiratory Syndrome During a College Cross Country Season. *Sports Med. Int. Open* **2017**, *1*, E188–E194. [CrossRef] [PubMed]
14. Walsh, N.P.; Gleeson, M.; Shephard, R.J.; Gleeson, M.; Woods, J.A.; Bishop, N.C.; Fleshner, M.; Green, C.; Pedersen, B.K.; Hoffman-Goetz, L.; et al. Position statement. Part one: Immune function and exercise. *Exerc. Immunol. Rev.* **2011**, *17*, 6–63.
15. Greenham, G.; Buckley, J.D.; Garrett, J.; Eston, R.; Norton, K. Biomarkers of Physiological Responses to Periods of Intensified, Non-Resistance-Based Exercise Training in Well-Trained Male Athletes: A Systematic Review and Meta-Analysis. *Sports Med.* **2018**, *48*, 2517–2548. [CrossRef] [PubMed]
16. Svendsen, I.S.; Gleeson, M.; Haugen, T.A.; Tønnessen, E. Effect of an intense period of competition on race performance and self-reported illness in elite cross-country skiers. *Scand. J. Med. Sci. Sports* **2015**, *25*, 846–853. [CrossRef]
17. Hamamcilar, O.; Kocahan, T.; Akınoğlu, B.; Hasanoğlu, A. Effect of dental caries and the consequential variation in blood parameters on the anaerobic performance of rowing athletes. *Med. J. Islamic World Acad. Sci.* **2019**, *27*, 55–60. [CrossRef]
18. Gallagher, J.; Ashley, P.; Petrie, A.; Needleman, I. Oral health and performance impacts in elite and professional athletes. *Community Dent. Oral Epidemiol.* **2018**, *46*, 563–568. [CrossRef]
19. Needleman, I.; Ashley, P.; Petrie, A.; Fortune, F.; Turner, W.; Jones, J.; Niggli, J.; Engebretsen, L.; Budgett, R.; Donos, N.; et al. Oral health and impact on performance of athletes participating in the London 2012 Olympic Games: A cross-sectional study. *Br. J. Sports Med.* **2013**, *47*, 1054–1058. [CrossRef]
20. Von Elm, E.; Altman, D.G.; Egger, M.; Pocock, S.J.; Gøtzsche, P.C.; Vandenbroucke, J.P. The Strengthening the Reporting of Observational Studies in Epidemiology (STROBE) statement: Guidelines for reporting observational studies. *J. Clin. Epidemiol.* **2008**, *61*, 344–349. [CrossRef]
21. Keul, J.; Dickhuth, H.H.; Lehmann, M.; Staiger, J. The athlete's heart–haemodynamics and structure. *Int. J. Sports Med.* **1982**, *3* (Suppl. S1), 33–43. [CrossRef] [PubMed]
22. Rexhepi, A.M.; Brestovci, B. Prediction of vo2max based on age, body mass, and resting heart rate. *Hum. Mov.* **2014**, *15*, 56–59. [CrossRef]
23. Lange, D.E.; Plagmann, H.C.; Eenboom, A.; Promesberger, A. Clinical methods for the objective evaluation of oral hygiene. *Dtsch. Zahnarztl. Z* **1977**, *32*, 44–47. (In German) [PubMed]
24. Landry, R.G.; Jean, M. Periodontal Screening and Recording (PSR) Index: Precursors, utility and limitations in a clinical setting. *Int. Dent. J.* **2002**, *52*, 35–40. [CrossRef]
25. Loos, B.G.; Craandijk, J.; Hoek, F.J.; Wertheim-van Dillen, P.M.; van der Velden, U. Elevation of systemic markers related to cardiovascular diseases in the peripheral blood of periodontitis patients. *J. Periodontol.* **2000**, *71*, 1528–1534. [CrossRef]
26. Machado, V.; Botelho, J.; Escalda, C.; Hussain, S.B.; Luthra, S.; Mascarenhas, P.; Orlandi, M.; Mendes, J.J.; D'Aiuto, F. Serum C-Reactive Protein and Periodontitis: A Systematic Review and Meta-Analysis. *Front. Immunol.* **2021**, *12*, 706432. [CrossRef]

27. Finoti, L.S.; Nepomuceno, R.; Pigossi, S.C.; Corbi, S.C.; Secolin, R.; Scarel-Caminaga, R.M. Association between interleukin-8 levels and chronic periodontal disease: A PRISMA-compliant systematic review and meta-analysis. *Medicine* **2017**, *96*, e6932. [CrossRef] [PubMed]
28. Torrungruang, K.; Ongphiphadhanakul, B.; Jitpakdeebordin, S.; Sarujikumjornwatana, S. Mediation analysis of systemic inflammation on the association between periodontitis and glycaemic status. *J. Clin. Periodontol.* **2018**, *45*, 548–556. [CrossRef] [PubMed]
29. Botelho, J.; Machado, V.; Hussain, S.B.; Zehra, S.A.; Proença, L.; Orlandi, M.; Mendes, J.J.; D'Aiuto, F. Periodontitis and circulating blood cell profiles: A systematic review and meta-analysis. *Exp. Hematol.* **2021**, *93*, 1–13. [CrossRef]
30. Koidou, V.P.; Cavalli, N.; Hagi-Pavli, E.; Nibali, L.; Donos, N. Expression of inflammatory biomarkers and growth factors in gingival crevicular fluid at different healing intervals following non-surgical periodontal treatment: A systematic review. *J. Periodontal Res.* **2020**, *55*, 801–809. [CrossRef]
31. Simpson, T.C.; Clarkson, J.E.; Worthington, H.V.; MacDonald, L.; Weldon, J.C.; Needleman, I.; Iheozor-Ejiofor, Z.; Wild, S.H.; Qureshi, A.; Walker, A.; et al. Treatment of periodontitis for glycaemic control in people with diabetes mellitus. *Cochrane Database Syst. Rev.* **2022**, *4*, CD004714. [CrossRef] [PubMed]
32. Catunda, R.Q.; Levin, L.; Kornerup, I.; Gibson, M.P. Prevalence of Periodontitis in Young Populations: A Systematic Review. *Oral Health Prev. Dent.* **2019**, *17*, 195–202. [CrossRef] [PubMed]
33. Eberhard, J.; Grote, K.; Luchtefeld, M.; Heuer, W.; Schuett, H.; Divchev, D.; Scherer, R.; Schmitz-Streit, R.; Langfeldt, D.; Stumpp, N.; et al. Experimental gingivitis induces systemic inflammatory markers in young healthy individuals: A single-subject interventional study. *PLoS ONE* **2013**, *8*, e55265. [CrossRef]
34. Li, W.; Shi, D.; Song, W.; Xu, L.; Zhang, L.; Feng, X.; Lu, R.; Wang, X.; Meng, H. A novel U-shaped relationship between BMI and risk of generalized aggressive periodontitis in Chinese: A cross-sectional study. *J. Periodontol.* **2019**, *90*, 82–89. [CrossRef] [PubMed]
35. Mountjoy, M.; Sundgot-Borgen, J.; Burke, L.; Carter, S.; Constantini, N.; Lebrun, C.; Meyer, N.; Sherman, R.; Steffen, K.; Budgett, R.; et al. The IOC consensus statement: Beyond the Female Athlete Triad–Relative Energy Deficiency in Sport (RED-S). *Br. J. Sports Med.* **2014**, *48*, 491–497. [CrossRef]
36. Ziebolz, D.; Jäger, G.C.; Hornecker, E.; Mausberg, R.F. Periodontal findings and blood analysis of blood donors: A pilot study. *J. Contemp. Dent. Pract.* **2007**, *8*, 43–50. [PubMed]
37. Solleveld, H.; Goedhart, A.; Vanden Bossche, L. Associations between poor oral health and reinjuries in male elite soccer players: A cross-sectional self-report study. *BMC Sports Sci. Med. Rehabil.* **2015**, *7*, 11. [CrossRef]
38. Gay-Escoda, C.; Vieira-Duarte-Pereira, D.-M.; Ardèvol, J.; Pruna, R.; Fernandez, J.; Valmaseda-Castellón, E. Study of the effect of oral health on physical condition of professional soccer players of the Football Club Barcelona. *Med. Oral Patol. Oral Cir. Bucal.* **2011**, *16*, 436–439. [CrossRef] [PubMed]
39. Rothman, K.J. No adjustments are needed for multiple comparisons. *Epidemiology* **1990**, *1*, 43–46. [CrossRef]
40. Chapple, I.L.C.; Mealey, B.L.; van Dyke, T.E.; Bartold, P.M.; Dommisch, H.; Eickholz, P.; Geisinger, M.L.; Genco, R.J.; Glogauer, M.; Goldstein, M.; et al. Periodontal health and gingival diseases and conditions on an intact and a reduced periodontium: Consensus report of workgroup 1 of the 2017 World Workshop on the Classification of Periodontal and Peri-Implant Diseases and Conditions. *J. Clin. Periodontol.* **2018**, *45* (Suppl. S20), S68–S77. [CrossRef]
41. Nesse, W.; Abbas, F.; van der Ploeg, I.; Spijkervet, F.K.L.; Dijkstra, P.U.; Vissink, A. Periodontal inflamed surface area: Quantifying inflammatory burden. *J. Clin. Periodontol.* **2008**, *35*, 668–673. [CrossRef] [PubMed]
42. Benigeri, M.; Brodeur, J.M.; Payette, M.; Charbonneau, A.; Ismaïl, A.I. Community periodontal index of treatment needs and prevalence of periodontal conditions. *J. Clin. Periodontol.* **2000**, *27*, 308–312. [CrossRef] [PubMed]
43. Baelum, V.; Manji, F.; Wanzala, P.; Fejerskov, O. Relationship between CPITN and periodontal attachment loss findings in an adult population. *J. Clin. Periodontol.* **1995**, *22*, 146–152. [CrossRef] [PubMed]

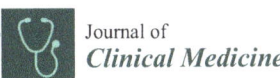

Article

Predictive Modeling of Injury Risk Based on Body Composition and Selected Physical Fitness Tests for Elite Football Players

Francisco Martins [1,2], **Krzysztof Przednowek** [3], **Cíntia França** [1,2], **Helder Lopes** [1], **Marcelo de Maio Nascimento** [4], **Hugo Sarmento** [5], **Adilson Marques** [6,7], **Andreas Ihle** [8,9,10], **Ricardo Henriques** [11] and **Élvio Rúbio Gouveia** [1,2,9,*]

1. Department of Physical Education and Sport, University of Madeira, 9020-105 Funchal, Portugal
2. Laboratory of Robotics and Engineering Systems, Interactive Technologies Institute, 9020-105 Funchal, Portugal
3. Institute of Physical Culture Sciences, Medical College, University of Rzeszów, 35-959 Rzeszów, Poland
4. Department of Physical Education, Federal University of Vale do São Francisco, Petrolina 56304-917, Brazil
5. University of Coimbra, Research Unit for Sport and Physical Activity (CIDAF), Faculty of Sport Sciences and Physical Education, 3004-504 Coimbra, Portugal
6. CIPER, Faculty of Human Kinetics, University of Lisbon, 1495-751 Lisbon, Portugal
7. ISAMB, Faculty of Medicine, University of Lisbon, 1649-020 Lisbon, Portugal
8. Department of Psychology, University of Geneva, 1205 Geneva, Switzerland
9. Center for the Interdisciplinary Study of Gerontology and Vulnerability, University of Geneva, 1205 Geneva, Switzerland
10. Swiss National Centre of Competence in Research LIVES—Overcoming Vulnerability: Life Course Perspectives, 1015 Lausanne, Switzerland
11. Marítimo da Madeira—Futebol, SAD, 9020-208 Funchal, Portugal
* Correspondence: erubiog@staff.uma.pt

Abstract: Injuries are one of the most significant issues for elite football players. Consequently, elite football clubs have been consistently interested in having practical, interpretable, and usable models as decision-making support for technical staff. This study aimed to analyze predictive modeling of injury risk based on body composition variables and selected physical fitness tests for elite football players through a sports season. The sample comprised 36 male elite football players who competed in the First Portuguese Soccer League in the 2020/2021 season. The models were calculated based on 22 independent variables that included players' information, body composition, physical fitness, and one dependent variable, the number of injuries per season. In the net elastic analysis, the variables that best predicted injury risk were sectorial positions (defensive and forward), body height, sit-and-reach performance, 1 min number of push-ups, handgrip strength, and 35 m linear speed. This study considered multiple-input single-output regression-type models. The analysis showed that the most accurate model presented in this work generates an error of RMSE = 0.591. Our approach opens a novel perspective for injury prevention and training monitorization. Nevertheless, more studies are needed to identify risk factors associated with injury prediction in elite soccer players, as this is a rising topic that requires several analyses performed in different contexts.

Keywords: sports injuries; machine learning; injury prediction; sports monitorization; elite football

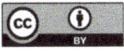

1. Introduction

Injuries are one of the most significant hampering issues for elite football players [1]. Football is known for its fast-paced and powerful actions [2,3], which might contribute to players' increased risk of injuries [4]. Due to their effects on individuals' mental states and overall teams' performances, elite players' injuries significantly impact the sports business [5,6]. Consequently, elite football clubs have been consistently interested in having practical, interpretable, and usable models as decision-making support for coaches and their technical staff members [7].

From the clinical standpoint, the literature describes the lower limbs as the most affected body zone by sports injuries [4,8–14], particularly for muscle injuries in the thigh area, the quadriceps, and the groin [4,10,15,16]. Since injuries in professional soccer are an increasingly problem, it is crucial that the work done in training sessions reflects the demands of competition, aiming at the development of athletes' performance, which includes injury prevention [17–19].

Machine learning or statistical learning methods are currently tools that can significantly support decision-making in various aspects of the training process. For instance, it has been reported in the literature that some models can optimize training loads [20], which reinforces the applicability of machine learning in improving injury prediction [21,22].

Researchers, managers, and coaches are becoming increasingly involved in injury forecasting, using regular data collection that will allow them to act consciously and intervene on time on this global issue [23]. An investigation conducted over 18 years showed that the total injury rate in practice and competition has dropped during the past years [24]. Although the cause leading to this decrease is still unknown, one potential explanation for this decrease may be related to the effectiveness of injury prevention. If so, it is likely that the motivation of the medical staff at elite football teams is increasing, in terms of implementing and overseeing preventive injury programs [24].

Machine learning offers a modern statistical method that uses algorithms mainly created to deal with unbalanced data sets and enable the modeling of interactions between a large number of variables [25]. In the football context, machine learning has been used in injury prediction, physical performance prediction, training load and monitoring, players' career trajectories, clubs' performance, and match attendance [26].

There has been some research done on elite-football-injury prediction up to this point [23,25,27–31]. In 2019, 96 male elite football players participated in a study throughout a season, with hamstring-strain injuries being the primary anticipated consequence. In that study, the prediction model showed moderate to high accuracy for identifying players at risk of hamstring-strain injuries during pre-season testing [31]. Another example involved 26 elite football players participating in year-long research to forecast non-contact injuries. The authors reported that machine learning was far more accurate than baselines and modern injury-risk-estimating approaches, detecting roughly 80% of injuries with about 50% accuracy [23]. In another study conducted with 132 male elite football and handball players, the prediction model accurately identified elite players at risk of developing muscular injuries [25].

Two types of variables are highlighted in the previous research on predictive modeling of injury risk [30]. The first block of predictor variables is modifiable variables, i.e., training loads or physiological and physical fitness tests. The second type is non-modifiable variables, including demographic variables, anthropometric parameters, and injury histories. Indeed, body composition and physical fitness tests are the most commonly assessed by sports staff given their close relationship with game performance and players' health. Moreover, evaluating and monitoring players' characteristics during the season provides valuable information to understand better players' behavioral changes and support coaches' decision-making in the training and match process. In the sports injury literature, most of the investigation conducted aimed to assess one specific variable at a time to predict injury risk. However, this approach limits the correlation of injury risk and a global interpretation of players' performance in professional football [23]. Therefore, this study aimed to analyze predictive modeling of injury risk based on body composition variables and selected physical fitness tests for elite football players across a sports season.

2. Materials and Methods

2.1. Participants

Thirty-six players from a professional football team participated in this study. This team competed in the First Portuguese League during the 2020/2021 season.

A description of the variables together with the basic statistics (M—mean value, SD—standard deviation) is given in Table 1. The models were calculated based on 22 independent variables (x_1–x_{22}) and one dependent variable (y). Independent variables include players' information (sectorial position, age, experience, and number of previous injuries), anthropometric parameters with body composition, and components of physical fitness (flexibility, general strength, explosive strength, speed, agility, and aerobic endurance). The dependent variable is the number of injuries per season. The predictive analysis did not use the data of all athletes. Twenty-four players' data were used. This was due to the fact that some of the athletes were noted to have missing data related to not taking certain physical fitness tests.

Table 1. Description of the variables used to construct the predictive model (N = 24).

Variable	Description	M	sd
x_1–x_3	Sectorial Position *	-	-
x_4	Age (y)	25.45	3.34
x_5	Experience (y)	7.29	3.38
x_6	Body mass (kg)	80.09	7.07
x_7	Height (cm)	182.52	6.01
x_8	TBW (L)	51.93	4.66
x_9	BFM (kg)	8.2	2.41
x_{10}	FFM (kg)	71.2	6.50
x_{11}	Previous injury (n)	1.29	1.63
x_{12}	Sit and reach (cm)	34.52	6.79
x_{13}	Push-ups (n)	43.63	8.68
x_{14}	Handgrip right (kg)	50.87	9.62
x_{15}	Handgrip left (kg)	48.92	8.67
x_{16}	CMJ height (cm)	40.14	4.58
x_{17}	SJ height (cm)	39.64	4.26
x_{18}	LS 5 m (s)	1.16	0.13
x_{19}	LS 10 m (s)	1.88	0.16
x_{20}	LS 35 m (s)	4.85	0.27
x_{21}	Estimated VO2 max (L/kg/min)	50.82	3.98
x_{22}	Yoyo (m)	1720	476
y	Injury frequency (n)	0.79	0.72

*—qualitative variable, M (mean value), sd (standard deviation), Me (median), TBW (total body water), BFM (body fat mass), FFM (fat free mass), CMJ (countermovement jump), SJ (squat jump), LS (linear speed), y (years), kg (kilograms), cm (centimeters), L (liters), n (number), s (speed), min (minutes), m (meters).

All procedures applied were approved by the Ethics Committee of the Faculty of Human Kinetics, CEIFMH No. 34/2021. The investigation was conducted following the Declaration of Helsinki, and informed consent was obtained from all participants.

2.2. Body-Composition Assessment

Body-composition variables were assessed using hand-to-foot bioelectrical impedance analysis (InBody 770, Cerritos, CA, USA). Height was measured to the nearest 0.1 cm using a stadiometer (SECA 213, Hamburg, Germany). The measurements occurred in the early morning, with participants fasting and wearing only their underwear. During the assessment, participants were barefoot, standing with both arms 45° apart from the trunk, with both feet bare on the spots of the platform. A total of 26 evaluations of body composition were considered during the season. Body mass, total body water (TBW), body fat mass (BFM), and fat-free mass (FFM) were retained for analysis.

2.3. Physical Fitness Assessment

The sit-and-reach bilateral test was used to evaluate flexibility measurement. A box (32.4 cm high and 53.3 cm long) with a 23 cm heel line mark was used. The participants sat barefoot in front of the box, with both knees fully extended and heels against the box. The research team held one hand lightly against each participant's knees to ensure complete leg extension. Then, participants placed their hands on top of each other, palms down, and slowly bent forward along the measuring scale. The forward-hold position was repeated twice. The third and final forward stretch was held for three seconds, and the score was recorded to the nearest 0.1 cm.

The push-ups test protocol consisted in performing the highest number of push-ups in one minute, respecting the success criteria judged by the evaluator. The participants started the test in the down position to get correct hand placement and then assumed the up position, from which they did the maximum number of push-ups possible. No cadence was used, although participants were encouraged to execute push-ups with good form but fast enough to obtain the best possible score in a minute. The evaluator independently counted the number of push-ups correctly executed.

The handgrip protocol consisted of three alternated data collection trials for each arm, performed using a hand dynamometer (Jamar Plus+, Chicago, IL, USA). Participants were instructed to hold a dynamometer in one hand, laterally to the trunk with the elbow at a 90° position [32]. From this position, participants were instructed to squeeze as hard as possible, progressively and continuously squeezing the hand dynamometer for about two seconds. The dynamometer could not contact the participant's body; otherwise, the trial was repeated. The best score of the three trials was retained for analysis.

The countermovement jump (CMJ) and the squat jump (SJ) were used to assess lower-body explosive strength [33]. Both protocols included four data collection trials and were performed using the Optojump Next (Microgate, Bolzano, Italy) system of analysis and measurement. In both tests, participants were encouraged to jump to their maximum height. Before data collection, three experimental trials were performed by each participant to ensure correct execution. For the CMJ, participants began in a tall standing position, with feet placed hip-width to shoulder-width apart. Then, participants dropped into the countermovement position to a self-selected depth, followed by a maximal-effort vertical jump. Hands remained on the hips for the entire movement to eliminate any influence of arm swing. If the hands were removed from the hips at any point, or excessive knee flexion was exhibited during the countermovement, the trial was repeated. The participants reset to the starting position after each jump. The SJ protocol testing began with the participant in a squat position at a self-selected depth of approximately 90° of knee flexion, holding this position for the researchers' count of three before jumping. If a dipping movement of the hips was evident, then the trial was repeated. The participants reset to the starting position after each jump.

Linear speed was assessed with maximal sprints at 5, 10, and 35 m, starting from a stationary position. Sprint time was recorded using Witty-Gate photocells (Microgate, Bolzano, Italy). Participants were allowed two trials for each sprinting distance, and the best time was used for analysis.

A yoyo intermittent recovery test was applied to evaluate the athlete's maximum oxygen uptake under repeated high-intensity aerobic exercise [34,35]. The test consists of a 2 × 20 m shuttle run at increasing speeds, interspersed with 10 s of active recovery, controlled by audio signals. The test terminated when the subject was no longer able to maintain the required speed. The total distance and VO2 maximum record were used as results [36]. The results used were based on the athletes' performance in the yoyo test, which is an indirect method of measuring such variables.

All tests were performed on the same day within a 4 h period in the morning (8 a.m.–12 p.m.). They were conducted by trained staff from the research team, who were familiar with each protocol. All protocols were followed with the utmost rigor, and the organization of the sequence of physical tests was designed to reduce the fatigue factor throughout all tests.

2.4. Injury Report

This study followed the Union of European Football Association (UEFA)'s recommendations for epidemiological investigations. An injury was defined as an event during a scheduled training session or match, resulting in an absence from the next training session or match [37]. Regarding the variables under analysis, the type, zone, and specific location of the injury are complementary variables that identify the part of the body that suffered structural and/or functional changes. The mechanism of injury is intended to understand if the injury was traumatic or if it was contracted by overload. The severity of the injury considers the period, in days, from the athlete's stoppage until resuming field work with the consent of the clinical department. Finally, an injury was marked as recurrent when a player was injured in the same place and type where they were previously affected by an injury. Injury records during the season, including in training and competitive moments, were made daily by the clinical department.

2.5. Predictive Modeling

In this analysis, multiple-input single-output models for prediction were used. The output of the model is a continuous variable and represents the number of occurrences of potential injuries. Therefore, we consider regression-type models, not classifiers. Classic regression models (OLS), shrinkage regression, and stepwise regression were used in the models' calculations. All predictive models were calculated using R Software version 4.2.0 (R Foundation for Statistical Computing, Vienna, Austria, 2022). The implemented methods included:

- The ordinary least squares regression (OLS) used a popular least-squares method, in which weights are calculated by minimizing the sum of the squared errors.
- The Ridge model was calculated using the criterion of performance, which includes a penalty for increased weights. Parameter λ decides the size of the penalty: the greater the value of λ is, the bigger the penalty. The value of lambda can vary from 0 to infinity [38].
- Lasso regression is the model where the mechanism facilitates assigning a penalty to variables, and, in this way, they are eliminated from equations. In Lasso regression [39], the parameter s (penalty) is used to optimize the model.
- Elastic net (ENET) [40] combines the features of ridge and LASSO regressions. The performance criterion is the so-called naive elastic net. To minimize the criterion, the LARS-EN algorithm was suggested [40], which is based on the LARS algorithm for LASSO regression. In elastic net regression, we have two parameters, penalty s and λ.
- Stepwise Forward Regression has a forward selection procedure (FS), which begins with an equation that contains only a free expression. The first variable in the equation is the one that has the highest correlation with the output variable. If the coefficient of regression of the variable differs significantly from zero, the variable remains in the equation and another variable is added. The second variable introduced into the equation is the one that has the highest correlation with output, which has been adjusted for the effect of the first variable. If the regression coefficient is statistically significant (using F-test), adding the next variable is implemented in the same way [41,42].

The presented methods were used to calculate models from all variables (Table 1). Additionally, OLS, Ridge, LASSO, and elastic net models have been reimplemented for the best subset of input variables computed from stepwise regression. All models calculated in the study were tested by leave-one-out cross validation (LOOCV). In this method, the data set is divided into two subsets: learning and testing (validation). In LOOCV, the test set is composed of a selected pair of data (x_i, y_i), and the number of tests is equal to the number of data n. During the cross-validation, $RMSE_{CV}$ error was calculated:

$$RMSE_{CV} = \sqrt{\frac{1}{n} \sum_{i=1}^{n} (y_i - \hat{y}_{-i})^2}$$

where n—number of patterns, y_{-i}—the output value of the model built in the i-th step of cross-validation based on a data set containing no testing pair (x_i, y_i), $\hat{y}_i$—the output value of the model built in the i-th step based on the full data set, and $RMSE_{CV}$—root mean square error of prediction.

3. Results

Table 2 summarizes the data regarding the participants and injuries characterization of Club Sport Marítimo in the 2020/2021 season. Of the 36 players participating in the study, 23 contracted at least one injury over the 2020/2021 season. Injured players missed an average of 14.3 days per injury. There were 0.9 injuries contracted by the number of participants (34 injuries/36 players) over the study period. Most injuries were classified as traumatic (52.9%). About 50% of the injuries were, according to their severity, moderate, since the athletes missed between 8 and 28 days of training and/or competition. Finally, four of the injuries counted were classified as recurrent.

Table 2. Characterization of participants and injuries of CS Marítimo in the 2020/2021 season.

No. of Players	36
No. of Injured Players	23
Total Injuries	34
Average Days Missed Due to Injury	14.3
Injury per Player	0.9
Injury Mechanism	
Traumatic	18 (52.9%)
Overload	16 (47.1%)
Injury Severity *	
Minimal (1–3 days)	4 (11.7%)
Mild (4–7 days)	7 (20.5%)
Moderate	17 (50%)
Severe (+28 days)	6 (17.6%)
Injury Recurrence	
Yes	4 (11.8%)
No	30 (88.2%)

* Number of days missed by a player due to a sports injury contracted in training or match.

Figures 1–3 summarize the type, area, and specific location of injuries. The lower limbs were the body area most affected by injuries (85.2%). Sprains (35.2%) and muscle injuries (35.2%) were the most recurrent type of injuries throughout the study period, particularly in the ankles (29.4%), quadriceps (11.7%), and hamstrings (11.7%).

Table 3 presents the errors for each model and the sets of predictors calculated by the variable selection methods. The classical OLS regression model has the worst predictive ability, for which the error of RMSE = 18.57. Such a large error shows that the injury-prediction problem is complex and needs to be regularized by, among other things, using shrinkage regression. The use of shrinkage models (Ridge, LASSO, and elastic net) resulted in a sharp decrease in error and, thus, an improvement in the predictive ability of the model. The best model performing injury-prediction tasks for all predictors is the Ridge model, in which the RMSE error was 0.698. The optimal Ridge model was calculated for $\lambda = 82.2$. Optimizations of all shrinkage models are presented in Figure 4. The LASSO model for all predictors was not calculated because the algorithm does not work properly for such a configuration of the number of variables and patterns. Therefore, the following model used was the elastic net regression model. For elastic net regression, a very small prediction error was obtained (RMSE = 0.633), and the number of predictors was reduced due to the properties of this method. The result of the elastic net analysis was that the best set of input variables is the set of seven variables: x_1—sectorial position 1, x_3—sectorial position 3, x_7—body height, x_{12}—sit and reach, x_{13}—n push-ups, x_{15}—handgrip (l), and x_{20}—V35 m.

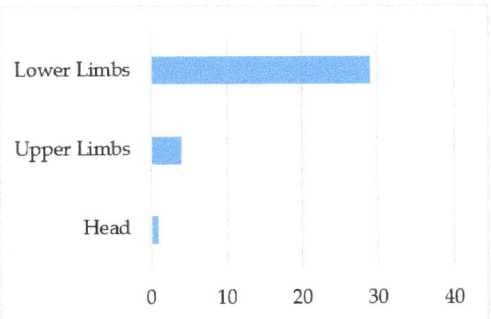

Figure 1. Injury frequency by zone (n).

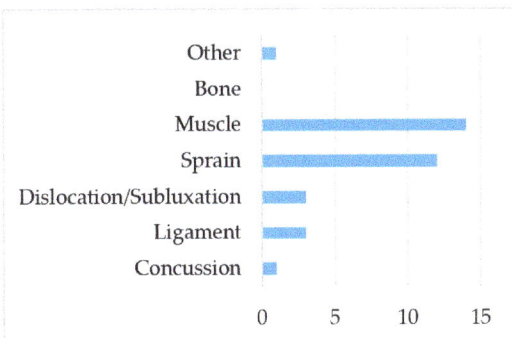

Figure 2. Injury frequency by type (n).

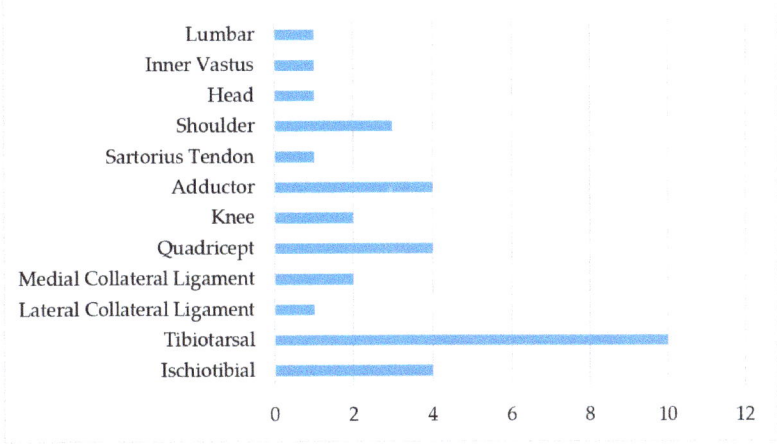

Figure 3. Injury frequency by specific location (n).

Table 3. Predictive errors for calculated models.

Method	Predictors	RMSECV	Parameter
OLS	$x_1, x_2, x_3, \ldots, x_{23}$	18.57	-
Ridge	$x_1, x_2, x_3, \ldots, x_{23}$	0.698	$\lambda = 82.2$
LASSO	$x_1, x_2, x_3, \ldots, x_{23}$	0.737	$s = 0$
Elastic net (EN)	$x_1, x_3, x_7, x_{12}, x_{13}, x_{15}, x_{20}$	0.633	$\lambda = 0.1, s = 0.22$
Forward (F)	$x_1, x_{12}, x_{13}, x_{15}$	0.618	-
Ridge (EN)	$x_1, x_3, x_7, x_{12}, x_{13}, x_{15}, x_{20}$	**0.592**	$\lambda = 17.5$
Ridge (F)	$x_1, x_{12}, x_{13}, x_{15}$	**0.591**	$\lambda = 7$
LASSO (EN)	$x_1, x_3, x_7, x_{12}, x_{13}, x_{15}, x_{20}$	0.635	$s = 0.55$
LASSO (F)	$x_1, x_{12}, x_{13}, x_{15}$	0.613	$s = 0.87$

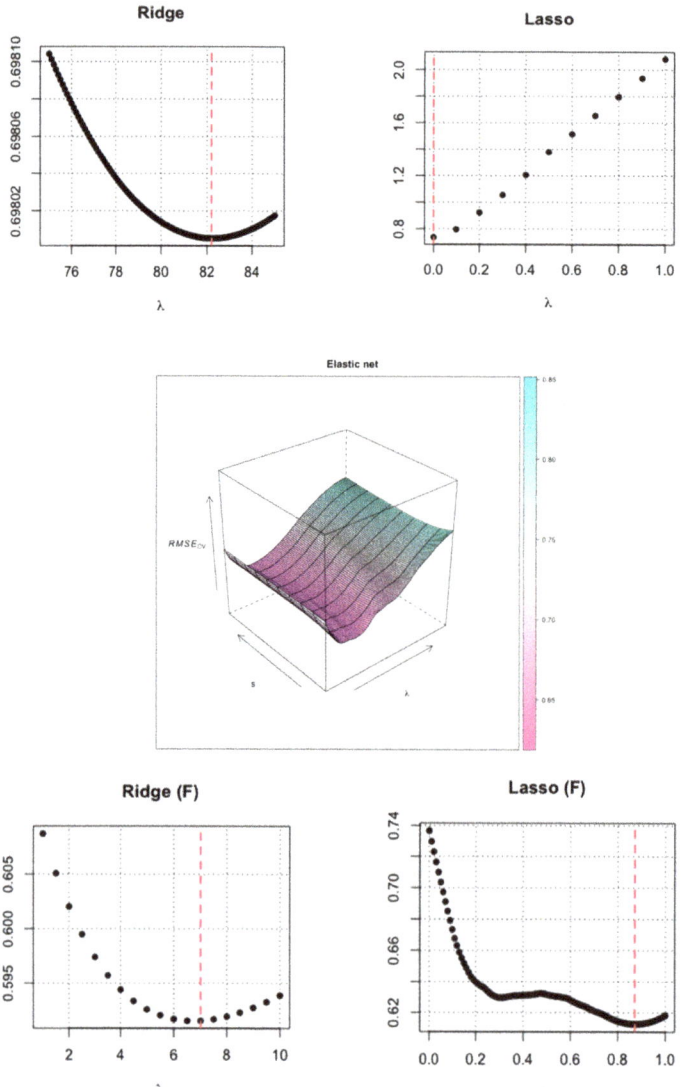

Figure 4. *Cont.*

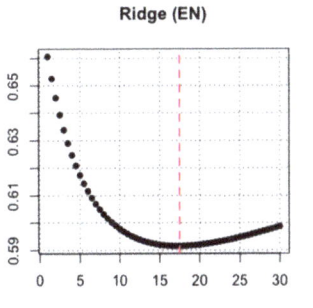
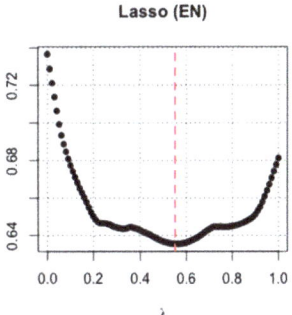

Figure 4. Optimization of predictive models (the red line indicates the optimal model).

The forward regression showed that the significant predictors are x_1 – sectorial position 1, x_{12}—sit and reach, x_{13}—n push-ups, and x_{15}—handgrip l). All the predictors determined by forward regression are contained in the set determined by elastic net regression. The model determined by forward regression generates an error of RMSE = 0.618. The predictors obtained using elastic net (E) and forward regression (F) were used in further predictive analysis. Both sets were used to recalculate the Ridge and LASSO models. The Ridge model with the set calculated by elastic net generates an error of RMSE = 0.592, and a very similar error was obtained for the Ridge model, with the set calculated by forward regression, with RMSE = 0.591. Both Ridge models with new sets of predictors show the best ability. LASSO models for enumerated sets of predictors showed worse predictive abilities than Ridge models. In the case of the best model, the model predicts the number of injury occurrences with an error of 0.59. This means that if a player has three injuries, the model would predict a value from the range of 2.41 to 3.59. The equations for the best models are presented in Table 4.

Table 4. Predictive errors for calculated models.

Method	Equation
Ridge (EN)	$y = 0.01 + 0.10 \oplus x_1 - 0.27 \oplus x_3 + 0.01 \oplus x_7 - 0.01 \oplus x_{12} - 0.01 \oplus x_{13} - 0.03 \oplus x_{15} - 0.45 \oplus x_{20}$
Ridge (F)	$y = -0.28 + 0.35 \oplus x_1 - 0.02 \oplus x_{12} \oplus -0.01 x_{13} + 0.04 \oplus x_{15}$

4. Discussion

This study aimed to analyze predictive modeling of injury risk based on players' sectorial position, body composition variables (i.e., weight, height, TBW, FAT, and FFM), and selected physical fitness tests, which include sit-and-reach, push-ups, handgrip, CMJ, SJ, 5 m, 10 m, 35 m, and yoyo tests.

This study considered multiple-input single-output regression-type models. It allowed us to select the best model to perform injury prediction tasks, considering all predictors. Previous work on predictive injury risk models is mostly based on classification learning models [31,43,44]. These models' predictive accuracy ranged from 75% to 82.9% [30]. The present study did not use a categorical variable but rather a continuous variable. A similar solution was presented in another work, where a continuous variable was also placed in the output [45]. A direct comparison of the models' predictive ability with those presented by other authors is complex because different quality criteria were used.

The value of cross-validation error is important, but a more critical element of the analysis presented was the identification of significant predictors of injury risk. An important part of the analysis was the variable-selection methods, resulting in a very clear and simplified model structure. The simple structure of the model and the linear nature of the methods made it possible to interpret the impact of individual variables on injury risk. Data-selection mechanisms were also used by other authors who have also used LASSO [44].

According to the data collected for this study, a professional football team can experience 0.9 injuries for every player on the field. This number is noticeably lower than that reported in a study following the analysis of three sports seasons, averaging 1.5 injuries per player [4]. In reality, training load and competitive load—both internal and external—are variables that are related to muscle injuries and that change depending on the situation and level of competition. In this study, sprains and muscular injuries were the most common types of injuries in the lower limbs. The quadriceps and hamstrings were the next most afflicted muscles, followed by the ankles. These results are consistent with the previous findings in the literature [10,12–14,16]. In reality, the lower limbs are under more pressure in this activity because of the tactical–technical maneuvers needed, which justifies their increased risk of damage. Overload injuries were more common than traumatic injuries. A recent investigation also established the existence of such prevalence [4]. In contrast, a different article discovered that overload was the cause of two out of every three injuries in their study [12]. Since there is a strong link between training load and the likelihood of injury, it is imperative to emphasize the significance of appropriately structuring the training cycles according to the players' attributes and physical condition. When individual training loads are measured using the right tools, this process happens more reliably and consistently. Coaches, players, and their technical-support personnel increasingly monitor and evaluate the sports load using a scientific method [46]. In reality, keeping an eye on the training process is essential for assessing the level of athlete weariness, which may help to lower the risk of injury. Soccer involves physical contact and high intensity. Therefore, injury-prevention procedures should take both overload and traumatic injuries into account. Each athlete missed 14.3 days of practice or competition after suffering an injury, on average. This finding differs from that seen in the literature, with players missing an average of seven to eight days owing to injury [4,8,12]. On the other hand, we draw the conclusion that more serious injuries result in a longer period of player absence. This demonstrates the necessity of strengthening all preventative and rehabilitation efforts, while taking into consideration the predictive variables of injury as well as more frequent medical checkups and physical testing. Some authors claim that muscle injuries in soccer are the most common [9,10], converging with our findings. The injury-recurrence rate in our study is consistent with the rates reported in the literature, which range from 8% to 22% [9,47,48]. According to earlier research, these percentage discrepancies may result from the resources available in the individual clinical departments as well as a particular club's infrastructure and material-resource capabilities to respond quickly, in order to maximize the injury prevention and healing process.

Regarding the impact of selected predictors included in the models, first of all, for sectorial position, the defensive and forward sectors were the ones that presented a higher risk of injury. A previous study conducted across three consecutive seasons with 123 Chilean elite male football players also reported that the defensive and forward sectors were the ones that contracted more injuries over the study period [4]. Among 71 Spanish elite male players, forwards were the ones who presented the highest rates in both incidence and severity of injury [14]. Indeed, the literature has described that certain positions, such as fullbacks and forwards, have more demanding tasks both in-game and during training sessions, such as covering greater distances and running with higher intensity than their peers. Overall, fullbacks and forwards perform a total of 29–35 sprints, which is higher than other positions (approx. 17–23 sprints) [49], which may justify their higher injury rates (i.e., hamstring injuries) [50,51]. Therefore, managing training loads appropriately following the physical demands of different sectors and playing positions might be a helpful method to lower the risk of injury in football [52]. Sports agents and coaches should consider load exposure according to players' position, particularly when designing training sessions [52]. Moreover, our results consolidate the need to consider the players' position as a variable to be included in the definition of injury-risk programs.

Another important predictor identified in our study was lower-limb flexibility. The sit-and-reach test is one of the physical fitness tests mostly used to predict the injury risk of elite football players across a sports season. In the literature, several studies have concluded that reduced flexibility in the lower limbs is related to the increased risk of injuries in elite football players [53–56]. Some studies report that it is essential to develop and introduce a standard battery assessment of flexibility in preseason tests, contributing to the awareness of the players' profile [56,57]. The newest Guidelines for Exercise Testing and Prescription from the American College of Sports Medicine reported that maintaining good flexibility in all joints depends on many specific variables, including distensibility of the joint capsule and muscle viscosity, which facilitates movement and may prevent injuries [58]. However, we must acknowledge some limitations on the topic. First, it is not entirely understood if pre-activity stretching unequivocally reduces injuries associated with training load. Secondly, the most recent guidelines recommend direct measures of range of motion (i.e., goniometer and inclinometer) rather than indirect methods, such as sit-and-reach tests assessing flexibility. This means that most of the indirect measures that we most often use in various sports context are coming into disuse. It is recommended that direct measures of range of motion should be used more regularly. In general, the important focus will be that future studies continue to investigate this topic, so we can draw more reliable and valid conclusions regarding the relationship between flexibility and sports injuries.

According to our analyses, the push-up, handgrip, and 35 m linear sprint tests may be reliable predictors of injury risk among elite football players. Besides, height was also one of the variables significantly integrated into injury-prediction models in elite football players. Those variables can be related to each other, since they all end up influencing the players' sports performance. In fact, the main value of this study is directed towards sports monitoring and injury prevention, as we analyzed the relationship between overall strength and height in elite soccer players as predictors of injury, and this is a topic on the rise. In the literature, we identified two studies conducted with youth footballers that have determined that injured players were significantly stronger, bigger, and more experienced than non-injured players [59,60]. This aspect becomes even more relevant when we talk about elite football players, since their demands are higher. The slightest physical differences can make all the difference in the outcome of individual action, dictating the outcome of crucial moments of games and seasons. We believe that these achievements can support future research on the topic to disentangle this complex net of variables that may affect the injury profile.

There are some limitations to this study that need to be acknowledged. The sample size and the fact that we only evaluated the elite players for 26 weeks across 42 weeks of the season are the main limitations of this study. The sample size is related to the number of patterns teaching predictive models. The greater the amount of recorded-injury information is, the better the material for calculating predictive models. Continued collection of learning patterns will improve the predictive ability of the models. Moreover, this is a cross-sectional study, which does not allow a cause–effect of the presented results. However, these results bring important and specific practical implications for those involved in the elite football context, mainly for the topics of injury prevention and training monitorization, since these are issues that are gaining significant attention in the sports business.

5. Conclusions

Addressing the need for further studies to identify risk factors for predicting injuries in elite football players, our approach opens a novel perspective on injury prevention and training monitorization, providing a methodology for evaluating and interpreting the complex relations between injury risk and players' performance in elite football. Players' sectorial position, body-composition variables, and physical fitness tests (sit-and-reach, push-up, handgrip, countermovement jump, squat jump, linear speed, and yoyo tests), were all important predictors that may be considered in the injury-risk prevention in elite football players. It would be an added value if future studies analyzed the influence of body-composition factors and physical fitness tests in elite football teams across different seasons.

Author Contributions: Conceptualization, F.M., É.R.G., K.P. and C.F.; methodology, F.M., É.R.G., K.P., C.F. and R.H.; validation, K.P., H.L. and R.H.; formal analysis, F.M., É.R.G., K.P. and C.F.; investigation, F.M., C.F. and R.H.; resources, É.R.G. and H.L.; writing—original draft preparation, F.M., É.R.G., K.P. and C.F.; writing—review and editing, M.d.M.N., H.S., A.M. and A.I.; visualization, M.d.M.N., H.S., A.M. and A.I.; project administration, É.R.G. and H.L.; funding acquisition, É.R.G. and H.L. All authors have read and agreed to the published version of the manuscript.

Funding: C.F., F.M. and E.R.G. acknowledge support from LARSyS—the Portuguese national funding agency for science, research, and technology (FCT)—pluriannual funding 2020–2023 (Reference: UIDB/50009/2020). This study is framed in the Marítimo Training Lab Project. The project received funding under application no. M1420-01-0247-FEDER-000033 in the System of Incentives for the Production of Scientific and Technological Knowledge in the Autonomous Region of Madeira—PROCiência 2020.

Institutional Review Board Statement: This study was conducted according to the guidelines of the Declaration of Helsinki, was approved by the Ethics Committee of the Faculty of Human Kinetics (CEIFMH N°34/2021), and followed the ethical standards of the Declaration of Helsinki for Medical Research in Humans (2013) and the Oviedo Convention (1997).

Informed Consent Statement: Informed consent was obtained from all subjects involved in the study. Written informed consent has been obtained from all players to publish this paper.

Data Availability Statement: The data presented in this study are available upon request from the corresponding author.

Acknowledgments: The authors would like to thank all players and their respective legal guardians for participating in this study.

Conflicts of Interest: The authors declare no conflict of interest.

References

1. Smpokos, E.; Mourikis, C.; Theos, C.; Manolarakis, G.; Linardakis, M. Injuries and risk factors in professional football players during four consecutive seasons. *Sport Sci. Health* **2021**, 1–8. [CrossRef]
2. Konefał, M.; Chmura, P.; Kowalczuk, E.; Figueiredo, A.J.; Sarmento, H.; Rokita, A.; Chmura, J.; Andrzejewski, M. Modeling of relationships between physical and technical activities and match outcome in elite German soccer players. *J. Sports Med. Phys. Fit.* **2019**, *59*, 752–759. [CrossRef] [PubMed]
3. Rice, S.M.; Purcell, R.; De Silva, S.; Mawren, D.; McGorry, P.D.; Parker, A.G. The mental health of elite athletes: A narrative systematic review. *Sports Med.* **2016**, *46*, 1333–1353. [CrossRef] [PubMed]
4. Yáñez, S.; Yáñez, C.; Martínez, M.; Núñez, M.; De la Fuente, C. Lesiones deportivas del plantel profesional de fútbol Santiago Wanderers durante las temporadas 2017, 2018 y 2019. *Arch. Soc. Chil. Med. Deporte* **2021**, *66*, 92–103.
5. Hägglund, M.; Waldén, M.; Magnusson, H.; Kristenson, K.; Bengtsson, H.; Ekstrand, J. Injuries affect team performance negatively in professional football: An 11-year follow-up of the UEFA Champions League injury study. *Br. J. Sports Med.* **2013**, *47*, 738–742. [CrossRef]
6. Hurley, O.A. Impact of player injuries on teams' mental states, and subsequent performances, at the Rugby World Cup 2015. *Front. Psychol.* **2016**, *7*, 807.
7. Kirkendall, D.T.; Dvorak, J. Effective injury prevention in soccer. *Physician Sportsmed.* **2010**, *38*, 147–157. [CrossRef]
8. Cohen, M.; Abdalla, R.J.; Ejnisman, B.; Amaro, J.T. Lesões ortopédicas no futebol. *Rev. Bras. Ortop.* **1997**, *32*, 940–944.
9. Ekstrand, J.; Hägglund, M.; Waldén, M. Epidemiology of muscle injuries in professional football (soccer). *Am. J. Sports Med.* **2011**, *39*, 1226–1232. [CrossRef]
10. Hoffman, D.T.; Dwyer, D.B.; Tran, J.; Clifton, P.; Gastin, P.B. Australian Football League injury characteristics differ between matches and training: A longitudinal analysis of changes in the setting, site, and time span from 1997 to 2016. *Orthop. J. Sports Med.* **2019**, *7*, 2325967119837641. [CrossRef]
11. Lee, I.; Jeong, H.S.; Lee, S.Y. Injury profiles in Korean youth soccer. *Int. J. Environ. Res. Public Health* **2020**, *17*, 5125. [CrossRef]
12. Noya Salces, J.; Gómez-Carmona, P.M.; Gracia-Marco, L.; Moliner-Urdiales, D.; Sillero-Quintana, M. Epidemiology of injuries in First Division Spanish football. *J. Sports Sci.* **2014**, *32*, 1263–1270. [CrossRef]
13. Raya-González, J.; de Ste Croix, M.; Read, P.; Castillo, D. A Longitudinal Investigation of muscle injuries in an elite spanish male academy soccer club: A hamstring injuries approach. *Appl. Sci.* **2020**, *10*, 1610. [CrossRef]

14. Torrontegui-Duarte, M.; Gijon-Nogueron, G.; Perez-Frias, J.C.; Morales-Asencio, J.M.; Luque-Suarez, A. Incidence of injuries among professional football players in Spain during three consecutive seasons: A longitudinal, retrospective study. *Phys. Ther. Sport* **2020**, *41*, 87–93. [CrossRef]
15. Jones, A.; Jones, G.; Greig, N.; Bower, P.; Brown, J.; Hind, K.; Francis, P. Epidemiology of injury in English Professional Football players: A cohort study. *Phys. Ther. Sport* **2019**, *35*, 18–22. [CrossRef]
16. Krutsch, W.; Memmel, C.; Alt, V.; Krutsch, V.; Tröß, T.; Meyer, T. Timing return-to-competition: A prospective registration of 45 different types of severe injuries in Germany's highest football league. *Arch. Orthop. Trauma Surg.* **2022**, *142*, 455–463. [CrossRef]
17. Bradley, P.S.; Noakes, T.D. Match running performance fluctuations in elite soccer: Indicative of fatigue, pacing or situational influences? *J. Sports Sci.* **2013**, *31*, 1627–1638. [CrossRef]
18. Harper, D.J.; Carling, C.; Kiely, J. High-intensity acceleration and deceleration demands in elite team sports competitive match play: A systematic review and meta-analysis of observational studies. *Sports Med.* **2019**, *49*, 1923–1947. [CrossRef]
19. Oliva-Lozano, J.M.; Gómez-Carmona, C.D.; Pino-Ortega, J.; Moreno-Pérez, V.; Rodríguez-Pérez, M.A. Match and training high intensity activity-demands profile during a competitive mesocycle in youth elite soccer players. *J. Hum. Kinet.* **2020**, *75*, 195–205. [CrossRef]
20. Przednowek, K.; Wiktorowicz, K.; Krzeszowski, T.; Iskra, J. A web-oriented expert system for planning hurdles race training programmes. *Neural Comput. Appl.* **2019**, *31*, 7227–7243. [CrossRef]
21. Stern, B.D.; Hegedus, E.J.; Lai, Y.-C. Injury prediction as a non-linear system. *Phys. Ther. Sport* **2020**, *41*, 43–48. [CrossRef] [PubMed]
22. Huang, C.; Jiang, L. Data monitoring and sports injury prediction model based on embedded system and machine learning algorithm. *Microprocess. Microsyst.* **2021**, *81*, 103654. [CrossRef]
23. Rossi, A.; Pappalardo, L.; Cintia, P.; Iaia, F.M.; Fernández, J.; Medina, D. Effective injury forecasting in soccer with GPS training data and machine learning. *PLoS ONE* **2018**, *13*, e0201264. [CrossRef] [PubMed]
24. Ekstrand, J.; Spreco, A.; Bengtsson, H.; Bahr, R. Injury rates decreased in men's professional football: An 18-year prospective cohort study of almost 12,000 injuries sustained during 1.8 million hours of play. *Br. J. Sports Med.* **2021**, *55*, 1084–1091. [CrossRef]
25. López-Valenciano, A.; Ayala, F.; Puerta, J.M.; Croix, M.D.S.; Vera-García, F.; Hernández-Sánchez, S.; Ruiz-Pérez, I.; Myer, G. A preventive model for muscle injuries: A novel approach based on learning algorithms. *Med. Sci. Sports Exerc.* **2018**, *50*, 915. [CrossRef]
26. Nassis, G.; Stylianides, G.; Verhagen, E.; Brito, J.; Figueiredo, P.; Krustrup, P. A review of machine learning applications in soccer with an emphasis on injury risk. *Biol. Sport* **2022**, *40*, 233–239. [CrossRef]
27. Brink, M.S.; Visscher, C.; Arends, S.; Zwerver, J.; Post, W.J.; Lemmink, K.A. Monitoring stress and recovery: New insights for the prevention of injuries and illnesses in elite youth soccer players. *Br. J. Sports Med.* **2010**, *44*, 809–815. [CrossRef]
28. Ehrmann, F.E.; Duncan, C.S.; Sindhusake, D.; Franzsen, W.N.; Greene, D.A. GPS and injury prevention in professional soccer. *J. Strength Cond. Res.* **2016**, *30*, 360–367. [CrossRef]
29. Venturelli, M.; Schena, F.; Zanolla, L.; Bishop, D. Injury risk factors in young soccer players detected by a multivariate survival model. *J. Sci. Med. Sport* **2011**, *14*, 293–298. [CrossRef]
30. Van Eetvelde, H.; Mendonça, L.D.; Ley, C.; Seil, R.; Tischer, T. Machine learning methods in sport injury prediction and prevention: A systematic review. *J. Exp. Orthop.* **2021**, *8*, 27. [CrossRef]
31. Ayala, F.; López-Valenciano, A.; Martín, J.A.G.; Croix, M.D.S.; Vera-Garcia, F.J.; García-Vaquero, M.D.P.; Ruiz-Pérez, I.; Myer, G.D. A preventive model for hamstring injuries in professional soccer: Learning algorithms. *Int. J. Sports Med.* **2019**, *40*, 344–353. [CrossRef]
32. Gerodimos, V. Reliability of handgrip strength test in basketball players. *J. Hum. Kinet.* **2012**, *31*, 25. [CrossRef]
33. Bosco, C.; Luhtanen, P.; Komi, P.V. A simple method for measurement of mechanical power in jumping. *Eur. J. Appl. Physiol. Occup. Physiol.* **1983**, *50*, 273–282. [CrossRef]
34. Schmitz, B.; Pfeifer, C.; Kreitz, K.; Borowski, M.; Faldum, A.; Brand, S.-M. The Yo-Yo intermittent tests: A systematic review and structured compendium of test results. *Front. Physiol.* **2018**, *9*, 870. [CrossRef]
35. Turner, A.; Walker, S.; Stembridge, M.; Coneyworth, P.; Reed, G.; Birdsey, L.; Barter, P.; Moody, J. A testing battery for the assessment of fitness in soccer players. *Strength Cond. J.* **2011**, *33*, 29–39. [CrossRef]
36. Bangsbo, J.; Iaia, F.M.; Krustrup, P. The Yo-Yo intermittent recovery test. *Sports Med.* **2008**, *38*, 37–51. [CrossRef]
37. Hägglund, M.; Waldén, M.; Bahr, R.; Ekstrand, J. Methods for epidemiological study of injuries to professional football players: Developing the UEFA model. *Br. J. Sports Med.* **2005**, *39*, 340–346. [CrossRef]
38. Hoerl, A.E.; Kennard, R.W. Ridge regression: Biased estimation for nonorthogonal problems. *Technometrics* **1970**, *12*, 55–67. [CrossRef]
39. Tibshirani, R. Regression shrinkage and selection via the lasso. *J. R. Stat. Soc. Ser. B* **1996**, *58*, 267–288. [CrossRef]
40. Zou, H.; Hastie, T. Regularization and variable selection via the elastic net. *J. R. Stat. Soc. Ser. B* **2005**, *67*, 301–320. [CrossRef]
41. Hastie, T.; Tibshirani, R.; Friedman, J. Unsupervised learning. In *The Elements of Statistical Learning*; Springer: Berlin/Heidelberg, Germany, 2009; pp. 485–585.
42. Chatterjee, S.; Hadi, A.S. *Regression Analysis by Example*; John Wiley & Sons: Hoboken, NJ, USA, 2015.
43. Carey, D.L.; Ong, K.-L.; Whiteley, R.; Crossley, K.M.; Crow, J.; Morris, M.E. Predictive modelling of training loads and injury in Australian football. *arXiv* **2017**, arXiv:170604336. [CrossRef]

44. Rodas, G.; Osaba, L.; Arteta, D.; Pruna, R.; Fernández, D.; Lucia, A. Genomic prediction of tendinopathy risk in elite team sports. *Int. J. Sports Physiol. Perform.* **2019**, *15*, 489–495. [CrossRef]
45. Ruddy, J.D.; Cormack, S.J.; Whiteley, R.; Williams, M.D.; Timmins, R.G.; Opar, D.A. Modeling the risk of team sport injuries: A narrative review of different statistical approaches. *Front. Physiol.* **2019**, *10*, 829. [CrossRef]
46. Halson, S. Monitorización de la carga de formación para conocer fatiga en los atletas. *Sports Med.* **2014**, *44*, 139–147. [CrossRef]
47. Stubbe, J.H.; van Beijsterveldt, A.-M.M.C.; van der Knaap, S.; Stege, J.; Verhagen, E.A.; van Mechelen, W.; Backx, F.J.G. Injuries in professional male soccer players in the Netherlands: A prospective cohort study. *J. Athl. Train.* **2015**, *50*, 211–216. [CrossRef]
48. Waldén, M.; Hägglund, M.; Ekstrand, J. Injuries in Swedish elite football—A prospective study on injury definitions, risk for injury and injury pattern during 2001. *Scand. J. Med. Sci. Sports* **2005**, *15*, 118–125. [CrossRef]
49. Di Salvo, V.; Baron, R.; González-Haro, C.; Gormasz, C.; Pigozzi, F.; Bachl, N. Sprinting analysis of elite soccer players during European Champions League and UEFA Cup matches. *J. Sports Sci.* **2010**, *28*, 1489–1494. [CrossRef]
50. Suarez-Arrones, L.; Torreño, N.; Requena, B.; De Villarreal, E.S.; Casamichana, D.; Barbero-Alvarez, J.C.; Munguía-Izquierdo, D. Match-play activity profile in professional soccer players during official games and the relationship between external and internal load. *J. Sports Med. Phys. Fit.* **2014**, *55*, 1417–1422.
51. Martín-García, A.; Díaz, A.G.; Bradley, P.S.; Morera, F.; Casamichana, D. Quantification of a professional football team's external load using a microcycle structure. *J. Strength Cond. Res.* **2018**, *32*, 3511–3518. [CrossRef] [PubMed]
52. Gabbett, T.J. The training—Injury prevention paradox: Should athletes be training smarter and harder? *Br. J. Sports Med.* **2016**, *50*, 273–280. [CrossRef] [PubMed]
53. Hrysomallis, C. Hip adductors' strength, flexibility, and injury risk. *J. Strength Cond. Res.* **2009**, *23*, 1514–1517. [CrossRef]
54. Arnason, A.; Sigurdsson, S.B.; Gudmundsson, A.; Holme, I.; Engebretsen, L.; Bahr, R. Risk factors for injuries in football. *Am. J. Sports Med.* **2004**, *32* (Suppl. S1), 5–16. [CrossRef]
55. Ekstrand, J.; Gillquist, J. Soccer injuries and their mechanisms: A prospective study. *Med. Sci. Sports Exerc.* **1983**, *15*, 267–270. [CrossRef]
56. Ibrahim, A.; Murrell, G.; Knapman, P. Adductor strain and hip range of movement in male professional soccer players. *J. Orthop. Surg.* **2007**, *15*, 46–49. [CrossRef]
57. Witvrouw, E.; Danneels, L.; Asselman, P.; D'Have, T.; Cambier, D. Muscle flexibility as a risk factor for developing muscle injuries in male professional soccer players: A prospective study. *Am. J. Sports Med.* **2003**, *31*, 41–46. [CrossRef]
58. Liguori, G.; American College of Sports Medicine (ACSM). *ACSM's Guidelines for Exercise Testing and Prescription*; Lippincott Williams & Wilkins: Philadelphia, PA, USA, 2016.
59. Turbeville, S.D.; Cowan, L.D.; Asal, N.R.; Owen, W.L.; Anderson, M.A. Risk factors for injury in middle school football players. *Am. J. Sports Med.* **2003**, *31*, 276–281. [CrossRef]
60. Turbeville, S.D.; Cowan, L.D.; Owen, W.L.; Asal, N.R.; Anderson, M.A. Risk factors for injury in high school football players. *Am. J. Sports Med.* **2003**, *31*, 974–980. [CrossRef]

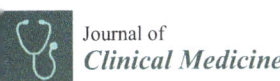

Journal of Clinical Medicine

Article

Exercise Hypertension in Athletes

Karsten Keller [1,2,3,*], Katharina Hartung [1], Luis del Castillo Carillo [1], Julia Treiber [1], Florian Stock [1], Chantal Schröder [1], Florian Hugenschmidt [1] and Birgit Friedmann-Bette [1]

1. Medical Clinic VII, Department of Sports Medicine, University Hospital Heidelberg, 69120 Heidelberg, Germany
2. Department of Cardiology, University Medical Center of the Johannes Gutenberg-University Mainz, 55131 Mainz, Germany
3. Center for Thrombosis and Hemostasis (CTH), University Medical Center of the Johannes Gutenberg-University Mainz, 55131 Mainz, Germany
* Correspondence: karsten.keller@med.uni-heidelberg.de

Abstract: Background: An exaggerated blood pressure response (EBPR) during exercise testing is not well defined, and several blood pressure thresholds are used in different studies and recommended in different guidelines. **Methods:** Competitive athletes of any age without known arterial hypertension who presented for preparticipation screening were included in the present study and categorized for EBPR according to American Heart Association (AHA), European Society of Cardiology (ESC), and American College of Sports Medicine (ACSM) guidelines as well as the systolic blood pressure/MET slope method. **Results:** Overall, 1137 athletes (mean age 21 years; 34.7% females) without known arterial hypertension were included April 2020–October 2021. Among them, 19.6%, 15.0%, and 6.8% were diagnosed EBPR according to ESC, AHA, and ACSM guidelines, respectively. Left ventricular hypertrophy (LVH) was detected in 20.5% of the athletes and was approximately two-fold more frequent in athletes with EBPR than in those without. While EBPR according to AHA (OR 2.35 [95%CI 1.66–3.33], $p < 0.001$) and ACSM guidelines (OR 1.81 [95%CI 1.05–3.09], $p = 0.031$) was independently (of age and sex) associated with LVH, EBPR defined according to ESC guidelines (OR 1.49 [95%CI 1.00–2.23], $p = 0.051$) was not. In adult athletes, only AHA guidelines (OR 1.96 [95%CI 1.32–2.90], $p = 0.001$) and systolic blood pressure/MET slope method (OR 1.73 [95%CI 1.08–2.78], $p = 0.023$) were independently predictive for LVH. **Conclusions:** Diverging guidelines exist for the screening regarding EBPR. In competitive athletes, the prevalence of EBPR was highest when applying the ESC (19.6%) and lowest using the ACSM guidelines (6.8%). An association of EBPR with LVH in adult athletes, independently of age and sex, was only found when the AHA guideline or the systolic blood pressure/MET slope method was applied.

Keywords: arterial hypertension; exercise hypertension; blood pressure; exercise testing

1. Introduction

Arterial hypertension is the most important and most common cardiovascular risk factor (CVRF) for morbidity and mortality worldwide [1–4]. The prevalence of arterial hypertension is high [5], affecting approximately 78 million adults in the United States of America [6]. While the prevalence of arterial hypertension increases substantially with age [7–10], its prevalence in athletes is low, at approximately 3% [11].

Diagnosis of arterial hypertension by resting blood pressure is well defined. In Europe, a systolic blood pressure (BP) value of ≥140 mmHg and a diastolic BP value of ≥90 mmHg are the defined thresholds of arterial hypertension [12–15]. In contrast, an exaggerated blood pressure response (EBPR) during treadmill and bicycle exercise testing is not well defined and poorly recognized, and several blood pressure thresholds were used in the different studies and are recommended in different guidelines [9,14,16–22]. While the American Heart Association (AHA) guideline [23] (EBPR threshold: systolic peak BP >210 mmHg

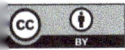

in men, >190 mmHg in women, and/or >90 mmHg diastolic peak BP in both sexes) and the European Society of Cardiology (ESC) guideline [22,24] (EBPR threshold: systolic peak BP >220 mmHg in men, >200 mmHg in women, and/or >85 mmHg in men and 80 mmHg in women for diastolic peak BP) used sex-specific EBPR thresholds, the American College of Sports Medicine (ACSM) guideline [20,21] (EBPR threshold: systolic peak BP >225 mmHg and/or >90 mmHg for diastolic peak BP in both sexes) recommends the same systolic and diastolic thresholds values for both sexes.

However, for arterial-hypertension-naïve individuals with EBPR during the exercise testing, it was shown that these individuals are at increased risk of developing both arterial hypertension as well as cardiovascular events in the future, underlining the importance of this phenomenon [1,4,17,25–37].

In the context of arterial hypertension, it is well known that an increase in left ventricular mass and left ventricular hypertrophy (LVH) are associated with cardiovascular disease (CVD) as well as an elevated number of cardiovascular events and mortality [37,38]. Despite the development of the heart in highly trained athletes, a septal thickness of ≥ 13 mm was observed in only a very small number of athletes and should be considered as LVH in athletes [22,39–41].

Thus, the objectives of the present study were to evaluate (I) how prevalent EBPR is in athletes and (II) which definition of an EBPR during exercise testing was best associated with LVH in athletes without known arterial hypertension.

2. Materials and Methods

We performed a retrospective analysis of athletes of any age without known arterial hypertension who presented at the Department of Sports Medicine (Medical Clinic VII) of the University Hospital Heidelberg (Germany) for their preparticipation screening examination between April 2020 and October 2021.

2.1. Enrolled Subjects

Athletes were eligible for this study if they performed regular training for competition, were able to perform an exercise test at our department, had no contraindications for exercise testing, and had no known diagnosis of arterial hypertension. Exclusion criteria were a known diagnosis of arterial hypertension and contraindications regarding performing exercise testing [22,23].

2.2. Ethical Aspects

The requirement for informed consent was waived as we used only anonymized retrospective data routinely collected during the health screening process. Studies in Germany involving a retrospective analysis of diagnostic standard data of anonymized patients do not require an ethics statement.

2.3. Definitions

Arterial hypertension at rest was defined according to the ESC guidelines [42]. In all athletes, a transthoracic echocardiography was performed. Investigated echocardiographic parameters were defined according to current guidelines [22,43].

LVH was defined as (I) septal or posterior left ventricular (LV) wall diameter ≥ 13 mm [22,40] or (II) LV mass >162 g in female or >224 g in male individuals [43]. LV mass was computed according the established 2D echocardiography area-length method: LV mass = 0.80 × (1.04 × [(septal LV wall thickness + LV end-diastolic diameter + posterior LV wall thickness)^3 − (LV end-diastolic diameter)^3]) + 0.6 g [43]. LVH was considered to be present if one or both of the definitions applied.

EBPR was defined on the basis of the peak BP values during exercise testing according to three different guidelines and the systolic BP/MET slope method:

- American Heart Association (AHA) guidelines [23]: systolic peak BP >210 mmHg in men, >190 mmHg in women, and/or >90 mmHg diastolic peak BP in both sexes.

- European Society of Cardiology (ESC) guidelines [22,24]: systolic peak BP >220 mmHg in men, >200 mmHg in women, and/or >85 mmHg in men and 80 mmHg in women for diastolic peak BP.
- The American College of Sports Medicine (ACSM) guidelines [20,21]: systolic peak BP >225 mmHg and/or >90 mmHg, for diastolic peak BP in both sexes.
- The systolic BP/MET slope method [44–47]: The Δ regarding systolic BP was calculated as maximum systolic BP during exercise—systolic BP at rest and was indexed by the increase in MET from rest (Δ regarding MET was calculated as peak MET-1) to obtain the systolic BP/MET slope [46]. In accordance with previous studies, a cutoff value > 6.2 mmHg/MET was used to define an EBPR [44,46]. The MET value was calculated based on the athletes' VO$_2$ maximum values during exercise testing as recommended by the ACSM guideline (MET = VO$_{2max}$/3.5 mL·kg^{-1}·min^{-1}) [48].
- Exercise testing was performed according to current guidelines with electrocardiogram (ECG) and BP measurements at the end of every load level. The exercise test was stopped if the athlete was at their maximum capacity or stopping criteria according to current guidelines [22,23].

Obesity was defined as body mass index (BMI) ≥30 kg/m^2 according to the World Health Organization.

2.4. Statistics

Athletes categorized as athletes with EBPR according to the three aforementioned guidelines and the systolic BP/MET slope method were compared to those athletes not categorized as EBPR (normal BP response during the exercise test) with the help of the Wilcoxon–Mann–Whitney U test for continuous variables and Fisher's exact or chi^2 test for categorical variables, as appropriate. Data of continuous variables were presented as median and interquartile range and categorical variables as absolute numbers with related percentages.

We performed univariate and multivariate logistic regression models to investigate the association between EBPR (defined according to the three guidelines) as well as BP values at rest and maximum values during exercise on the one hand and LVH on the other hand. Multivariate regression models were adjusted for age and sex in order to prove the independence of the statistical results of athletes' age and sex. Results of the logistic regressions are presented as odds ratio (OR) and 95% Confidence interval (CI).

All statistical analyses were carried out with the use of SPSS software (IBM Corp. Released 2017. IBM SPSS Statistics for Windows, Version 25.0. Armonk, NY, USA). Only the p values < 0.05 (two-sided) were considered to be statistically significant. No adjustment for multiple testing was applied to the present analysis.

3. Results

3.1. Athletes' Characteristics

Overall, 1137 athletes (mean age 21 years; median 18 years (IQR 15/25); 395 (34.7%) females) without known arterial hypertension were included in the present study between April 2020 and October 2021. Most included athletes were in the second or third decade of life (Figure 1A). Among them, CVRF were rare, with nicotine abuse reported in 34 (3.0%) and obesity detected in 14 (1.2%) athletes. LVH was diagnosed in 233 athletes (regardless of athletes' sex: 20.5%; 87 female athletes (22.0%); 146 male athletes (19.7%)). Median past training period was 8 (IQR 5/12) years.

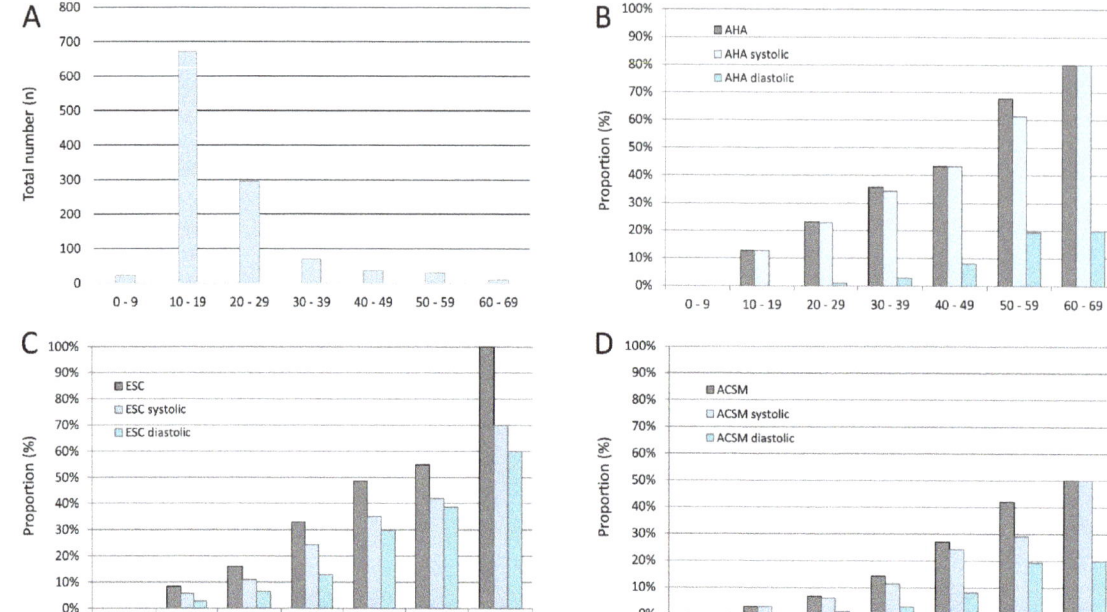

Figure 1. Included numbers of athletes and proportion of blood pressure deviations stratified for age by decade. Panel (**A**) Total numbers of included athletes stratified for age by decade. Panel (**B**) Proportion of athletes with exaggerated blood pressure response according to American Heart Association (AHA) guideline stratified for age by decade. Panel (**C**) Proportion of athletes with exaggerated blood pressure response according to European Society of Cardiology (ESC) guideline stratified for age by decade. Panel (**D**) Proportion of athletes with exaggerated blood pressure response according to American College of Sports Medicine (ACSM) guideline stratified for age by decade.

3.2. Prevalence of Exaggerated Blood Pressure Response (EBPR) during Exercise Testing

Overall, 223 athletes (regardless of athletes' sex: 19.6%; 74 female athletes (18.7%); 149 male athletes (20.1%)) had a diagnosis of EBPR according to AHA guidelines (Table 1), 171 (regardless of athletes' sex: 15.0%; 66 female athletes (16.7%); 105 male athletes (14.2%)) according to ESC guidelines (Table 2), and 77 (regardless of athletes' sex: 6.8%; 11 female athletes (2.8%); 66 male athletes (8.9%)) according to ACSM guidelines (Table 3).

Table 1. Patient characteristics of the 1137 examined athletes without known arterial hypertension stratified for exaggerated blood pressure response according to AHA guideline.

Parameters	Normal Blood Pressure Response According to AHA Classification (n = 914; 80.4%)	Exaggerated Blood Pressure Response According to AHA Classification (n = 223; 19.6%)	p-Value
Age (in years)	17.0 (15.0/22.0)	22.0 (18.0/33.0)	<0.001
Female sex	321 (35.1%)	74 (33.2%)	0.586
Body height (cm)	174.0 (166.9/181.0)	179.0 (173.0/184.0)	<0.001
Body weight (kg)	67.0 (57.6/77.7)	75.8 (68.0/85.8)	<0.001
Body mass index (kg/m^2)	22.0 (20.2/24.1)	23.4 (22.0/25.4)	<0.001
Body fat (%)	11.3 (8.5/16.4)	11.9 (9.0/16.3)	0.140

Table 1. *Cont.*

Parameters	Normal Blood Pressure Response According to AHA Classification (*n* = 914; 80.4%)	Exaggerated Blood Pressure Response According to AHA Classification (*n* = 223; 19.6%)	*p*-Value
Leading athletes at a regional or national level	707 (77.4%)	146 (65.5%)	<0.001
Training years	8.0 (5.0/11.0)	11.0 (6.0/15.0)	<0.001
Cardiovascular risk factors			
Nicotine abuse	20 (2.2%)	14 (6.3%)	0.003
Obesity	8 (0.9%)	6 (2.7%)	0.039
Blood pressure values			
Systolic blood pressure (mmHg)	115.0 (110.0/120.0)	120.0 (115.0/130.0)	<0.001
Diastolic blood pressure (mmHg)	70.0 (60.0/75.0)	70.0 (70.0/80.0)	<0.001
Maximum systolic blood pressure during exercise (mmHg)	180.0 (160.0/190.0)	220.0 (210.0/230.0)	<0.001
Maximum diastolic blood pressure during exercise (mmHg)	70.0 (70.0/80.0)	80.0 (70.0/85.0)	<0.001
Exercise parameters			
VO_2 maximum during exercise	45.5 (39.9/50.5)	44.0 (37.2/49.5)	0.031
Respiratory exchange ratio (RER)	1.15 (1.10/1.20)	1.15 (1.11/1.21)	0.864
Maximum lactate value	9.46 (7.79/11.2)	9.21 (7.61/11.24)	0.861
Echocardiographic parameters			
Left ventricular hypertrophy	151 (16.5%)	82 (36.8%)	<0.001
Left ventricular mass	158.8 (128.0/200.4)	194.2 (164.1/220.8)	<0.001
Aortic valve regurgitation	48 (5.3%)	26 (11.7%)	0.001
Mitral valve regurgitation	474 (51.9%)	153 (68.6%)	<0.001
Tricuspid valve regurgitation	115 (12.6%)	43 (19.3%)	0.027
Pulmonary valve regurgitation	91 (10.0%)	17 (7.6%)	0.311
Heart volume in total (mL)	760.5 (625.8/906.3)	910.3 (770.2/1004.5)	<0.001
Heart volume related to body weight (mL/kg)	11.4 (10.2/12.4)	11.7 (10.6/12.8)	0.003
Left ventricular ejection fraction (%)	65.0 (62.0/69.0)	66.0 (62.0/69.0)	0.140
Left ventricular end-diastolic diameter (cm)	49.0 (45.0/53.0)	51.0 (48.0/54.0)	<0.001
Left atrial area (cm^2)	13.5 (11.1/15.4)	15.2 (12.9/17.6)	<0.001
Right atrial area (cm^2)	13.2 (11.0/15.5)	15.1 (13.3/17.7)	<0.001
Tricuspid annular plane systolic excursion (TAPSE, cm)	2.46 (2.20/2.70)	2.6 (2.3/2.9)	<0.001
Systolic pulmonary artery pulmonary pressure (mmHg)	20.0 (17.0/23.0)	20.3 (17.0/23.6)	0.274
E/A quotient	2.7 (1.9/3.7)	2.6 (1.8/3.6)	0.215
E/E' quotient	4.7 (4.0/5.7)	4.8 (4.0/5.7)	0.606

Table 2. Patient characteristics of the 1137 examined athletes without known arterial hypertension stratified for exaggerated blood pressure response according to ESC guideline.

Parameters	Normal Blood Pressure Response According to ESC Classification (n = 966; 85.0%)	Exaggerated Blood Pressure Response According to ESC Classification (n = 171; 15.0%)	p-Value
Age (in years)	17.0 (15.0/22.0)	26.0 (18.0/42.0)	<0.001
Female sex	329 (34.1%)	66 (38.6%)	0.251
Body height (cm)	175.0 (167.0/182.0)	179.0 (171.0/184.0)	<0.001
Body weight (kg)	68.2 (58.3/78.5)	75.8 (66.4/84.0)	<0.001
Body mass index (kg/m^2)	22.1 (20.2/24.2)	23.7 (22.3/25.5)	<0.001
Body fat (%)	11.0 (8.5/16.0)	13.0 (9.5/17.2)	<0.001
Leading athletes at a regional or national level	754 (78.1%)	99 (57.9%)	<0.001
Training years	8.0 (5.0/11.0)	11.0 (7.0/16.0)	<0.001
Cardiovascular risk factors			
Nicotine abuse	19 (2.0%)	15 (8.8%)	<0.001
Obesity	8 (0.8%)	6 (3.5%)	0.011
Blood pressure values			
Systolic blood pressure (mmHg)	115.0 (110.0/120.0)	120.0 (110.0/130.0)	<0.001
Diastolic blood pressure (mmHg)	70.0 (60.0/75.0)	75.0 (70.0/80.0)	<0.001
Maximum systolic blood pressure during exercise (mmHg)	180.0 (160.0/195.0)	220.0 (210.0/230.0)	<0.001
Maximum diastolic blood pressure during exercise (mmHg)	70.0 (70.0/80.0)	85.0 (80.0/90.0)	<0.001
Exercise parameters			
VO$_2$ maximum during exercise	45.6 (40.1/50.6)	42.0 (35.1/49.1)	<0.001
Respiratory exchange ratio (RER)	1.15 (1.10/1.20)	1.15 (1.11/1.21)	0.497
Maximum lactate value	9.42 (7.71/11.2)	9.28 (7.96/11.07)	0.933
Echocardiographic parameters			
Left ventricular hypertrophy	177 (18.3%)	56 (32.7%)	<0.001
Left ventricular mass	164.3 (132.6/200.8)	188.0 (153.2/219.7)	<0.001
Aortic valve regurgitation	50 (5.2%)	24 (14.0%)	<0.001
Mitral valve regurgitation	506 (52.4%)	121 (70.8%)	<0.001
Tricuspid valve regurgitation	123 (12.7%)	35 (20.5%)	0.022
Pulmonary valve regurgitation	94 (9.7%)	14 (8.2%)	0.526
Heart volume in total (mL)	774.4 (634.6/919.0)	883.0 (728.4/982.6)	<0.001
Heart volume related to body weight (mL/kg)	11.5 (10.3/12.5)	11.5 (10.3/12.5)	0.790
Left ventricular ejection fraction (%)	65.0 (62.0/68.0)	66.0 (63.0/69.0)	0.012
Left ventricular end-diastolic diameter (cm)	50.0 (46.0/53.0)	51.0 (47.0/54.0)	0.004
Left atrial area (cm^2)	13.6 (11.3/15.6)	15.0 (12.6/15.6)	<0.001

Table 2. Cont.

Parameters	Normal Blood Pressure Response According to ESC Classification (n = 966; 85.0%)	Exaggerated Blood Pressure Response According to ESC Classification (n = 171; 15.0%)	p-Value
Right atrial area (cm^2)	13.4 (11.1/15.7)	15.0 (12.9/17.7)	<0.001
Tricuspid annular plane systolic excursion (TAPSE, cm)	2.50 (2.20/2.80)	2.6 (2.4/2.9)	<0.001
Systolic pulmonary artery pulmonary pressure (mmHg)	20.0 (17.0/23.0)	21.0 (18.0/24.1)	0.018
E/A quotient	2.7 (2.0/3.7)	2.2 (1.6/3.3)	<0.001
E/E' quotient	4.7 (4.0/5.7)	4.9 (4.1/6.0)	0.167

Table 3. Patient characteristics of the 1137 examined athletes without known arterial hypertension stratified for exaggerated blood pressure response according to ACSM guideline.

Parameters	Normal Blood Pressure Response According to ACSM Classification (n = 1060; 93.2%)	Exaggerated Blood Pressure Response According to ACSM Classification (n = 77; 6.8%)	p-Value
Age (in years)	18.0 (15.0/23.0)	29.0 (19.5/48.5)	<0.001
Female sex	384 (36.2%)	11 (14.3%)	<0.001
Body height (cm)	175.0 (167.0/182.0)	181.0 (175.3/186.5)	<0.001
Body weight (kg)	68.4 (58.8/78.5)	80.3 (75.0/87.9)	<0.001
Body mass index (kg/m^2)	22.2 (20.4/24.2)	24.4 (23.0/26.3)	<0.001
Body fat (%)	11.3 (8.6/16.7)	11.5 (9.2/14.0)	0.884
Leading athletes at a regional or national level	817 (77.1%)	36 (46.8%)	<0.001
Training years	8.0 (5.0/11.0)	13.0 (8.5/18.8)	<0.001
Cardiovascular risk factors			
Nicotine abuse	27 (2.5%)	7 (9.1%)	0.006
Obesity	10 (0.9%)	4 (5.2%)	0.012
Blood pressure values			
Systolic blood pressure (mmHg)	115.0 (110.0/120.0)	125.0 (120.0/135.0)	<0.001
Diastolic blood pressure (mmHg)	70.0 (60.0/75.0)	80.0 (70.0/80.0)	<0.001
Maximum systolic blood pressure during exercise (mmHg)	180.0 (160.0/200.0)	230.0 (230.0/240.0)	<0.001
Maximum diastolic blood pressure during exercise (mmHg)	75.0 (70.0/80.0)	80.0 (80.0/90.0)	<0.001
Exercise parameters			
VO$_2$ maximum during exercise	45.4 (39.8/50.4)	43.2 (35.8/49.5)	0.040
Respiratory exchange ratio (RER)	1.15 (1.11/1.20)	1.15 (1.11/1.21)	0.515
Maximum lactate value	9.40 (7.75/11.21)	9.41 (7.85/11.16)	0.974
Echocardiographic parameters			
Left ventricular hypertrophy	203 (19.2%)	30 (39.0%)	<0.001
Left ventricular mass	164.3 (132.8/200.8)	207.1 (181.4/227.7)	<0.001

Table 3. Cont.

Parameters	Normal Blood Pressure Response According to ACSM Classification (n = 1060; 93.2%)	Exaggerated Blood Pressure Response According to ACSM Classification (n = 77; 6.8%)	p-Value
Aortic valve regurgitation	60 (5.7%)	14 (18.2%)	<0.001
Mitral valve regurgitation	571 (53.9%)	56 (72.7%)	0.001
Tricuspid valve regurgitation	141 (13.3%)	17 (22.1%)	0.090
Pulmonary valve regurgitation	101 (9.5%)	7 (9.1%)	1.000
Heart volume in total (mL)	774.6 (642.5/919.0)	965.4 (829.4/1047.0)	<0.001
Heart volume related to body weight (mL/kg)	11.5 (10.3/12.5)	11.7 (10.4/12.6)	0.350
Left ventricular ejection fraction (%)	65.0 (62.0/69.0)	66.0 (62.0/72.0)	0.037
Left ventricular end-diastolic diameter (cm)	49.0 (46.0/53.0)	52.0 (49.5/54.5)	<0.001
Left atrial area (cm^2)	13.6 (11.4/15.7)	15.7 (14.4/18.2)	<0.001
Right atrial area (cm^2)	13.5 (11.2/15.8)	16.5 (14.0/18.5)	<0.001
Tricuspid annular plane systolic excursion (TAPSE, cm)	2.50 (2.20/2.80)	2.6 (2.3/2.9)	0.001
Systolic pulmonary artery pulmonary pressure (mmHg)	20.0 (17.0/23.0)	22.0 (20.0/25.0)	<0.001
E/A quotient	2.7 (1.9/3.7)	2.1 (1.5/3.2)	<0.001
E/E' quotient	4.7 (4.0/5.7)	5.1 (4.1/6.4)	0.080

3.3. Comparison of Athletes with and without Exaggerated Blood Pressure Response (EBPR) during Exercise Testing

While the proportions of female athletes with and without EBPR according to ESC and AHA guidelines were widely balanced, comprising approximately 1/3 of the athletes with EBPR, the proportion of male athletes with EBPR according to ACSM was distinctly higher, with 85.7% of all individuals with EBPR (Table 3). CVRF nicotine abuse and obesity were both more prevalent in athletes with EBPR regardless of which definition of EBPR was chosen (Tables 1–3). The criteria regarding full effort during the exercise test did not differ between athletes with and without EBPR (Tables 1–3).

The proportion of athletes with EBPR increased with inclining age regardless of the chosen definition. Notably, EBPR was more often diagnosed due to maximum systolic in comparison to maximum diastolic blood pressure values during exercise (Figure 1B–D).

3.4. Prevalence of Left Ventricular Hypertrophy (LVH) in Athletes

LVH was approximately two-fold more frequent in athletes with EBPR than in those without (risk ratios (RR) 2.2, 1.8, and 2.0 when using the definitions of AHA guidelines, ESC guidelines, and ACSM guidelines, respectively).

Interestingly, aortic valve regurgitation and mitral valve regurgitation were both more prevalent in athletes with EBPR (Tables 1–3).

3.5. Association of Exaggerated Blood Pressure Response (EBPR) during Exercise Testing and Left Ventricular Hypertrophy (LVH) in Athletes

In addition, we computed logistic regression models in order to analyse associations between EBPR defined according to the different guidelines on the one hand and LVH on the other hand. While EBPR according to the definition of the AHA guidelines (OR 2.35

(95%CI 1.66–3.33), $p < 0.001$) and the ACSM guidelines (OR 1.81 (95%CI 1.05–3.09), $p = 0.031$) were independently (of age and sex) associated with LVH, EBPR defined according to the ESC guidelines (OR 1.49 (95%CI 1.00–2.23), $p = 0.051$) was not independently associated with LVH (Figure 2B, Table 4).

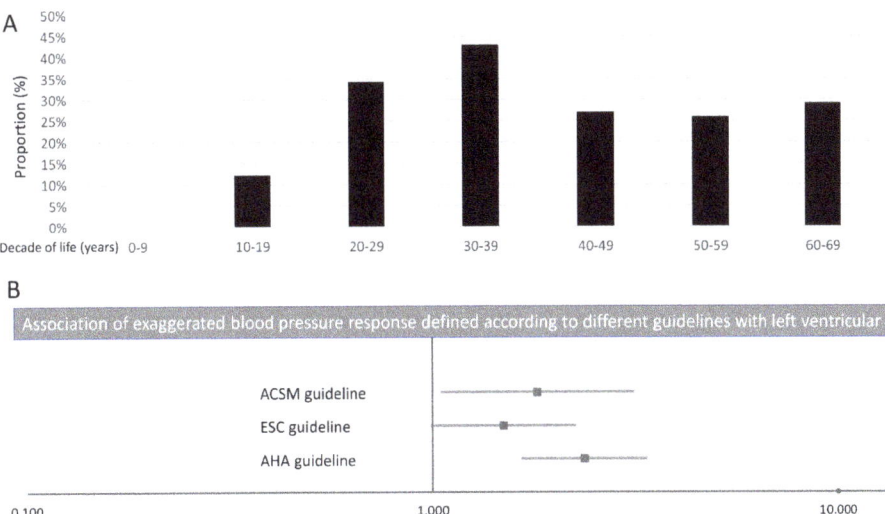

Figure 2. Exaggerated blood pressure response and left ventricular hypertrophy. Panel (**A**) Proportion of left ventricular hypertrophy stratified for age by decades. Panel (**B**) Association of exaggerated blood pressure response according to AHA, ESC, and ACSM guidelines with left ventricular hypertrophy.

Table 4. Association between of exaggerated blood pressure response, blood pressure values at rest, and maximum value during exercise on the one hand and left ventricular hypertrophy on the other hand (univariate and multivariate logistic regression model).

	Left Ventricular Hypertrophy			
	Univariate Regression Model		Multivariate Regression Model (Adjusted for Age and Sex)	
	OR (95% CI)	*p*-Value	OR (95% CI)	*p*-Value
AHA guideline classification of exaggerated blood pressure response	2.939 (2.127–4.060)	<0.001	2.351 (1.660–3.328)	<0.001
ESC guideline classification of exaggerated blood pressure response	2.171 (1.517–3.107)	<0.001	1.493 (0.998–2.232)	0.051
ACSM guideline classification of exaggerated blood pressure response	2.695 (1.663–4.367)	<0.001	1.805 (1.054–3.093)	0.031
Systolic blood pressure/MET slope (>6.2 mmHg/MET)	2.120 (1.449–3.101)	<0.001	2.257 (0.403–12.655)	0.355
Systolic blood pressure at rest (mmHg)	1.023 (1.010–1.036)	<0.001	1.016 (1.001–1.030)	0.033
Diastolic blood pressure at rest (mmHg)	1.025 (1.007–1.043)	0.005	1.011 (0.992–1.030)	0.253
Maximum systolic blood pressure during exercise (mmHg)	1.024 (1.018–1.030)	<0.001	1.026 (1.019–1.033)	<0.001
Maximum diastolic blood pressure during exercise (mmHg)	1.023 (1.007–1.040)	0.005	1.006 (0.989–1.024)	0.470

In addition, LVH was associated with systolic BP at rest and maximum systolic BP during exercise, but not with diastolic BP values (Table 4).

3.6. Prevalence of Exaggerated Blood Pressure Response (EBPR) during Exercise Testing and Left Ventricular Hypertrophy (LVH) in Adult Athletes

When focusing on the adult athletes only, 598 athletes (33.1% females; median age 23.0 (19.0–29.0) years) aged 18 years or older remained in the analysis. Among these, 180 (30.1%) had an LVH.

According to the guideline definitions, 170 (regardless of athletes' sex: 28.4%; 54 female athletes (27.3%); 116 male athletes (29.0%)) athletes were classified as EBPR according to AHA guidelines, 137 (regardless of athletes' sex: 22.9%; 54 female athletes (27.3%); 83 male athletes (20.8%)) according to ESC guidelines, and 65 (regardless of athletes' sex: 10.9%; 11 female athletes (5.6%); 54 male athletes (13.5%)) according to ACSM guidelines.

3.7. Association of Exaggerated Blood Pressure Response (EBPR) during Exercise Testing and Left Ventricular Hypertrophy (LVH) in Adult Athletes

In adult athletes, only the definition of EBPR according to AHA guidelines was independently predictive for LVH (univariate: OR 1.88 (95%CI 1.29–2.74), $p = 0.001$; multivariate: OR 1.96 (95% CI 1.32–2.90), $p = 0.001$). EBPR according to the ESC (univariate: OR 1.40 (95% CI 0.94–2.10), $p = 0.100$; multivariate: OR 1.44 (95%CI 0.93–2.22), $p = 0.104$) as well as ACSM guidelines (univariate: OR 1.64 (95% CI 0.97–2.79), $p = 0.067$; multivariate: OR 1.73 (95% CI 0.98–3.07), $p = 0.060$) were not associated with LVH independently of age and sex.

3.8. Prevalence of Exaggerated Blood Pressure Response (EBPR) during Exercise Testing Identified by Systolic BP/MET Slope Method with a Cutoff Value > 6.2 mmHg/MET

When using the systolic BP/MET slope method with a cutoff value > 6.2 mmHg/MET to define an EBPR in those 639 athletes, who underwent spiroergometric testing, we detected 386 athletes (60.4%) with normal BP response and 253 athletes with EBPR (regardless of athletes' sex: 39.6%; 80 female athletes (36.5%); 173 male athletes (41.2%)) (Table 5). LVH was more prevalent in athletes with than without EBPR (29.6% vs. 16.6%, $p < 0.001$).

Table 5. Patient characteristics of the 639 examined athletes with spiroergometry and without known arterial hypertension stratified for exaggerated blood pressure response according to systolic blood pressure/MET slope.

Parameters	Normal Blood Pressure Response According to Systolic Blood Pressure/MET Slope (≤6.2 mmHg/MET) (n = 386; 60.4%)	Exaggerated Blood Pressure Response According to Systolic Blood Pressure/MET Slope (>6.2 mmHg/MET) (n = 253; 39.6%)	p-Value
Age (in years)	18.0 (15.0/22.0)	24.0 (18.0/36.5)	<0.001
Female sex	139 (36.0%)	80 (31.6%)	0.253
Body height (cm)	175.0 (168.0/182.0)	178.0 (170.0/184.0)	0.014
Body weight (kg)	66.8 (58.0/77.7)	76.0 (66.0/85.9)	<0.001
Body mass index (kg/m^2)	21.7 (20.2/24.0)	23.8 (22.3/26.0)	<0.001
Body fat (%)	12.4 (8.2/16.6)	12.2 (9.2/17.1)	0.003
Leading athletes at a regional or national level	295 (76.4%)	135 (53.4%)	<0.001
Training years	7.0 (5.0/10.0)	10.0 (5.0/14.0)	<0.001
Cardiovascular risk factors			
Nicotine abuse	8 (2.1%)	18 (7.1%)	0.003
Obesity	1 (0.3%)	9 (3.6%)	0.001

Table 5. *Cont.*

Parameters	Normal Blood Pressure Response According to Systolic Blood Pressure/MET Slope (≤6.2 mmHg/MET) (n = 386; 60.4%)	Exaggerated Blood Pressure Response According to Systolic Blood Pressure/MET Slope (>6.2 mmHg/MET) (n = 253; 39.6%)	p-Value
Blood pressure values			
Systolic blood pressure (mmHg)	120.0 (110.0/125.0)	120.0 (110.0/125.0)	0.908
Diastolic blood pressure (mmHg)	70.0 (60.0/75.0)	70.0 (65.0/80.0)	0.003
Maximum systolic blood pressure during exercise (mmHg)	170.0 (155.0/180.0)	210.0 (190.0/220.0)	<0.001
Maximum diastolic blood pressure during exercise (mmHg)	70.0 (65.0/80.0)	80.0 (70.0/80.0)	<0.001
Exercise parameters			
VO_2 maximum during exercise	47.5 (42.1/51.5)	41.9 (36.2/47.0)	<0.001
Respiratory exchange ratio (RER)	1.15 (1.10/1.19)	1.15 (1.11/1.21)	0.037
Maximum lactate value	9.36 (7.67/11.24)	9.51 (7.89/11.24)	0.533
Echocardiographic parameters			
Left ventricular hypertrophy	64 (16.6%)	75 (29.6%)	<0.001
Left ventricular mass	163.6 (132.3/199.3)	188.1 (153.4/220.6)	<0.001
Aortic valve regurgitation	20 (5.2%)	22 (8.7%)	0.080
Mitral valve regurgitation	203 (52.6%)	169 (66.8%)	<0.001
Tricuspid valve regurgitation	46 (12.0%)	51 (20.2%)	0.010
Pulmonary valve regurgitation	34 (8.8%)	25 (9.9%)	0.647
Heart volume in total (mL)	772.0 (639.0/908.5)	896.4 (732.9/1000.0)	<0.001
Heart volume related to body weight (mL/kg)	11.4 (10.2/12.4)	11.4 (10.2/12.3)	0.803
Left ventricular ejection fraction (%)	65.0 (62.0/69.0)	66.0 (63.0/69.0)	0.041
Left ventricular end-diastolic diameter (cm)	50.0 (46.0/53.0)	51.0 (47.0/54.0)	<0.001
Left atrial area (cm^2)	13.5 (11.0/15.3)	14.9 (12.6/17.4)	<0.001
Right atrial area (cm^2)	13.3 (11.1/15.5)	14.9 (12.8/17.9)	<0.001
Tricuspid annular plane systolic excursion (TAPSE, cm)	2.40 (2.20/2.70)	2.60 (2.40/2.90)	<0.001
Systolic pulmonary artery pulmonary pressure (mmHg)	20.0 (16.5/23.0)	21.5 (18.0/24.0)	0.002
E/A quotient	2.5 (1.9/3.4)	2.4 (1.6/3.6)	0.111
E/E' quotient	4.7 (4.0/5.7)	4.9 (4.1/5.9)	0.193

3.9. Association of Exaggerated Blood Pressure Response (EBPR) during Exercise Testing Identified by Systolic BP/MET Slope Method with a Cutoff Value > 6.2 mmHg/MET and Left Ventricular Hypertrophy (LVH) in Athletes

Systolic BP/MET slope > 6.2 mmHg/MET was associated with LVH in the univariate regression analysis (OR 2.12 (95% CI 1.45–3.10), $p < 0.001$), but this association remained not significant after adjustment for age and sex (OR 2.26 (95% CI 0.40–12.66),

$p = 0.355$). Sex-specific analyses revealed a significant association of systolic BP/MET slope > 6.2 mmHg/MET with LVH in male (OR 2.348 (95%CI 1.472–3.746), $p < 0.001$) in contrast to female athletes (OR 1.706 (95%CI 0.878–3.315), $p = 0.115$).

In contrast, in the 398 adult athletes with spiroergometric evaluation, systolic BP/MET slope > 6.2 mmHg/MET was associated with LVH in both, the univariate (OR 1.67 (95% CI 1.07–2.60), $p = 0.023$) as well as multivariate logistic regression analysis adjusted for age and sex (OR 1.73 (95% CI 1.08–2.78), $p = 0.023$). However, sex-specific analyses also revealed sex-specific differences in adult athletes. While systolic BP/MET slope > 6.2 mmHg/MET was associated with LVH in male adult athletes (OR 1.848 (95% CI 1.079–3.166), $p = 0.025$), in females, no association was seen (OR 1.325 (95% CI 0.603–2.913), $p = 0.484$).

4. Discussion

Arterial hypertension is accompanied by substantially increased cardiovascular morbidity and mortality [2,4,7,9,17,49–51].

Among individuals who were not categorized as patients with arterial hypertension [12–15] a number of individuals revealed EBPR during exercise testing. The consequences of this phenomenon are not well elucidated, and study results are inconsistent. In previous investigations, a large number of different definitions of EBPR were used, hampering a clear interpretation of study results [1,4,17,25–37]. However, several studies have shown that individuals without known arterial hypertension who present with EBPR during the exercise testing are at increased risk to develop arterial hypertension in the future and might also be prone to develop cardiovascular events [1,4,17,25–37]. Three guideline definitions are currently available and valid: the AHA [23], the ESC [22,24], and the ACSM guidelines [20,21]. In this context, it is widely unclear from which study sample these definitions were derived and whether these definitions were able to predict cardiovascular morbidity, e.g., LVH, in athletes.

Thus, the objectives of our present study were to evaluate the prevalence of EBPR in athletes and which definition regarding EBPR during exercise testing was best/strongest associated with LVH in athletes without known arterial hypertension.

The main results of the study can be summarized as follows:

(I) EBPR was diagnosed between 6.8% and 19.6% of all athletes in our study according to the different guideline recommendations. Prevalence was highest when categorized according to the ESC guidelines (19.6%) and lowest according to the ACSM guidelines (6.8%).
(II) CVRF, such as nicotine abuse and obesity, were more prevalent in athletes with EBPR.
(III) The proportion of athletes with EBPR increased with inclining age regardless of the chosen definition.
(IV) EBPR was more often diagnosed due to maximum systolic in comparison to maximum diastolic BP values during exercise.
(V) Only the EBPR definition of the AHA guideline was able to predict LVH independently of age and sex in both the overall sample as well as in adult athletes as the only guideline recommended threshold.
(VI) In addition, the recently implemented systolic BP/MET slope method with a cutoff value > 6.2 mmHg/MET to define an EBPR, was able to predict LVH in adult athletes independently of age and sex.

Our study results reveal a large variation regarding the prevalence of EBPR according to the different guideline definitions in athletes without known arterial hypertension (variation of 12.8% according to different guideline recommendations). The prevalence was highest when categorized according to the ESC guidelines [22,24] (19.6%) and lowest when classified according to the ACSM guidelines [20,42] (6.8%). In contrast to the study of Caselli at al. [24], who reported that only a rate of 7.5% of the 1876 investigated athletes had an EBPR defined according to the ESC guidelines, we identified a frequency of 19.6% in the athletes presenting with EBPR according the ESC guidelines' definition. However, the differences between our results and the aforementioned study might be based on differences regarding the performance level of the examined athletes and athletes' ages in both studies.

As expected, CVRF, such as nicotine abuse and obesity, were in our study more prevalent in those athletes with EBPR. This finding is in line with the literature, reporting a close relation between obesity and elevated blood pressure [52,53]. Arterial hypertension is frequently observed in individuals who are obese [53]. In addition, smoking was strongly associated with arterial hypertension in several studies [54,55].

The proportion of athletes with EBPR increased significantly with inclining age regardless of the chosen definition. In this context, studies underlined a physiological increase in BP with age [4,56–58]. While at birth, the systolic and diastolic BP values are on average at levels of 70 mmHg and 50 mmHg, respectively [4,56,58], BP values rise progressively throughout childhood and adolescence [4,56–58]. As aforementioned, BP is substantially determined by body weight, and it is of key interest that BP in childhood has a strong impact on adult BP levels [4,57,58]. Individuals aged ≥70 years reach an average systolic BP of approximately 140 mmHg. Diastolic BP tends also to rise with the aging process but the intense of this increase is less steep and after the 50th life year, diastolic mean BP either inclines only slightly or even declines [4,56]. These changes in BP reflect normal age-dependent development, while BP deviations due to arterial hypertension could be detected in every period of life [4,56]. The association between a growing burden of arterial hypertension with increasing age is well known and described [4,6,56,59]. While in Germany, 10–35% of the citizens aged between 30 and 60 were diagnosed with arterial hypertension, the frequency increases to higher than 65% in people aged 60 years and older [8]. In light of the quoted literature, an age-dependent increase regarding the proportion of athletes with EBPR might be expected but could also be interpreted as an increasing number of athletes who might have undiagnosed or masked arterial hypertension.

In stress situations, the BP rises from resting to stress level depending on the exercise intensity and the affecting stressor [4,17,19,60]. The BP responses to exercise are a result of cardiac output and peripheral vascular resistance [61]. Cardiac output is elevated to provide oxygenated blood and nutrition for the active regions of the body according to increased demand [62]. During physical activity, BP values increase, whereby the rise in systolic BP values becomes more pronounced compared to diastolic BP. BP values generally increase to an exercise dependent and predetermined individual limit [1,4,17,61]. Normal systolic BP response in progressive exercise testing on a bicycle stress test comprise a systolic BP increase of approximately 7 to 10 mmHg per 25 watt workload incline [19]. Expected maximal BP values in bicycle testing are approximately 200/100 mmHg in healthy untrained adults in the general population and approximately 215/105 mmHg in those individuals who are older than 50 years [16]. Notably, only systolic BP values, not diastolic values, could be reliably measured with the standardly used non-invasive methods [1].

Thus, in our present study, it is of outstanding importance that EBPR was more often diagnosed due to maximum systolic in comparison to maximum diastolic BP values during exercise, although all of the guideline recommendations defined a diastolic threshold regarding EBPR [20–24].

Although three different guideline recommendations for the definition of EBPR are available, only the EBPR definition of the AHA guidelines [23] was able to predict LVH independently of age and sex in both the overall sample as well as in adult athletes only in our study. Nevertheless, despite this result, we do not think that the definition of EBPR as systolic BP > 210 mmHg in men, > 190 mmHg in women, and/or > 90 mmHg diastolic peak BP in both sexes [23] is well suited to identify individuals at risk and deduce further consequences as a singular diagnostic tool in athletes. From the experiences of daily routine in sports medicine, the defined systolic BP values regarding EBPR are too low for exercise testing in male and female athletes. In accordance with these experiences of daily practice, it has been reported in the literature that very fit and powerful athletes reach physiologically higher BP values during competition as well as exercise testing [4,16,19,63]. Although, systolic BP values ≥ 250 mmHg and diastolic BP values ≥ 120 mmHg were defined as stopping criteria for bicycle ergometry exercise testing [16,63,64]—especially in young athletes, who exceed these thresholds within their normal sports practice—a stop of the exercise testing even at this higher and rigid recommended thresholds (250/120 mmHg) seems limited in its usefulness and the decision to stop should be made individually [16,19,63].

In order to encounter these only-in-part useful definitions of EBPR for athletes, a workload-indexed EBPR definition was introduced by different authors with promising results [44–47]. Our study confirmed these results—that an EBPR defined according to the systolic BP/MET slope method with a cutoff value >6.2 mmHg/MET was able to predict LVH in adult athletes independently of age and sex. A threshold of 6.2 mmHg/MET was chosen since a systolic BP/MET slope >6.2 mmHg/MET was in the study of Hedman et al. associated with a 27% higher risk for mortality during a 20-year observational period in males compared to those with <4.3 mmHg/MET [44,46]. However, we detected sex-specific differences regarding this associations between EBPR defined according to the systolic BP/MET slope method with a cutoff value >6.2 mmHg/MET and LVH with significant associations in males and missing associations in females. In accordance, several studies revealed sex-specific differences regarding blood pressure response in males and females [65–67]. In studies, men had significantly higher systolic BP values at 50%, 75%, and 100% of maximum exercise efforts [67].

Nevertheless, although these recommended EBPR thresholds—defined by the three guidelines—seem only in part to be suitable for athletes (but more for the general untrained population), an identified EBPR and especially a prolonged and delayed decline in blood pressure after exercise testing could provide clues regarding a masked arterial hypertension or development of a manifest arterial hypertension in the future [4,63].

In athletes with EBPR and/or a prolonged and delayed decline in blood pressure after exercise testing, a 24 h blood pressure measurement could give important and valuable additional diagnostic information [15]. Where the threshold regarding EBPR in athletes from which further diagnostic procedures should be implemented is still controversial [16,19,63].

5. Conclusions

EBPR was diagnosed in between 6.8% and 19.6% of all athletes without known arterial hypertension. Prevalence was highest when athletes were categorized according to ESC guidelines (19.6%) and lowest when categorized according to ACSM guidelines (6.8%). The proportion of athletes with EBPR increased with inclining age regardless of the chosen definition. Only the EBPR definition of the AHA guidelines and the systolic blood pressure/MET slope method were associated with LVH independently of age and sex in adult athletes. However, the prognostic value of this association remains to be elucidated by sufficiently powered in-depth long-term studies. Such studies are also necessary to further evaluate the importance of the identification of EBPR in athletes and the significance of actual EBPR guidelines as diagnostic tools in young athletes.

Author Contributions: Conceptualization, K.K. and B.F.-B.; Data curation, K.K. and J.T.; Formal analysis, K.K.; Investigation, K.K.; Methodology, K.K.; Project administration, K.K.; Supervision, K.K.; Visualization, K.K.; Writing—original draft, K.K.; Writing—review & editing, K.K., K.H., L.d.C.C., J.T., F.S., C.S., F.H. and B.F.-B. All authors have read and agreed to the published version of the manuscript.

Funding: This research received no external funding.

Institutional Review Board Statement: The requirement for informed consent was waived as we used only anonymized retrospective data routinely collected during the health screening process. Studies in Germany involving a retrospective analysis of diagnostic standard data of anonymized patients do not require an ethics statement.

Informed Consent Statement: The requirement for informed consent was waived as we used only anonymized retrospective data routinely collected during the health screening process. Studies in Germany involving a retrospective analysis of diagnostic standard data of anonymized patients do not require an ethics statement.

Data Availability Statement: The data presented in this study are available upon request from the corresponding author.

Conflicts of Interest: The authors declare no conflict of interest.

References

1. Mancia, G.; Fagard, R.; Narkiewicz, K.; Redon, J.; Zanchetti, A.; Bohm, M.; Christiaens, T.; Cifkova, R.; De Backer, G.; Dominiczak, A.; et al. 2013 ESH/ESC guidelines for the management of arterial hypertension: The Task Force for the Management of Arterial Hypertension of the European Society of Hypertension (ESH) and of the European Society of Cardiology (ESC). *Eur. Heart J.* **2013**, *34*, 2159–2219. [CrossRef] [PubMed]
2. Schmieder, R.E. End organ damage in hypertension. *Dtsch. Arztebl. Int.* **2010**, *107*, 866–873. [CrossRef] [PubMed]
3. Kearney, P.M.; Whelton, M.; Reynolds, K.; Muntner, P.; Whelton, P.K.; He, J. Global burden of hypertension: Analysis of worldwide data. *Lancet* **2005**, *365*, 217–223. [CrossRef]
4. Keller, K.; Stelzer, K.; Ostad, M.A.; Post, F. Impact of exaggerated blood pressure response in normotensive individuals on future hypertension and prognosis: Systematic review according to PRISMA guideline. *Adv. Med. Sci.* **2017**, *62*, 317–329. [CrossRef]
5. Wolf-Maier, K.; Cooper, R.S.; Banegas, J.R.; Giampaoli, S.; Hense, H.W.; Joffres, M.; Kastarinen, M.; Poulter, N.; Primatesta, P.; Rodriguez-Artalejo, F.; et al. Hypertension prevalence and blood pressure levels in 6 European countries, Canada, and the United States. *JAMA* **2003**, *289*, 2363–2369. [CrossRef]
6. Go, A.S.; Mozaffarian, D.; Roger, V.L.; Benjamin, E.J.; Berry, J.D.; Borden, W.B.; Bravata, D.M.; Dai, S.; Ford, E.S.; Fox, C.S.; et al. Heart disease and stroke statistics–2013 update: A report from the American Heart Association. *Circulation* **2013**, *127*, e6–e245. [CrossRef]
7. Sacks, F.M.; Campos, H. Dietary therapy in hypertension. *N. Engl. J. Med.* **2010**, *362*, 2102–2112. [CrossRef]
8. Mahfoud, F.; Himmel, F.; Ukena, C.; Schunkert, H.; Bohm, M.; Weil, J. Treatment strategies for resistant arterial hypertension. *Dtsch. Arztebl. Int.* **2011**, *108*, 725–731. [CrossRef]
9. Mancia, G.; De Backer, G.; Dominiczak, A.; Cifkova, R.; Fagard, R.; Germano, G.; Grassi, G.; Heagerty, A.M.; Kjeldsen, S.E.; Laurent, S.; et al. 2007 ESH-ESC Practice Guidelines for the Management of Arterial Hypertension: ESH-ESC Task Force on the Management of Arterial Hypertension. *J. Hypertens.* **2007**, *25*, 1751–1762. [CrossRef]
10. Moebus, S.; Hanisch, J.; Bramlage, P.; Losch, C.; Hauner, H.; Wasem, J.; Jockel, K.H. Regional differences in the prevalence of the metabolic syndrome in primary care practices in Germany. *Dtsch. Arztebl. Int.* **2008**, *105*, 207–213. [CrossRef]
11. Niebauer, J.; Borjesson, M.; Carre, F.; Caselli, S.; Palatini, P.; Quattrini, F.; Serratosa, L.; Adami, P.E.; Biffi, A.; Pressler, A.; et al. Recommendations for participation in competitive sports of athletes with arterial hypertension: A position statement from the sports cardiology section of the European Association of Preventive Cardiology (EAPC). *Eur. Heart J.* **2018**, *39*, 3664–3671. [CrossRef]
12. Whelton, P.K.; Carey, R.M.; Aronow, W.S.; Casey, D.E., Jr.; Collins, K.J.; Dennison Himmelfarb, C.; DePalma, S.M.; Gidding, S.; Jamerson, K.A.; Jones, D.W.; et al. 2017 ACC/AHA/AAPA/ABC/ACPM/AGS/APhA/ASH/ASPC/NMA/PCNA Guideline for the Prevention, Detection, Evaluation, and Management of High Blood Pressure in Adults: Executive Summary: A Report of the American College of Cardiology/American Heart Association Task Force on Clinical Practice Guidelines. *J. Am. Coll. Cardiol.* **2018**, *71*, 2199–2269. [CrossRef]
13. Cuspidi, C. Is exaggerated exercise blood pressure increase related to masked hypertension? *Am. J. Hypertens.* **2011**, *24*, 861. [CrossRef]
14. Matthews, C.E.; Pate, R.R.; Jackson, K.L.; Ward, D.S.; Macera, C.A.; Kohl, H.W.; Blair, S.N. Exaggerated blood pressure response to dynamic exercise and risk of future hypertension. *J. Clin. Epidemiol.* **1998**, *51*, 29–35. [CrossRef]
15. Williams, B.; Mancia, G.; Spiering, W.; Agabiti Rosei, E.; Azizi, M.; Burnier, M.; Clement, D.L.; Coca, A.; de Simone, G.; Dominiczak, A.; et al. 2018 ESC/ESH Guidelines for the management of arterial hypertension. *Eur. Heart J.* **2018**, *39*, 3021–3104. [CrossRef]
16. Kindermann, W. Arterielle Hypertonie. In *Sportkardiologie*; Kindermann, W., Dickhuth, H.-H., Niess, A., Röcker, K., Urhausen, A., Eds.; Steinkopf-Verlag: Darmstadt, Germany, 2007; Volume 2, pp. 227–240.
17. Mancia, G.; De Backer, G.; Dominiczak, A.; Cifkova, R.; Fagard, R.; Germano, G.; Grassi, G.; Heagerty, A.M.; Kjeldsen, S.E.; Laurent, S.; et al. 2007 Guidelines for the management of arterial hypertension: The Task Force for the Management of Arterial Hypertension of the European Society of Hypertension (ESH) and of the European Society of Cardiology (ESC). *Eur. Heart J.* **2007**, *28*, 1462–1536. [CrossRef]
18. Le, V.V.; Mitiku, T.; Sungar, G.; Myers, J.; Froelicher, V. The blood pressure response to dynamic exercise testing: A systematic review. *Prog. Cardiovasc. Dis.* **2008**, *51*, 135–160. [CrossRef]
19. Sieira, M.C.; Ricart, A.O.; Estrany, R.S. Blood pressure response to exercise testing. *Apunts Med. Esport* **2010**, *45*, 191–200.
20. Lea & Febiger. *American College of Sports Medicine. ACSM's Guidelines for Exercise Testing and Prescription*; Wolters Kluwer: Philadelphia, PA, USA, 1991; Volume 4.
21. Currie, K.D.; Floras, J.S.; La Gerche, A.; Goodman, J.M. Exercise Blood Pressure Guidelines: Time to Re-evaluate What is Normal and Exaggerated? *Sports Med.* **2018**, *48*, 1763–1771. [CrossRef]
22. Pelliccia, A.; Sharma, S.; Gati, S.; Back, M.; Borjesson, M.; Caselli, S.; Collet, J.P.; Corrado, D.; Drezner, J.A.; Halle, M.; et al. 2020 ESC Guidelines on sports cardiology and exercise in patients with cardiovascular disease. *Eur. Heart J.* **2021**, *42*, 17–96. [CrossRef]

23. Fletcher, G.F.; Ades, P.A.; Kligfield, P.; Arena, R.; Balady, G.J.; Bittner, V.A.; Coke, L.A.; Fleg, J.L.; Forman, D.E.; Gerber, T.C.; et al. Exercise standards for testing and training: A scientific statement from the American Heart Association. *Circulation* **2013**, *128*, 873–934. [CrossRef]
24. Caselli, S.; Serdoz, A.; Mango, F.; Lemme, E.; Vaquer Segui, A.; Milan, A.; Attenhofer Jost, C.; Schmied, C.; Spataro, A.; Pelliccia, A. High blood pressure response to exercise predicts future development of hypertension in young athletes. *Eur. Heart J.* **2019**, *40*, 62–68. [CrossRef]
25. Laukkanen, J.A.; Kurl, S.; Rauramaa, R.; Lakka, T.A.; Venalainen, J.M.; Salonen, J.T. Systolic blood pressure response to exercise testing is related to the risk of acute myocardial infarction in middle-aged men. *Eur. J. Prev. Cardiol.* **2006**, *13*, 421–428. [CrossRef]
26. Laukkanen, J.A.; Rauramaa, R. Systolic blood pressure during exercise testing and the risk of sudden cardiac death. *Int. J. Cardiol.* **2013**, *168*, 3046–3047. [CrossRef]
27. Gupta, M.P.; Polena, S.; Coplan, N.; Panagopoulos, G.; Dhingra, C.; Myers, J.; Froelicher, V. Prognostic significance of systolic blood pressure increases in men during exercise stress testing. *Am. J. Cardiol.* **2007**, *100*, 1609–1613. [CrossRef]
28. Kjeldsen, S.E.; Mundal, R.; Sandvik, L.; Erikssen, G.; Thaulow, E.; Erikssen, J. Supine and exercise systolic blood pressure predict cardiovascular death in middle-aged men. *J. Hypertens.* **2001**, *19*, 1343–1348. [CrossRef]
29. Schultz, M.G.; Otahal, P.; Cleland, V.J.; Blizzard, L.; Marwick, T.H.; Sharman, J.E. Exercise-induced hypertension, cardiovascular events, and mortality in patients undergoing exercise stress testing: A systematic review and meta-analysis. *Am. J. Hypertens.* **2013**, *26*, 357–366. [CrossRef]
30. Allison, T.G.; Cordeiro, M.A.; Miller, T.D.; Daida, H.; Squires, R.W.; Gau, G.T. Prognostic significance of exercise-induced systemic hypertension in healthy subjects. *Am. J. Cardiol.* **1999**, *83*, 371–375. [CrossRef]
31. Kurl, S.; Laukkanen, J.A.; Rauramaa, R.; Lakka, T.A.; Sivenius, J.; Salonen, J.T. Systolic blood pressure response to exercise stress test and risk of stroke. *Stroke A J. Cereb. Circ.* **2001**, *32*, 2036–2041. [CrossRef]
32. Palatini, P. Blood pressure behaviour during physical activity. *Sports Med.* **1988**, *5*, 353–374. [CrossRef]
33. Syme, A.N.; Blanchard, B.E.; Guidry, M.A.; Taylor, A.W.; Vanheest, J.L.; Hasson, S.; Thompson, P.D.; Pescatello, L.S. Peak systolic blood pressure on a graded maximal exercise test and the blood pressure response to an acute bout of submaximal exercise. *Am. J. Cardiol.* **2006**, *98*, 938–943. [CrossRef]
34. Wilson, N.V.; Meyer, B.M. Early prediction of hypertension using exercise blood pressure. *Prev. Med.* **1981**, *10*, 62–68. [CrossRef]
35. Singh, J.P.; Larson, M.G.; Manolio, T.A.; O'Donnell, C.J.; Lauer, M.; Evans, J.C.; Levy, D. Blood pressure response during treadmill testing as a risk factor for new-onset hypertension. The Framingham heart study. *Circulation* **1999**, *99*, 1831–1836. [CrossRef] [PubMed]
36. Smith, R.G.; Rubin, S.A.; Ellestad, M.H. Exercise hypertension: An adverse prognosis? *J. Am. Soc. Hypertens. JASH* **2009**, *3*, 366–373. [CrossRef] [PubMed]
37. Levy, D.; Garrison, R.J.; Savage, D.D.; Kannel, W.B.; Castelli, W.P. Prognostic implications of echocardiographically determined left ventricular mass in the Framingham Heart Study. *N. Engl. J. Med.* **1990**, *322*, 1561–1566. [CrossRef] [PubMed]
38. Okwuosa, T.M.; Soliman, E.Z.; Lopez, F.; Williams, K.A.; Alonso, A.; Ferdinand, K.C. Left ventricular hypertrophy and cardiovascular disease risk prediction and reclassification in blacks and whites: The Atherosclerosis Risk in Communities Study. *Am. Heart J.* **2015**, *169*, 155–161. [CrossRef] [PubMed]
39. Scharhag, J.; Lollgen, H.; Kindermann, W. Competitive sports and the heart: Benefit or risk? *Dtsch. Arztebl. Int.* **2013**, *110*, 14–23. [CrossRef]
40. Galderisi, M.; Cardim, N.; D'Andrea, A.; Bruder, O.; Cosyns, B.; Davin, L.; Donal, E.; Edvardsen, T.; Freitas, A.; Habib, G.; et al. The multi-modality cardiac imaging approach to the Athlete's heart: An expert consensus of the European Association of Cardiovascular Imaging. *Eur. Heart J. Cardiovasc. Imaging* **2015**, *16*, 353. [CrossRef]
41. Marwick, T.H.; Gillebert, T.C.; Aurigemma, G.; Chirinos, J.; Derumeaux, G.; Galderisi, M.; Gottdiener, J.; Haluska, B.; Ofili, E.; Segers, P.; et al. Recommendations on the use of echocardiography in adult hypertension: A report from the European Association of Cardiovascular Imaging (EACVI) and the American Society of Echocardiography (ASE). *Eur. Heart J. Cardiovasc. Imaging* **2015**, *16*, 577–605. [CrossRef]
42. Williams, B.; Mancia, G.; Spiering, W.; Agabiti Rosei, E.; Azizi, M.; Burnier, M.; Clement, D.L.; Coca, A.; de Simone, G.; Dominiczak, A.; et al. 2018 ESC/ESH Guidelines for the management of arterial hypertension: The Task Force for the management of arterial hypertension of the European Society of Cardiology and the European Society of Hypertension: The Task Force for the management of arterial hypertension of the European Society of Cardiology and the European Society of Hypertension. *J. Hypertens.* **2018**, *36*, 1953–2041. [CrossRef]
43. Lang, R.M.; Badano, L.P.; Mor-Avi, V.; Afilalo, J.; Armstrong, A.; Ernande, L.; Flachskampf, F.A.; Foster, E.; Goldstein, S.A.; Kuznetsova, T.; et al. Recommendations for cardiac chamber quantification by echocardiography in adults: An update from the American Society of Echocardiography and the European Association of Cardiovascular Imaging. *J. Am. Soc. Echocardiogr.* **2015**, *28*, 1–39.e14. [CrossRef]
44. Bauer, P.; Kraushaar, L.; Hoelscher, S.; Weber, R.; Akdogan, E.; Keranov, S.; Dorr, O.; Nef, H.; Hamm, C.W.; Most, A. Blood Pressure Response and Vascular Function of Professional Athletes and Controls. *Sports Med. Int. Open* **2021**, *5*, E45–E52. [CrossRef]
45. Bauer, P.; Kraushaar, L.; Dorr, O.; Nef, H.; Hamm, C.W.; Most, A. Workload-indexed blood pressure response to a maximum exercise test among professional indoor athletes. *Eur. J. Prev. Cardiol.* **2021**, *28*, 1487–1494. [CrossRef]

46. Hedman, K.; Cauwenberghs, N.; Christle, J.W.; Kuznetsova, T.; Haddad, F.; Myers, J. Workload-indexed blood pressure response is superior to peak systolic blood pressure in predicting all-cause mortality. *Eur. J. Prev. Cardiol.* **2020**, *27*, 978–987. [CrossRef]
47. Hedman, K.; Lindow, T.; Elmberg, V.; Brudin, L.; Ekstrom, M. Age- and gender-specific upper limits and reference equations for workload-indexed systolic blood pressure response during bicycle ergometry. *Eur. J. Prev. Cardiol.* **2021**, *28*, 1360–1369. [CrossRef]
48. *ACSM's Guidelines for Exercise Testing: American College of Sports Medicine*; Wolters Kluwer: Philadelphia, PA, USA, 2010.
49. MacMahon, S.; Peto, R.; Cutler, J.; Collins, R.; Sorlie, P.; Neaton, J.; Abbott, R.; Godwin, J.; Dyer, A.; Stamler, J. Blood pressure, stroke, and coronary heart disease. Part 1, Prolonged differences in blood pressure: Prospective observational studies corrected for the regression dilution bias. *Lancet* **1990**, *335*, 765–774. [CrossRef]
50. Lewington, S.; Clarke, R.; Qizilbash, N.; Peto, R.; Collins, R. Age-specific relevance of usual blood pressure to vascular mortality: A meta-analysis of individual data for one million adults in 61 prospective studies. *Lancet* **2002**, *360*, 1903–1913.
51. Middeke, M. Antihypertensive drug therapy: Where do we stand? *Der. Internist.* **2015**, *56*, 230–239. [CrossRef]
52. Rocchini, A.P.; Key, J.; Bondie, D.; Chico, R.; Moorehead, C.; Katch, V.; Martin, M. The effect of weight loss on the sensitivity of blood pressure to sodium in obese adolescents. *N. Engl. J. Med.* **1989**, *321*, 580–585. [CrossRef]
53. Heymsfield, S.B.; Wadden, T.A. Mechanisms, Pathophysiology, and Management of Obesity. *N. Engl. J. Med.* **2017**, *376*, 254–266. [CrossRef]
54. Carter, B.D.; Abnet, C.C.; Feskanich, D.; Freedman, N.D.; Hartge, P.; Lewis, C.E.; Ockene, J.K.; Prentice, R.L.; Speizer, F.E.; Thun, M.J.; et al. Smoking and mortality—beyond established causes. *N. Engl. J. Med.* **2015**, *372*, 631–640. [CrossRef] [PubMed]
55. Bowman, T.S.; Gaziano, J.M.; Buring, J.E.; Sesso, H.D. A prospective study of cigarette smoking and risk of incident hypertension in women. *J. Am. Coll. Cardiol.* **2007**, *50*, 2085–2092. [CrossRef] [PubMed]
56. Whelton, P.K. Epidemiology of hypertension. *Lancet* **1994**, *344*, 101–106. [CrossRef]
57. Jackson, L.V.; Thalange, N.K.; Cole, T.J. Blood pressure centiles for Great Britain. *Arch. Dis. Child.* **2007**, *92*, 298–303. [CrossRef] [PubMed]
58. Lee, J.; Rajadurai, V.S.; Tan, K.W. Blood pressure standards for very low birthweight infants during the first day of life. *Arch. Dis. Child. Fetal Neonatal Ed.* **1999**, *81*, F168–F170. [CrossRef] [PubMed]
59. Hajjar, I.; Kotchen, T.A. Trends in prevalence, awareness, treatment, and control of hypertension in the United States, 1988-2000. *JAMA J. Am. Med. Assoc.* **2003**, *290*, 199–206. [CrossRef] [PubMed]
60. Jordan, J. Pathophysiology of hypertension: What are our current concepts? *Der. Internist.* **2015**, *56*, 219–223. [CrossRef] [PubMed]
61. Balady, G.J.; Arena, R.; Sietsema, K.; Myers, J.; Coke, L.; Fletcher, G.F.; Forman, D.; Franklin, B.; Guazzi, M.; Gulati, M.; et al. Clinician's Guide to cardiopulmonary exercise testing in adults: A scientific statement from the American Heart Association. *Circulation* **2010**, *122*, 191–225. [CrossRef]
62. Schultz, M.G.; Sharman, J.E. Exercise Hypertension. *Pulse* **2014**, *1*, 161–176. [CrossRef]
63. Gibbons, R.J.; Balady, G.J.; Bricker, J.T.; Chaitman, B.R.; Fletcher, G.F.; Froelicher, V.F.; Mark, D.B.; McCallister, B.D.; Mooss, A.N.; O'Reilly, M.G.; et al. ACC/AHA 2002 guideline update for exercise testing: Summary article. A report of the American College of Cardiology/American Heart Association Task Force on Practice Guidelines (Committee to Update the 1997 Exercise Testing Guidelines). *J. Am. Coll. Cardiol.* **2002**, *40*, 1531–1540. [CrossRef]
64. Löllgen, H.; Gerke, R. Belastungs-EKG (Ergometrie). *Herzschr. Elektrophys.* **2008**, *19*, 98–106. [CrossRef]
65. Bauer, P.; Kraushaar, L.; Dorr, O.; Nef, H.; Hamm, C.W.; Most, A. Sex differences in workload-indexed blood pressure response and vascular function among professional athletes and their utility for clinical exercise testing. *Eur. J. Appl. Physiol.* **2021**, *121*, 1859–1869. [CrossRef]
66. Reckelhoff, J.F. Gender differences in the regulation of blood pressure. *Hypertension* **2001**, *37*, 1199–1208. [CrossRef]
67. Gleim, G.W.; Stachenfeld, N.S.; Coplan, N.L.; Nicholas, J.A. Gender differences in the systolic blood pressure response to exercise. *Am. Heart J.* **1991**, *121*, 524–530. [CrossRef]

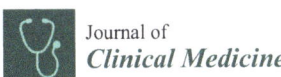

Article

Albumin-to-Alkaline Phosphatase Ratio as a Prognostic Biomarker for Spinal Fusion in Lumbar Degenerative Diseases Patients Undergoing Lumbar Spinal Fusion

Youfeng Guo [1], Haihong Zhao [1], Haowei Xu [1], Huida Gu [1], Yang Cao [1], Kai Li [2], Ting Li [3], Tao Hu [1,*], Shanjin Wang [1], Weidong Zhao [1] and Desheng Wu [1,*]

[1] Department of Spine Surgery, Shanghai East Hospital, School of Medicine, Tongji University, Shanghai 200092, China
[2] Key Laboratory of Inorganic Coating Materials CAS, Shanghai Institute of Ceramics, Chinese Academy of Sciences, Shanghai 200050, China
[3] Institute of Biomedical Engineering, Chinese Academy of Medical Sciences and Peking Union Medical College, Tianjin 300192, China
* Correspondence: dr_hutao@tongji.edu.cn (T.H.); 1300116@tongji.edu.cn (D.W.)

Abstract: Objective: To determine if preoperative albumin-alkaline phosphatase ratio (AAPR) is predictive of clinical outcomes in patients with degenerative lumbar diseases undergoing lumbar fusion. Method: 326 patients undergoing posterior lumbar decompression and fusion were retrospectively analyzed. The cumulative grade was calculated by summing the Pfirrmann grades of all lumbar discs. Grouping was based on the 50th percentile of cumulative grade. The relationship between AAPR, intervertebral disc degeneration (IDD) severity, and fusion rate was explored using correlation analyses and logistic regression models. Meanwhile, the ROC curve evaluated the discrimination ability of AAPR in predicting severe degeneration and non-fusion. Results: High AAPR levels were significantly negatively correlated with severe degeneration and non-fusion rate. A multivariate binary logistic analysis revealed that high preoperative AAPR was an independent predictor of severe degeneration and postoperative non-fusion (OR: 0.114; 95% CI: 0.027–0.482; p = 0.003; OR: 0.003; 95% CI: 0.0003–0.022; p < 0.001). The models showed excellent discrimination and calibration. The areas under the curve (AUC) of severe degeneration and non-fusion identified by AAPR were 0.635 and 0.643. Conclusion: The AAPR can help predict the severity of disc degeneration and the likelihood of non-fusion.

Keywords: degenerative lumbar diseases; albumin-to-alkaline phosphatase ratio; spinal fusion rate; prognostic marker

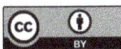

1. Introduction

The spine is the central axis bone of the human body and the pillar of the body. It serves as a weight-bearing, shock-absorbing, protective, and moving device and regulates various activities of the upper and lower limbs to maintain body balance. Many patients suffer from severe pain and dysfunction due to degenerative spinal diseases, and their motor ability will be further limited, which is a severe issue in sports medicine. Intervertebral Disc Degeneration (IDD) is a common cause of low back pain and discogenic low back pain, which places a heavy financial burden on families and society [1]. IDD is characterized by extensive morphological and mechanical changes in the disc, decreased intervertebral space height, disc structure destruction, reduced spinal mobility, and loss of disc biomechanical function [2,3]. These changes ultimately lead to low back pain and clinical symptoms. Among the primary biochemical changes associated with IDD are the diminished number and function of nucleus pulposus cells and the loss of matrix macromolecules such as type II collagen and proteoglycan in the extracellular matrix, causing the destruction of cells' conditions for survival [4,5]. Inflammatory mediators play a crucial role in this process [6]. Research has shown that inflammatory factors promote disc degeneration mainly by triggering an inflammatory response and apoptosis [7]. The inflammatory factors in intervertebral disc tissues interact in a cascade reaction, further aggravating the inflammatory response of intervertebral disc tissue and ultimately accelerating IDD. Spinal fusion is a classic treatment option for those who suffer from degenerative spinal diseases [8]. Some patients, however, suffer from spinal fusion failure after surgery, which leads to a loss of spinal stability and chronic pain caused by local abnormalities, directly affecting the patients' movement ability. Spinal fusion is a multifaceted and complex process that requires the involvement of many different cells, molecules, extracellular matrix (ECM) components, and growth factors. It is imperative for a successful spinal fusion to undergo the initial phase of the inflammatory process within the first two weeks [9]. Angiogenesis and osteogenesis may be disrupted by repeated excessive inflammation, however, posing a negative impact on bone formation.

The serum albumin (ALB) synthesized in the liver serves various physiological functions, including free radical scavenging, antioxidant, and vascular permeability [10]. Recent reports indicate that ALB is an accurate biomarker of underlying systemic inflammatory responses in organisms [9–11]. Additionally, alkaline phosphatase (ALP) is widely expressed in the liver, bones, and kidney and is involved in many physiological processes, such as bone mineralization, vascular calcification, and immune system function [12–14]. Studies suggest that biochemical analysis of peripheral blood and whole blood count extraction parameters can aid in the prognosis of diseases such as breast cancer and colorectal cancer [14,15]. The albumin to alkaline phosphatase ratio (AAPR), also based on serum albumin and alkaline phosphatase, can provide insights into systemic inflammation and nutritional status. AAPR has been studied in the context of many different diseases, including non-small cell lung cancer and cholangiocarcinoma, and a low AAPR was associated with a poor prognosis [16,17]. In addition, the activity or mass concentration of bone-specific ALP is closely related to the metabolism of pre-bone cells and forms a chemically classifiable bone matrix. The level of serum ALP activity is a commonly used marker for the evaluation of bone formation rather than the amount of a functional enzyme affecting osteogenesis. Fauran Clavel et al. found that the slowdown of osteogenesis could be demonstrated by the decrease of serum ALP activity [18]. Moreover, serum albumin has been shown to enhance osteogenic differentiation and bone formation in bone defect models [19,20]. Khalooeifard et al. found that increasing protein intake can improve vertebral fusion rate and enhance the recovery ability of patients after spinal fusion [21]. There was also a study showing that ALB decreased the risk of non-fusion rate [22]. As described above, AAPR can be derived or calculated with these two indicators. Moreover, the inflammatory reaction may affect bone metabolism, disrupt the dynamic balance between osteogenesis and osteoclasts, and result in poor bone healing. Hence, AAPR, an indicator reflecting the body systemic inflammatory response, also has the theoretical potential to be an osteogenic marker.

However, there has not been any research on the role of AAPR in degenerative lumbar discs. Therefore, the study of whether AAPR can be applied to lumbar disc degeneration patients is intriguing. Consequently, we conducted a retrospective study to study AAPR's correlation with the extent of lumbar disc degeneration before surgery and its prognostic value for postoperative fusion rate.

2. Materials and Methods

2.1. Study Design and Patient Characteristics

Prior to its implementation, ethical approval was obtained from the Shanghai East Hospital Ethics Committee. We enrolled all participants retrospectively and obtained informed consent in accordance with our institutional guidelines.

Three hundred and twenty-six lumbar spinal stenosis patients accompanied with lumbar disc herniation who received lumbar fusion surgery were retrospectively analyzed from May 2019 to May 2020. The following criteria were used to select participants:

(1) lower back pain symptoms of lumbar disc herniation and lumbar spinal stenosis; (2) a positive straight leg elevation test or neurological dysfunction (lack of movement, numbness, or lack of reflexes in the lower extremities); (3) MRI findings of disc herniation or spinal stenosis should also correspond to the findings of all participating participants; (4) patients intending to undergo single segmental fusion. Participants who met the following criteria were excluded from the study: (1) a history of spinal deformity, spinal infection, injury, or tumor; (2) the corresponding disc segment had been surgically fused; (3) known history of chronic diseases of lungs, kidneys, or liver; (4) Known inflammatory conditions (such as osteomyelitis, polychondritis, rheumatoid arthritis, etc.).

We collected data on routine clinical variables such as demographics, radiographic findings (intervertebral disc calcification and disc degeneration), and biochemical tests such as uric acid (UA). The presence of intervertebral disc calcification was assessed by lumbar CT. The above information is obtained from our center's electronic record-keeping system and imaging system. A standard posterior lumbar posterior decompression and fusion was performed in all cases, including instrumentation and bone grafting. Moreover, follow-up radiography was prescribed for the patients after discharge. The imaging system collected lumbar CT data from patients two years after spinal fusion surgery to assess fusion rate. Spinal fusion rate was evaluated by an experienced radiologist without prior knowledge of clinical information through CT images according to the evaluation system proposed by Siepe [23].

2.2. Albumin-to-Alkaline Phosphatase Ratio (AAPR) and Disc Degeneration Assessment

We performed routine blood tests on the patient within three days before surgery and recorded relevant data. AAPR is defined as the serum albumin/serum alkaline phosphatase ratio. The Pfirrmann grading system was used by magnetic resonance imaging (MRI) to evaluate the degree of disc degeneration [24], and the cumulative grade is calculated by summarizing the five discs' grades. All MRI images were read blindly by three experienced spine surgeons. Grouping was based on the median of cumulative grade.

2.3. Statistical Analysis

The continuous data were expressed as mean ± standard deviation (SD) and categorical data were presented as frequencies and percentages. The Chi-square and nonparametric tests were used to compare baseline characteristics between groups. Univariate and multivariate analyses were performed by binary logistic regression models to assess the prognostic effect of variables and estimate odds ratios (OR) with 95% confidence intervals (CI). Hosmer–Lemeshow goodness of fit test was used to assess the model fit (Hosmer-Lemeshow statistic ≥ 0.05). The receiver operating characteristic (ROC) curve and the area under the ROC curve (AUC) were also performed to assess the predictive ability of the built models. At the same time, ROC analysis determined AAPR's predictive power and the optimal cut-off value. p-values for linear trends were calculated using the quartile median values. Collected data were encoded into SPSS 26.0 and analyzed.

3. Results

3.1. Patient Demographics and Outcomes

The baseline characteristics of study participants are shown in Table 1. There were 185 women (56.7%) among the patients with an average age of 63.48. The mean BMI of the patients was 24.80 kg/m^2. There were significant differences in the following factors: age ($p < 0.001$), ALP ($p < 0.001$), RBP ($p < 0.001$), AST ($p = 0.048$), lumbar CT value ($p < 0.001$), AAPR ($p < 0.001$), fusion rate ($p = 0.001$), and the prevalence of hypertension ($p = 0.042$), disc calcification ($p < 0.001$) and osteoporosis ($p = 0.018$) between the high score group (accumulative grade > 18) and the low score group (accumulative grade ≤ 18). No significant differences were observed among the two groups regarding gender distribution, BMI, VAS, the length of hospital stay, hematological indicators other than ALP, AST and RBP, smoking history, etc.

Table 1. Demographic characteristics of patients with disc degeneration disease.

	All	Low Score Group (Accumulative Grade ≤ 18)	High Score Group (Accumulative Grade > 18)	p-Value
Subjects, n (%)	326	179	147	
Age (year)	63.48 ± 13.38	60.49 ± 14.93	67.11 ± 10.13	<0.001
Gender				0.562
Male, n (%)	141 (43.3)	80 (44.7)	61 (41.5)	
Female, n (%)	185 (56.7)	99 (55.3)	86 (58.5)	
BMI (kg/m^2)	24.80 ± 3.54	24.96 ± 3.49	24.60 ± 3.60	0.371
Smoking (y)	42 (12.9)	22 (12.3)	20 (13.6)	0.724
Alcohol abuse (y)	27 (8.3)	11 (6.1)	16 (10.9)	0.122
Hypertension (y)	155 (47.5)	76 (42.5)	79 (53.7)	0.042
DM (y)	57 (17.5)	30 (16.8)	27 (18.4)	0.704
CHD (y)	40 (12.3)	24 (13.4)	16 (10.9)	0.490
Osteoporosis (y)	115 (35.3)	53 (29.6)	62 (42.2)	0.018
Calcification (y)	164 (50.3)	60 (33.5)	104 (70.7)	<0.001
ALB (g/L)	42.49 ± 3.29	42.56 ± 3.19	42.41 ± 3.41	0.923
ALP (U/L)	74.18 ± 27.27	68.65 ± 24.02	80.90 ± 29.47	<0.001
AAPR	0.64 ± 0.22	0.69 ± 0.24	0.58 ± 0.17	<0.001
Calcium (mmol/L)	2.26 ± 0.10	2.25 ± 0.09	2.27 ± 0.10	0.092
Phosphorus (mmol/L)	1.14 ± 0.17	1.15 ± 0.16	1.14 ± 0.17	0.505
FBG (mmol/L)	5.54 ± 1.47	5.45 ± 1.36	5.65 ± 1.60	0.394
BUN (mmol/L)	6.04 ± 1.77	6.05 ± 1.73	6.02 ± 1.82	0.547
Scr (μmol/L)	72.33 ± 23.22	72.09 ± 21.65	72.62 ± 25.06	0.779
UA (μmol/L)	320.44 ± 82.57	323.42 ± 80.03	316.82 ± 85.69	0.597
ALT (U/L)	19.51 ± 14.34	20.12 ± 16.06	18.77 ± 11.92	0.549
AST (U/L)	19.12 ± 8.64	18.75 ± 9.80	19.56 ± 6.99	0.048
RBP (mg/L)	41.26 ± 9.54	42.83 ± 9.49	39.35 ± 9.27	<0.001
Fusion (y)	230 (70.6)	140 (78.2)	90 (61.2)	0.001
VAS	3.91 ± 1.84	3.73 ± 1.84	4.13 ± 1.84	0.067
Hospital stay (day)	12.21 ± 4.39	12.20 ± 4.36	12.21 ± 4.45	0.854
CT value (HU)	131.26 ± 49.20	140.51 ± 52.51	120.01 ± 42.35	<0.001

Values are expressed as n (%) or mean ± SD. BMI, body mass index; VAS, visual analogue scale; AAPR, albumin-to-alkaline phosphatase ratio; FBG, fasting blood glucose; CHD, coronary heart disease; DM, diabetes mellitus; ALT, alanine transaminase; AST, aspartate transaminase; RBP, retinol-binding Protein; UA, uric acid; BUN, blood urea nitrogen; Scr, serum creatinine.

3.2. IDD Severity Classification and Association with AAPR

Table 2 illustrates the distribution of disc grades among the target population. There were 41.7%, 35.9%, and 32.5% of grades for L1/2, L2/3, and L3/4, respectively, which were smaller than 4 (2, 3, and 3). For L4/5 and L5/S1, however, the majority (38.0% and 43.9%) were equal to or greater than 4. At the same time, the low score group showed the same trend as the whole population. On the other hand, all discs except L1/2 scored more than or equal to 4 in the high score group.

We defined mild to moderate degeneration as a score of less than 4 and severe degeneration as a score of more than or equal to 4. As shown in Table 3, the mean levels of LMR were substantially lower in the severe degeneration group (Pfirrmann grade ≥ 4) compared with the mild to moderate degeneration group (Pfirrmann grade < 4) in all lumbar discs except L5/S1. In addition, correlation analysis showed that LMR was significantly correlated with age, osteoporosis, calcification, Scr, VAS, CT value, non-fusion rate, and accumulative grade in all demographic and clinical parameters in Table 4. It is worth mentioning that there is a borderline positive correlation between LMR and UA. The LMR did not show any significant correlation with the length of hospital stay.

Table 2. The Pfirrmann grading system for lumbar disc degeneration.

	1	2	3	4	5
All (n = 326)					
L1/2	0	136 (41.7)	106 (32.5)	50 (15.3)	34 (10.4)
L2/3	0	79 (24.2)	117 (35.9)	78 (23.9)	52 (16.0)
L3/4	1 (0.3)	49 (15.0)	106 (32.5)	105 (32.2)	65 (19.9)
L4/5	0	24 (7.4)	82 (25.2)	124 (38.0)	96 (29.4)
L5/S1	0	27 (8.3)	53 (16.3)	103 (31.6)	143 (43.9)
Low score group (n = 179)					
L1/2	0	114 (63.7)	47 (26.3)	14 (7.8)	4 (2.2)
L2/3	0	77 (43.0)	81 (45.3)	19 (10.6)	2 (1.1)
L3/4	1 (0.6)	49 (27.4)	90 (50.3)	37 (20.7)	2 (1.1)
L4/5	0	24 (13.4)	64 (35.8)	74 (41.3)	17 (9.5)
L5/S1	0	27 (15.1)	42 (23.5)	65 (36.3)	45 (25.1)
High score group (n = 147)					
L1/2	0	22 (15.0)	59 (40.1)	36 (24.5)	30 (20.4)
L2/3	0	2 (1.4)	36 (24.5)	59 (40.1)	50 (34.0)
L3/4	0	0	16 (10.9)	68 (46.3)	63 (42.9)
L4/5	0	0	18 (12.2)	50 (34.0)	79 (53.7)
L5/S1	0	0	11 (7.5)	38 (25.9)	98 (66.7)

Values are expressed as n (%).

Table 3. The relationship between the severity of individual disc degeneration and AAPR/.

		AAPR	p
L1/2	Pfirrmann grade < 4	0.65 ± 0.21	0.003
	Pfirrmann grade ≥ 4	0.59 ± 0.22	
L2/3	Pfirrmann grade < 4	0.68 ± 0.23	<0.001
	Pfirrmann grade ≥ 4	0.58 ± 0.18	
L3/4	Pfirrmann grade < 4	0.70 ± 0.25	<0.001
	Pfirrmann grade ≥ 4	0.58 ± 0.17	
L4/5	Pfirrmann grade < 4	0.68 ± 0.19	<0.001
	Pfirrmann grade ≥ 4	0.62 ± 0.23	
L5/S1	Pfirrmann grade < 4	0.67 ± 0.23	0.181
	Pfirrmann grade ≥ 4	0.63 ± 0.21	

Values are expressed as mean ± SD; AAPR, albumin-to-alkaline phosphatase ratio.

3.3. Univariable and Multivariable Analysis on Predictive Factors of Severe Disc Degeneration

Univariable binary logistic regression analysis based on the entire patient cohort showed that each additional unit of age ($p < 0.001$), hypertension ($p = 0.043$), osteoporosis ($p = 0.019$), calcification ($p < 0.001$), RBP ($p = 0.001$), and AAPR ($p < 0.001$) was significantly associated with severe disc degeneration (Table 5). ROC analysis was performed by defining severe disc degeneration as an endpoint, with the AUC(AAPR) being 0.652 (95% CI: 0.593–0.712) and the difference being statistically significant ($p < 0.001$) (Figure 1a). It is found that the optimal critical value for AAPR is 0.68, while the maximum approximate index is calculated at this point (0.251). Multivariable binary logistic regression model 1 built on clinical parameters further demonstrated that every one unit of increase in RBP (OR: 0.948; 95% CI: 0.919-0.977; $p = 0.001$), AAPR (OR: 0.114; 95% CI: 0.027-0.482; $p = 0.003$), and the occurrence of CHD (OR: 0.360; 95% CI: 0.155-0.834; $p = 0.017$) and disc calcification (OR: 3.215; 95% CI: 1.848-5.594; $p < 0.001$) were determined to be independent predictors of severe disc degeneration. Moreover, AAPR did not interact significantly with calcification, CAD, or RBP in the one-way ANOVA ($p > 0.05$). This model is also capable of calibration and discrimination ($p > 0.05$ and $p < 0.05$, respectively). The area under ROC curve is 0.782 (Figure 1c). At the same time, trend analysis showed that the higher the AAPR, the lower the risk of severe disc degeneration ($p = 0.010$; Table 6).

Table 4. Correlation of AAPR with demographic and clinical parameters.

	r	p
Age	−0.110	0.046
Gender	0.070	0.210
BMI	0.028	0.611
Smoking	0.026	0.640
Alcohol abuse	−0.070	0.209
Hypertension	−0.045	0.417
DM	−0.014	0.796
CHD	−0.058	0.295
Osteoporosis	−0.167	0.002
Calcification	−0.422	<0.001
Calcium	0.025	0.656
phosphorus	0.080	0.150
FBG	−0.034	0.546
BUN	0.046	0.408
Scr	0.179	0.001
UA	0.108	0.052
ALT	−0.019	0.728
AST	−0.064	0.249
RBP	0.036	0.521
Non-fusion	−0.132	0.017
VAS	−0.132	0.017
Hospital stay, day	0.087	0.118
CT value	0.198	<0.001
Accumulative grade	−0.379	<0.001

BMI, body mass index; VAS, visual analogue scale; AAPR, albumin-to-alkaline phosphatase ratio; FBG, fasting blood glucose; CHD, coronary heart disease; DM, diabetes mellitus; ALT, alanine transaminase; AST, aspartate transaminase; RBP, retinol-binding protein; UA, uric acid; BUN, blood urea nitrogen; Scr, serum creatinine.

Table 5. Univariate and multivariate analysis model 1 of risk factors for severe degeneration.

Variables	Univariate		Multivariate	
	OR (95% CI)	p	OR (95% CI)	p
Age (year)	1.042 (1.023–1.062)	<0.001	1.027 (0.999–1.055)	0.062
Gender (male)	0.878 (0.565–1.364)	0.562	0.953 (0.478–1.903)	0.892
BMI	0.971 (0.913–1.034)	0.358	0.979 (0.903–1.061)	0.604
Smoking	1.124 (0.587–2.151)	0.724	1.492 (0.623–3.574)	0.369
Alcohol abuse	1.865 (0.837–4.155)	0.127	2.037 (0.735–5.646)	0.172
Hypertension	1.574 (1.015–2.443)	0.043	1.179 (0.649–2.141)	0.588
DM	1.117 (0.630–1.982)	0.704	0.935 (0.397–2.201)	0.877
CHD	0.789 (0.402–1.548)	0.490	0.360 (0.155–0.834)	0.017
Osteoporosis	1.734 (1.096–2.742)	0.019	1.045 (0.581–1.880)	0.883
Calcification	4.797 (2.993–7.689)	<0.001	3.215 (1.848–5.594)	<0.001
AAPR	0.055 (0.015–0.194)	<0.001	0.114 (0.027–0.482)	0.003
Calcium	6.241 (0.649–59.996)	0.113	14.486 (0.796–263.562)	0.071
phosphorus	0.618 (0.166–2.308)	0.474	1.456 (0.296–7.161)	0.644
FBG	1.096 (0.944–1.274)	0.229	1.080 (0.868–1.344)	0.489
BUN	0.988 (0.873–1.118)	0.850	0.975 (0.822–1.157)	0.773
Scr	1.001 (0.992–1.010)	0.839	1.004 (0.988–1.021)	0.590
UA	0.999 (0.996–1.002)	0.472	1.001 (0.997–1.004)	0.755
ALT	0.993 (0.977–1.009)	0.405	0.996 (0.961–1.032)	0.832
AST	1.011 (0.985–1.038)	0.408	1.003 (0.947–1.061)	0.928
RBP	0.960 (0.937–0.984)	0.001	0.948 (0.919–0.977)	0.001

BMI, body mass index; AAPR, albumin-to-alkaline phosphatase ratio; FBG, fasting blood glucose; CHD, coronary heart disease; DM, diabetes mellitus; ALT, alanine transaminase; AST, aspartate transaminase; RBP, retinol-binding protein; UA, uric acid; BUN, blood urea nitrogen; Scr, serum creatinine.

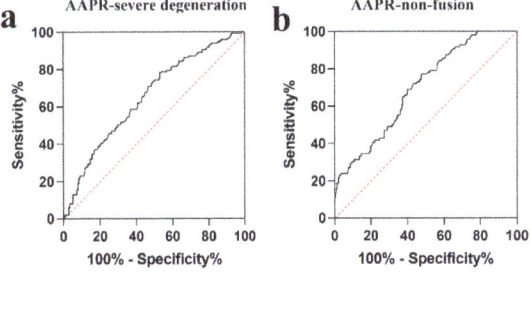

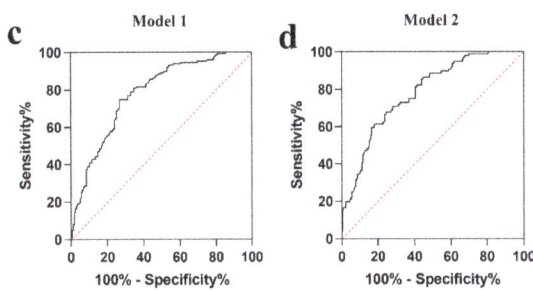

Figure 1. Receiver operating characteristic (ROC) curve to determine the predictive performance of AAPR for severe degeneration (**a**) and non-fusion (**b**). ROC curve analysis of severe degeneration (**c**) and non-fusion models (**d**) (see Tables 5 and 7 for included variables).

Table 6. Association of severe degeneration and non-fusion with AAPR.

Variable	Cases	Model 1 (Degeneration Model)		Model 2 (Non-Fusion Model)	
		OR [95% CI]	p for Trend	OR [95% CI]	p for Trend
		AAPR (Median [Range])			
Q1 (0.42 [≤0.49])	82	Reference		Reference	
Q2 (0.56 [0.49–0.61])	81	0.632 [0.306–1.306]		0.653 [0.320–1.334]	
Q3 (0.67 [0.61–0.75])	82	0.731 [0.342–1.563]		0.400 [0.184–0.873]	
Q4 (0.85 [>0.75])	81	0.316 [0.139–0.719]	0.010	0.103 [0.038–0.277]	<0.001

AAPR, albumin-to-alkaline phosphatase ratio.

3.4. Univariable and Multivariable Analysis on Risk Factors of Non-Fusion

Univariable binary logistic regression analysis based on the entire patient cohort showed that each additional unit of AAPR ($p < 0.001$) and phosphorus ($p = 0.002$) were significantly associated with postoperative non-fusion rate, as shown in Table 7. ROC analysis was performed by defining non-fusion as an endpoint, with the AUC(AAPR) being 0.695 (95% CI: 0.636–0.755) and the difference being statistically significant ($p < 0.001$) (Figure 1b). The optimal cut-off value for AAPR is 0.63. After adjustment by all covariable estimates, multivariate binary logistic regression analysis model 2 showed that for every one unit increase in UA (OR: 1.005; 95% CI: 1.001-1.010; $p = 0.014$), phosphorus (OR: 16.677; 95% CI: 2.794–99.552; $p = 0.002$), AAPR (OR: 0.003; 95% CI: 0.0003–0.022; $p < 0.001$), and the prevalence of CHD (OR: 0.357; 95% CI: 0.128–0.998; $p = 0.049$) could be independent prognostic factors for non-fusion in patients with lumbar disease undergoing lumbar fusion surgery. At the time, the one-way ANOVA showed no significant interactions between AAPR and UA, CHD, or phosphorus. In addition, this model has effective calibration and discrimination ($p > 0.05$ and $p < 0.05$, respectively). The area under ROC curve of the model is 0.781 (Figure 1d). Trend analysis showed that the higher the AAPR, the lower the risk of a non-fusion rate ($p < 0.001$; Table 6).

Table 7. Univariate and multivariate analysis model 2 of risk factors for non-fusion.

Variables	Univariate		Multivariate	
	OR (95% CI)	p	OR (95% CI)	p
Age (year)	0.995 (0.977–1.013)	0.569	0.987 (0.960–1.014)	0.345
Gender (male)	0.630 (0.385–1.031)	0.066	0.570 (0.261–1.247)	0.159
BMI	0.973 (0.909–1.042)	0.432	0.959 (0.880–1.046)	0.345
Smoking	1.086 (0.538–2.191)	0.819	1.915 (0.743–4.936)	0.179
Alcohol abuse	0.826 (0.337–2.023)	0.675	0.808 (0.262–2.489)	0.710
Hypertension	0.855 (0.530–1.379)	0.520	1.101 (0.582–2.081)	0.767
DM	0.742 (0.385–1.432)	0.374	0.666 (0.237–1.873)	0.441
CHD	0.470 (0.200–1.102)	0.082	0.357 (0.128–0.998)	0.049
Osteoporosis	1.222 (0.746–2.002)	0.426	1.129 (0.591–2.156)	0.713
Calcification	1.581 (0.977–2.559)	0.062	0.834 (0.439–1.586)	0.580
AAPR	0.009 (0.002–0.047)	<0.001	0.003 (0.0003–0.022)	<0.001
Calcium	1.616 (0.144–18.189)	0.697	0.397 (0.017–9.500)	0.569
phosphorus	9.892 (2.270–43.106)	0.002	16.677 (2.794–99.552)	0.002
FBG	1.024 (0.873–1.201)	0.770	1.104 (0.868–1.405)	0.418
BUN	0.985 (0.859–1.128)	0.823	1.007 (0.837–1.212)	0.938
Scr	0.988 (0.976–1.001)	0.062	0.996 (0.976–1.016)	0.673
UA	1.001 (0.998–1.004)	0.531	1.005 (1.001–1.010)	0.014
ALT	1.002 (0.986–1.018)	0.808	0.988 (0.952–1.025)	0.510
AST	1.014 (0.987–1.041)	0.318	1.016 (0.959–1.076)	0.595
RBP	0.988 (0.963–1.014)	0.356	0.986 (0.956–1.016)	0.344

BMI, body mass index; AAPR, albumin-to-alkaline phosphatase ratio; FBG, fasting blood glucose; CHD, coronary heart disease; DM, diabetes mellitus; ALT, alanine transaminase; AST, aspartate transaminase; RBP, retinol-binding protein; UA, uric acid; BUN, blood urea nitrogen; Scr, serum creatinine.

4. Discussion

In this study, we evaluated the prognostic value of AAPR after spinal fusion in patients with lumbar degenerative disease. According to analyses of patient characteristics, AAPR was closely related to non-fusion rate and severe disc degeneration. Binary logistic regression analysis showed that AAPR was an independent predictor of fusion rate and severe disc degeneration in the entire cohorts. Additionally, the levels of AAPR in the severe degeneration group were lower than that in the mild to moderate degeneration group, which verified the close relationship between AAPR and the severity of IDD to a certain extent. In addition, previous studies found that L4/5 or L5/S1 levels are the prone sites for lumbar diseases. In this study, we observed that the degree of disc degeneration was more severe at L4/5 and L5/S1 levels, and the cumulative grade was higher than L1/2, L2/3, and L3/4. At the same time, the ROC curve demonstrated that circulation AAPR levels could be used to predict severe IDD. Therefore, the low AAPR appeared to be an independent risk factor for severe disc degeneration. Additionally, AAPR is not the only factor contributing to disc degeneration and fusion rate. In the logistic regression analysis, serum phosphorus, UA, and CHD were also predictive factors for non-fusion, while the occurrence of CHD, disc calcification, and retinol-binding proteins appeared to have an impact on degeneration.

AAPR incorporates the two basic laboratory parameters, ALB and ALP, which are easily accessible and not too expensive. There is a high concentration of albumin in serum, which serves as a storage and transport system for many endogenous and exogenous substances [25]. It can reflect the human nutritional status and inflammatory state and be related to the severity of many diseases [26,27]. Several studies have demonstrated that ALB regulates inflammatory responses by binding to lipopolysaccharides and reactive oxygen species [28]. Moreover, data have been accumulating on the utility of albumin as a prognostic marker, including the prognostic value of different albumin parameters alone or when combined [29,30]. ALP catalyzes the hydrolysis of phosphate esters and is responsible for transferring phosphate groups, which are mainly produced in the liver and bone. ALP activity could reflect the metabolism and immunity of the body and be used as an immunometric [31,32]. ALP activity is increased in various hepatobiliary diseases, rickets, osteogenesis imperfecta, osteomalacia, etc. [33,34]. A higher level of ALP alone has been associated with a poor prognosis. It has become increasingly important to determine the level of alkaline phosphatase in serum in clinical medicine for the detection and monitoring of many diseases. However, there is no study on the correlation between serum ALP and disc degeneration. It is worth mentioning that we separately analyzed the effects of ALB and ALP on severe disc degeneration and fusion rate (see the Supplementary Materials). The results showed that ALP was an independent predictor of non-fusion (OR: 1.047, 95% CI: 1.031–1.063, $p < 0.001$; Supplementary Materials Table S3), not severe disc degeneration (OR: 1.011, 95% CI: 0.999–1.022, $p = 0.079$; Supplementary Materials Table S1). However, Inose et al. found no significant correlation between serum ALP and non-fusion rate [22]. In sharp contrast, ALB is not significantly associated with severe degeneration (OR: 0.976, 95% CI: 0.889–1.072, $p = 0.612$; Supplementary Materials Table S2) and non-fusion rate (OR: 1.020, 95% CI: 0.927–1.122, $p = 0.685$; Supplementary Materials Table S4), which may be related to the sample size. Furthermore, this could be related to the nutritional status of the population included in this study, and there are no primary diseases such as liver and kidney disease, so the groups do not differ significantly. AAPR was applied in patients undergoing surgery for hepatocellular carcinoma for the first time by Chan et al.; this conclusion has been confirmed in the following studies [35,36]. Furthermore, previous research has shown that low levels of this indicator are associated with poor outcomes [37,38]. Despite varying cutoff values, these studies confirm that patients with high AAPR have a better prognosis than those with low AAPR. Therefore, we believe this ratio can provide insight into the microenvironment of local tissue inflammation and can be utilized to measure inflammation status in peripheral blood. It is undeniable that AAPR, a composite index, still has a particular clinical value, even though the effect of AAPR on fusion rate may be due to the mediating effect of ALP.

There were also other factors associated with fusion rate and disc degeneration identified. Multiple binary logistic regression showed that RBP acted as a protective factor against severe disc degeneration, while disc calcification as a risk factor. RBP, a vitamin transporter, is synthesized in the liver and is widely distributed in the blood, cerebrospinal fluid, urinary fluid, and other body fluids. RBP has a complex mechanism of action that exhibits both pro-oxidant and antioxidant effects [39,40]. However, no studies have been conducted on the relationship between RBP and IDD. In addition, intervertebral disc calcification occurs as a result of IDD, and it further aggravates the degeneration [41]. At the same time, the occurrence of calcification was positively correlated with advancing age and a reduced intervertebral height [42]. Calcium deposits in the cellular and extracellular space may cause cell death and decreased activity, resulting in disc degeneration, consistent with this study. A fascinating finding was that although CHD was negatively associated with severe disc degeneration, the effect of CHD on disc degeneration was not significant in models with only CHD and calcification. Furthermore, this study showed that preoperative high serum phosphorus levels were associated with fusion rate, while Shih et al. found no correlation between the fusion rate and the serum levels of calcium or phosphorus [43]. Additionally, we note that UA can enhance fusion rate, which may be related to its antioxidant abilities. Lastly, no significant influence of factors such as age or BMI on disc degeneration or fusion rate was detected, which may be the result of the small sample size.

However, this study has some limitations. Due to the fact that our cohort was a single-center retrospective one containing only Chinese patients, these results may not be generalizable to other populations. Therefore, it is suggested that further multicenter prospective studies be conducted. Additionally, the applicability of the current AAPR cut-off value to other conditions needs to be further examined. At the same time, we investigated the relationship between only one AAPR value and the severity of disc degeneration and fusion rate. Considering that serum AAPR may be affected by other factors, such as liver disease and diet, continuous monitoring may be necessary [44]. Third, larger sample sizes are necessary to test our results, primarily to determine whether or not the statistical significance of results is clinically significant and to measure the smallest clinically meaningful differences. A further research issue is how to exclude the effects of non-steroidal anti-inflammatory drugs, which have been taken by patients before surgery, on AAPR levels in vivo. In addition, since the included population mainly consisted of the elderly with the poor osteogenic ability and the follow-up period was two years, the fusion rate did not meet the expected results. Therefore, we will extend the follow-up period and examine more subtle characteristics of the elderly to verify the validity of this study.

5. Conclusions

The results of our study suggest that preoperative AAPR may be a prognostic predictor of postoperative fusion rate. At the same time, AAPR was related to severe disc degeneration, helping clinicians identify high-risk patients and guide individualized treatment.

Supplementary Materials: The following supporting information can be downloaded at: https://www.mdpi.com/article/10.3390/jcm11164719/s1, Table S1. Univariate and multivariate analysis model 3 (ALP) of risk factors for severe degeneration. Table S2. Univariate and multivariate analysis model 4 (ALB) of risk factors for severe degeneration. Table S3. Univariate and multivariate analysis model 5 (ALP) of risk factors for non-fusion. Table S4. Univariate and multivariate analysis model 6 (ALB) of risk factors for non-fusion.

Author Contributions: Y.G.: conceptualization, methodology, material preparation, data collection, analysis, and original draft preparation. H.Z., H.G., Y.C. and H.X.: investigation, data collection, and visualization. W.Z., T.L. and S.W.: development or design of methodology and creation of models. D.W., T.H. and K.L.: supervision and writing-reviewing and editing. All authors have read and agreed to the published version of the manuscript.

Funding: This study was supported by Shanghai East Hospital Xuri Young Excellent Talents Program 2019xrrcjh04 and Key Laboratory of Inorganic Coating Materials, Chinese Academy of Sciences (HX-2020-027).

Institutional Review Board Statement: The study was conducted in accordance with the Declaration of Helsinki and approved by the Shanghai East Hospital Ethics Committee (approval number EC. D (BG). 016. 02. 1).

Informed Consent Statement: Informed consent was obtained from all subjects involved in the study.

Data Availability Statement: The datasets generated and/or analyzed during the present study are available from the corresponding author upon reasonable request.

Conflicts of Interest: The authors have no relevant financial or non-financial interest to disclose.

References

1. Luoma, K.; Riihimäki, H.; Luukkonen, R.; Raininko, R.; Viikari-Juntura, E.; Lamminen, A. Low Back Pain in Relation to Lumbar Disc Degeneration. *Spine* **2000**, *25*, 487–492. [CrossRef] [PubMed]
2. Costi, J.J.; Stokes, I.; Gardner-Morse, M.; Iatridis, J. Frequency-Dependent Behavior of the Intervertebral Disc in Response to Each of Six Degree of Freedom Dynamic Loading. *Spine* **2008**, *33*, 1731–1738. [CrossRef] [PubMed]
3. Suthar, P. MRI Evaluation of Lumbar Disc Degenerative Disease. *J. Clin. Diagn. Res.* **2015**, *9*, TC04–TC09. [CrossRef] [PubMed]
4. Wang, S.; Rui, Y.; Lu, J.; Wang, C. Cell and molecular biology of intervertebral disc degeneration: Current understanding and implications for potential therapeutic strategies. *Cell Prolif.* **2014**, *47*, 381–390. [CrossRef] [PubMed]
5. Vergroesen, P.-P.; Kingma, I.; Emanuel, K.; Hoogendoorn, R.; Welting, T.; van Royen, B.; van Dieën, J.; Smit, T. Mechanics and biology in intervertebral disc degeneration: A vicious circle. *Osteoarthr. Cartil.* **2015**, *23*, 1057–1070. [CrossRef]
6. Molinos, M.; Almeida, C.R.; Caldeira, J.; Cunha, C.; Gonçalves, R.M.; Barbosa, M.A. Inflammation in intervertebral disc degeneration and regeneration. *J. R. Soc. Interface* **2015**, *12*, 20150429. [CrossRef] [PubMed]

7. Taniguchi, K.; Karin, M. NF-κB, inflammation, immunity and cancer: Coming of age. *Nat. Rev. Immunol.* **2018**, *18*, 309–324. [CrossRef] [PubMed]
8. Eck, J.C.; Sharan, A.; Ghogawala, Z.; Resnick, D.K.; Watters, W.C.; Mummaneni, P.V.; Dailey, A.T.; Choudhri, T.F.; Groff, M.W.; Wang, J.C.; et al. Guideline update for the performance of fusion procedures for degenerative disease of the lumbar spine. Part 7: Lumbar fusion for intractable low-back pain without stenosis or spondylolisthesis. *J. Neurosurg. Spine* **2014**, *21*, 42–47. [CrossRef] [PubMed]
9. Loi, F.; Córdova, L.A.; Pajarinen, J.; Lin, T.; Yao, Z.; Goodman, S.B. Inflammation, fracture and bone repair. *Bone* **2016**, *86*, 119–130. [CrossRef]
10. Małkowski, P.; Rozga, J.; Piątek, T. Human albumin: Old, new, and emerging applications. *Ann. Transplant.* **2013**, *18*, 205–217. [CrossRef] [PubMed]
11. Eckart, A.; Struja, T.; Kutz, A.; Baumgartner, A.; Baumgartner, T.; Zurfluh, S.; Neeser, O.; Huber, A.; Stanga, Z.; Mueller, B.; et al. Relationship of Nutritional Status, Inflammation, and Serum Albumin Levels during Acute Illness: A Prospective Study. *Am. J. Med.* **2020**, *133*, 713–722.e7. [CrossRef] [PubMed]
12. Vimalraj, S. Alkaline phosphatase: Structure, expression and its function in bone mineralization. *Gene* **2020**, *754*, 144855. [CrossRef]
13. Demer, L.L.; Tintut, Y. Inflammatory, Metabolic, and Genetic Mechanisms of Vascular Calcification. *Arter. Thromb. Vasc. Biol.* **2014**, *34*, 715–723. [CrossRef]
14. Estaki, M.; DeCoffe, D.; Gibson, D.L. Interplay between intestinal alkaline phosphatase, diet, gut microbes and immunity. *World J. Gastroenterol.* **2014**, *20*, 15650–15656. [CrossRef]
15. Bottini, A.; Berruti, A.; Brizzi, M.P.; Bersiga, A.; Generali, D.; Allevi, G.; Aguggini, S.; Bolsi, G.; Bonardi, S.; Bertoli, G.; et al. Pretreatment haemoglobin levels significantly predict the tumour response to primary chemotherapy in human breast cancer. *Br. J. Cancer* **2003**, *89*, 977–982. [CrossRef]
16. Li, D.; Yu, H.; Li, W. Albumin-to-alkaline phosphatase ratio at diagnosis predicts survival in patients with metastatic non-small-cell lung cancer. *OncoTargets Ther.* **2019**, *12*, 5241–5249. [CrossRef]
17. Nie, M.; Sun, P.; Chen, C.; Bi, X.; Wang, Y.; Yang, H.; Liu, P.; Li, Z.; Xia, Y.; Jiang, W. Albumin-to-Alkaline Phosphatase Ratio: A Novel Prognostic Index of Overall Survival in Cisplatin-based Chemotherapy-treated Patients with Metastatic Nasopharyngeal Carcinoma. *J. Cancer* **2017**, *8*, 809–815. [CrossRef]
18. Fauran-Clavel, M.; Oustrin, J. Alkaline phosphatase and bone calcium parameters. *Bone* **1986**, *7*, 95–99. [CrossRef]
19. Skaliczki, G.; Schandl, K.; Weszl, M.; Major, T.; Kovács, M.; Skaliczki, J.; Szendrői, M.; Dobó-Nagy, C.; Lacza, Z. Serum albumin enhances bone healing in a nonunion femoral defect model in rats: A computer tomography micromorphometry study. *Int. Orthop.* **2013**, *37*, 741–745. [CrossRef]
20. Horváthy, D.B.; Schandl, K.; Schwarz, C.M.; Renner, K.; Hornyák, I.; Szabó, B.T.; Niculescu-Morzsa, E.; Nehrer, S.; Dobó-Nagy, C.; Doros, A.; et al. Serum albumin-coated bone allograft (BoneAlbumin) results in faster bone formation and mechanically stronger bone in aging rats. *J. Tissue Eng. Regen. Med.* **2019**, *13*, 416–422. [CrossRef]
21. Khalooeifard, R.; Oraee-Yazdani, S.; Keikhaee, M.; Shariatpanahi, Z.V. Protein Supplement and Enhanced Recovery after Posterior Spine Fusion Surgery: A Randomized, Double-blind, Placebo-controlled Trial. *Clin. Spine Surg.* **2022**, *35*, E356–E362. [CrossRef] [PubMed]
22. Inose, H.; Yamada, T.; Mulati, M.; Hirai, T.; Ushio, S.; Yoshii, T.; Kato, T.; Kawabata, S.; Okawa, A. Bone Turnover Markers as a New Predicting Factor for Nonunion After Spinal Fusion Surgery. *Spine* **2018**, *43*, E29–E34. [CrossRef] [PubMed]
23. Siepe, C.J.; Stosch-Wiechert, K.; Heider, F.; Amnajtrakul, P.; Krenauer, A.; Hitzl, W.; Szeimies, U.; Stäbler, A.; Mayer, H.M. Anterior stand-alone fusion revisited: A prospective clinical, X-ray and CT investigation. *Eur. Spine J.* **2015**, *24*, 838–851. [CrossRef]
24. Pfirrmann, C.; Metzdorf, A.; Zanetti, M.; Hodler, J.; Boos, N. Magnetic Resonance Classification of Lumbar Intervertebral Disc Degeneration. *Spine* **2001**, *26*, 1873–1878. [CrossRef] [PubMed]
25. Farrugia, A. Albumin Usage in Clinical Medicine: Tradition or Therapeutic? *Transfus. Med. Rev.* **2010**, *24*, 53–63. [CrossRef]
26. Don, B.R.; Kaysen, G. Poor Nutritional Status and Inflammation: Serum Albumin: Relationship to Inflammation and Nutrition. *Semin. Dial.* **2004**, *17*, 432–437. [CrossRef] [PubMed]
27. Deveci, B.; Gazi, E. Relation Between Globulin, Fibrinogen, and Albumin with the Presence and Severity of Coronary Artery Disease. *Angiology* **2021**, *72*, 174–180. [CrossRef] [PubMed]
28. Belcher, D.A.; Williams, A.T.; Palmer, A.F.; Cabrales, P. Polymerized albumin restores impaired hemodynamics in endotoxemia and polymicrobial sepsis. *Sci. Rep.* **2021**, *11*, 10834. [CrossRef]
29. Galata, C.; Busse, L.; Birgin, E.; Weiß, C.; Hardt, J.; Reissfelder, C.; Otto, M. Role of Albumin as a Nutritional and Prognostic Marker in Elective Intestinal Surgery. *Can. J. Gastroenterol. Hepatol.* **2020**, *2020*, 7028216. [CrossRef]
30. Kawashima, A.; Yamamoto, Y.; Sato, M.; Nakata, W.; Kakuta, Y.; Ishizuya, Y.; Yamaguchi, Y.; Yamamoto, A.; Yoshida, T.; Takayama, H.; et al. FAN score comprising fibrosis-4 index, albumin–bilirubin score and neutrophil–lymphocyte ratio is a prognostic marker of urothelial carcinoma patients treated with pembrolizumab. *Sci. Rep.* **2021**, *11*, 21199. [CrossRef]
31. Singh, S.B.; Lin, H.C. Role of Intestinal Alkaline Phosphatase in Innate Immunity. *Biomolecules* **2021**, *11*, 1784. [CrossRef] [PubMed]
32. Vercalsteren, E.; Vranckx, C.; Lijnen, H.R.; Hemmeryckx, B.; Scroyen, I. Adiposity and metabolic health in mice deficient in intestinal alkaline phosphatase. *Adipocyte* **2018**, *7*, 149–155. [CrossRef]
33. Gutman, A.B. Serum alkaline phosphatase activity in diseases of the skeletal and hepatobiliary systems: A consideration of the current status. *Am. J. Med.* **1959**, *27*, 875–901. [CrossRef]

34. Peach, H.; Compston, J.E.; Vedi, S.; Horton, L.W. Value of plasma calcium, phosphate, and alkaline phosphatase measurements in the diagnosis of histological osteomalacia. *J. Clin. Pathol.* **1982**, *35*, 625–630. [CrossRef] [PubMed]
35. Chen, Z.-H.; Zhang, X.-P.; Cai, X.-R.; Xie, S.-D.; Liu, M.-M.; Lin, J.-X.; Ma, X.-K.; Chen, J.; Lin, Q.; Dong, M.; et al. The Predictive Value of Albumin-to-Alkaline Phosphatase Ratio for Overall Survival of Hepatocellular Carcinoma Patients Treated with Trans-Catheter Arterial Chemoembolization Therapy. *J. Cancer* **2018**, *9*, 3467–3478. [CrossRef] [PubMed]
36. Li, H.; Li, J.; Wang, J.; Liu, H.; Cai, B.; Wang, G.; Wu, H. Assessment of Liver Function for Evaluation of Long-Term Outcomes of Intrahepatic Cholangiocarcinoma: A Multi-Institutional Analysis of 620 Patients. *Front. Oncol.* **2020**, *10*, 525. [CrossRef] [PubMed]
37. Acikgoz, Y.; Bal, O.; Dogan, M. Albumin-to-Alkaline Phosphatase Ratio: Does It Predict Survival in Grade 1 and Grade 2 Neuroendocrine Tumors? *Pancreas* **2021**, *50*, 111–117. [CrossRef]
38. Li, J.; Zuo, M.; Zhou, X.; Xiang, Y.; Zhang, S.; Feng, W.; Liu, Y. Prognostic Significance of Preoperative Albumin to Alkaline Phosphatase Ratio in Patients with Glioblastoma. *J. Cancer* **2021**, *12*, 5950–5959. [CrossRef]
39. Chen, J.; Shao, Y.; Sasore, T.; Moiseyev, G.; Zhou, K.; Ma, X.; Du, Y.; Ma, J.-X. Interphotoreceptor Retinol-Binding Protein Ameliorates Diabetes-Induced Retinal Dysfunction and Neurodegeneration through Rhodopsin. *Diabetes* **2021**, *70*, 788–799. [CrossRef]
40. Wang, J.; Chen, H.; Liu, Y.; Zhou, W.; Sun, R.; Xia, M. Retinol binding protein 4 induces mitochondrial dysfunction and vascular oxidative damage. *Atherosclerosis* **2015**, *240*, 335–344. [CrossRef]
41. Rutges, J.; Duit, R.; Kummer, J.; Oner, F.; van Rijen, M.; Verbout, A.; Castelein, R.; Dhert, W.; Creemers, L. Hypertrophic differentiation and calcification during intervertebral disc degeneration. *Osteoarthr. Cartil.* **2010**, *18*, 1487–1495. [CrossRef] [PubMed]
42. Hawellek, T.; Hubert, J.; Hischke, S.; Rolvien, T.; Krause, M.; Püschel, K.; Rüther, W.; Niemeier, A. Microcalcification of lumbar spine intervertebral discs and facet joints is associated with cartilage degeneration, but differs in prevalence and its relation to age. *J. Orthop. Res.* **2017**, *35*, 2692–2699. [CrossRef]
43. Shih, T.-Y.; Wu, Y.-C.; Tseng, S.-C.; Chen, K.-H.; Pan, C.-C.; Lee, C.-H. Correlation between Preoperative Serum Levels of Calcium, Phosphate, and Intact Parathyroid Hormone and Radiological Outcomes in Spinal Interbody Fusion among End-Stage Renal Disease Patients. *J. Clin. Med.* **2021**, *10*, 5447. [CrossRef] [PubMed]
44. Sheng, G.; Peng, N.; Hu, C.; Zhong, L.; Zhong, M.; Zou, Y. The albumin-to-alkaline phosphatase ratio as an independent predictor of future non-alcoholic fatty liver disease in a 5-year longitudinal cohort study of a non-obese Chinese population. *Lipids Health Dis.* **2021**, *20*, 50. [CrossRef] [PubMed]

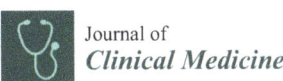

Article

The Modified Longitudinal Capsulotomy by Outside-In Approach in Hip Arthroscopy for Femoroplasty and Acetabular Labrum Repair—A Cohort Study

Shuang Cong [†], Jianying Pan [†], Guangxin Huang, Denghui Xie and Chun Zeng *

Department of Joint Surgery, Center for Orthopedic Surgery, The Third Affiliated Hospital of Southern Medical University, Guangzhou 510630, China
* Correspondence: 16624664320@163.com
† These authors contributed equally to this work.

Abstract: Hip arthroscopy is difficult to perform due to the limited arthroscopic view. To solve this problem, the capsulotomy is an important technique. However, the existing capsulotomy approaches were not perfect in the surgical practice. Thus, this study aimed to propose a modified longitudinal capsulotomy by outside-in approach and demonstrate its feasibility and efficacy in arthroscopic femoroplasty and acetabular labrum repair. A retrospective cohort study was performed and twenty-two postoperative patients who underwent hip arthroscopy in our hospital from January 2019 to December 2021 were involved in this study. The patients (14 females and 8 males) had a mean age of 38.26 ± 12.82 years old. All patients were diagnosed cam deformity and labrum tear in the operation and underwent arthroscopic femoroplasty and labrum repair by the modified longitudinal capsulotomy. The mean follow-up time was 10.4 months with a range of 6–12 months. There were no major complications, including infection, neurapraxias, hip instability or revision in any patients. The average mHHS were 74.4 ± 15.2, 78.2 ± 13.7 and 85.7 ± 14.5 in 3 months, 6 months and 12 months after surgery, respectively, which were all better than that before surgery (44.9 ± 8.6) ($p < 0.05$). The average VAS were 2.8 ± 1.2, 1.5 ± 0.6 and 1.2 ± 0.7 in 3 months, 6 months and 12 months after surgery, respectively, which were all lower than that before surgery (5.5 ± 2.0) ($p < 0.05$). The modified longitudinal capsulotomy by outside-in approach is proved to be a safe and feasible method for hip arthroscopy considering to the feasibility, efficacy and security. The arthroscopic femoroplasty and labrum repair can be performed conveniently by this approach and the patient reported outcomes after surgery were better that before surgery in short-term follow-up. This new method is promising and suggested to be widely used clinically.

Keywords: femoroacetabular impingement; hip arthroscopy; longitudinal capsulotomy; femoroplasty; labrum repair

Citation: Cong, S.; Pan, J.; Huang, G.; Xie, D.; Zeng, C. The Modified Longitudinal Capsulotomy by Outside-In Approach in Hip Arthroscopy for Femoroplasty and Acetabular Labrum Repair—A Cohort Study. *J. Clin. Med.* **2022**, *11*, 4548. https://doi.org/10.3390/jcm11154548

Academic Editors: Jiwu Chen and Yaying Sun

Received: 20 May 2022
Accepted: 26 July 2022
Published: 4 August 2022

Publisher's Note: MDPI stays neutral with regard to jurisdictional claims in published maps and institutional affiliations.

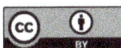

Copyright: © 2022 by the authors. Licensee MDPI, Basel, Switzerland. This article is an open access article distributed under the terms and conditions of the Creative Commons Attribution (CC BY) license (https://creativecommons.org/licenses/by/4.0/).

1. Introduction

Femoroacetabular impingement (FAI) is the most common disorder in young adults and patients with high activities, which can lead to inguinal pain and limited motion of hip joint [1]. Clinically, patients with symptom for more than 6 months, failure of conservative therapy and positive finding of labral tear on MRI were considered to be the indications of surgery. The surgical treatment of FAI was femoroplasty and/or acetabuloplasty under hip arthroscopy, to correct the osteophyte of cam deformity and/or pincer deformity, as well as repair the torn labrum [2]. However, only surgeons with high arthroscopic experience could product the hip arthroscopy, due to the hip's deep location, narrow joint space and high curvature of joint surface, which leading to a very limited arthroscopic view [3].

For the problems above, surgeons proposed many techniques to obtain satisfactory arthroscopic view, in which the most effective technique is the sufficient incision of the hip capsule [4]. In the previous reports, the typical approach is the interportal capsulotomy by the inside-out approach [5]. The hip joint is accessed through portals while the hip in traction and making a capsulotomy inside-out, which making the incision on hip capsule from lateral portal to anterior portal transversely [6].

However, the interportal capsulotomy by inside-out approach has some obvious limitations. Firstly, this approach is complicated to perform, especially in the case of severe pincer deformity. Secondly, the inside-out approach needs the guide of fluoroscopy, leading the patients and surgeons into radiation exposure. Finally, the arthroscopic view obtained by the interportal capsulotomy is not satisfactory enough for consequent femoroplasty and acetabular labrum repair.

Recently, some surgeons proposed a new approach for hip arthroscopy, the so-called outside-in approach [4,7–11]. By this approach, an extracapsular space anterior to the hip joint is established first. Then, surgeons perform the capsulotomy in this extracapsular space and enter the peripheral compartment of hip joint directly without hip traction and fluoroscopy. In the previous studies, many different kinds of capsulotomy were reported, including interportal capsulotomy and T-capsulotomy, as well as longitudinal capsulotomy [6,7].

In our surgical practice, the longitudinal capsulotomy was proved to obtain much better arthroscopic view than either interportal capsulotomy or T-capsulotomy, while it also has some limitations. In the longitudinal capsulotomy, the exposure of the head–neck junction is not enough for femoroplasty, and the acetabular rim is not enough for anchor insertion during the labrum repair. For this reason, we proposed a modified longitudinal capsulotomy which adding a small transverse incision at the proximal capsule to obtain a better arthroscopic view, to make the operating space large enough, and to let the consequent surgical procedure easy to perform.

This study aims to introduce our surgical procedures of the modified longitudinal capsulotomy by outside-in approach, and demonstrate its feasibility and efficacy in arthroscopic femoroplasty and acetabular labrum repair. The hypotheses of this study were the modified longitudinal capsulotomy by outside-in approach can obtain a better arthroscopic view than the traditional surgical approach, and femoroplasty and acetabular labrum repair can be achieved conveniently in the new approach.

2. Materials and Methods

2.1. Study Design and Participant

With institutional review board (IRB) approval, a retrospective cohort study was performed to collect the patients who underwent hip arthroscopy in our hospital from January 2019 to December 2021. The inclusion and exclusion criteria were as follows:

2.1.1. Inclusion Criteria

① Patients underwent hip arthroscopy in our hospital with diagnosis of FAI and acetabular labrum tear; ② patients underwent femoroplasty and labrum repair during surgery. For all the participants, the diagnosis of FAI and labrum tear were made according to the typical symptoms, physical examination, and radiologic information. Patients with symptom for more than 6 months, failure of conservative therapy, and positive finding of labral tear on MRI were considered to be the indications of the hip arthroscopic surgery.

2.1.2. Exclusion Criteria

① Patients with previous hip surgery history, avascular necrosis, traumatic history around the affected hip and other hip deformities; ② hip osteoarthritis as Tönnis grade > 1 on X-ray image; ③ autoimmune diseases or systemic inflammatory diseases, such as ankylosing spondylitis and rheumatic arthritis.

2.1.3. Sample Size Calculation

A post hoc power analysis was performed using G*Power software (version 3.1; Heinrich Heine University, North Rhine Westphalia, Germany; www.psychologie.hhu.de).

Based on the pre-analysis of mHHS before and after the surgery in this study, a minimum of 19 hips were needed to achieve a statistical power of 0.80 by setting $\alpha = 0.05$ and assuming an effect size of 0.5 to detect significant differences between pre and post operative mHHS.

2.2. Preoperative Assessment

For all the patients participating in our study, clinical and radiological assessment was performed in detail. The functional scores for clinical assessment included mHHS (modified Harris hip score) and VAS (Visual analogue score). The mHHS can provide an overall evaluation of the patient-reported clinical function, while the VAS can make a measurement for pain intensity. In the measurement of VAS, a 10-cm-long line is showed with the left end of the scale labeled 0 representing no pain, and the right end labeled 10 representing most severe pain. The patients mark the point on the line based on the severity of the pain they felt, ranging from 0 to 10 [12].

The radiological assessment included X-rays (anteroposterior view, frog view), 3D-CT and MRI (oblique axial view, oblique coronal view, and oblique sagittal view) [13–15]. The alpha angle and lateral center edge angle (LCEA) were measured in the X-rays according to previous studies [16,17]. Radiographic parameters were assessed by two surgeons separately blinded to each other (the first and the second authors) with Picture Archiving and Communication Systems (PACS), and the final result was made by a senior surgeon in cases of disagreement. If the alpha angle > 55° or LCEA > 40°, the femoroplasty or acetabuloplasty was performed in surgery [18,19]. The 3D-CT was used to identify the location and size of the cam and pincer deformity. The labrum and cartilage injuries were identified in MRI.

2.3. Surgical Procedure

2.3.1. Patient Positioning

All patients underwent hip arthroscopy in the supine position on the orthopedic traction bed, and all patients were under general anesthesia with full muscle relaxation. The perineal post was properly installed. The operative limb was positioned at 15° of internal rotation, neutral flexion/extension and abduction/adduction, while the contralateral limb was positioned at 45° of abduction. The feet were well-padded and fixed in traction boots.

2.3.2. Portal Placement

Before surgery, the outline of the anterior superior iliac spine (ASIS) and the great trochanter were marked before surgery. Three portals were used in all patients. The anterolateral (AL) portal was established between the gluteus minimus and the iliocapsularis muscles, located 1 cm anterior and 1 cm proximal to the great trochanter. The mid-anterior (MA) portal was established 5 cm distal and 1 cm lateral to the ASIS. Finally, the distal anterolateral accessory (DALA) portal was established 5 cm distal and 1 cm anterior to the great trochanter.

2.3.3. Capsulotomy

With the AL portal as an observation portal and MA portal as operation portal, an extracapsular space anterior to the hip joint is established first. After the pericapsular tissue cleared off from the hip capsule, the reflected head of the rectus femoris was located. The longitudinal capsulotomy was performed at the midpoint of the anterior femoral neck, 1 cm lateral and parallel to the rectus femoris using radiofrequency probes. Then, the arthroscopy was entered the hip joint and the femoral head–neck junction was exposed (Figure 1A). The longitudinal incision was extended proximally until the acetabular labrum was exposed (Figure 1B). A 1 cm transverse incision vertical to the longitudinal capsulotomy was performed in the proximal end of longitudinal incision (Figure 1C). A Wissinger rod was used to lift away the pericapsular tissue from DALA portal if necessary.

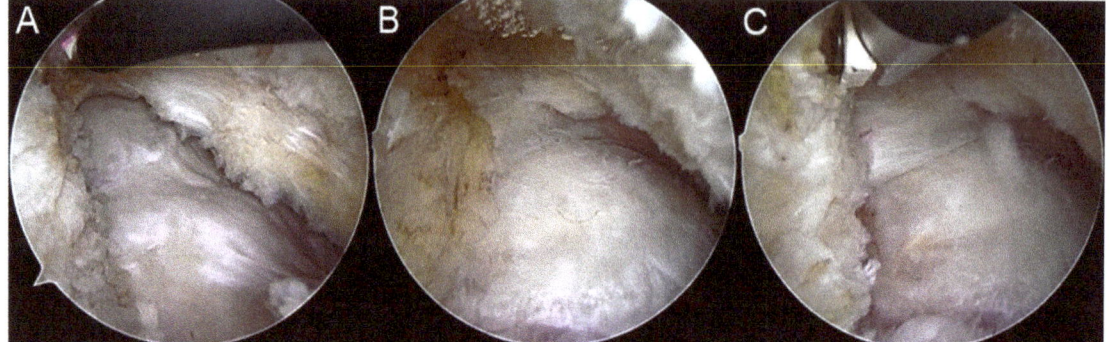

Figure 1. The procedures of modified longitudinal capsulotomy. (**A**) After the longitudinal capsulotomy was performed using radiofrequency probes, the arthroscopy was entered the hip joint and the femoral head–neck junction was exposed. (**B**) The longitudinal incision was extended proximally until the acetabular labrum was exposed. (**C**) A 1 cm transverse incision vertical to the longitudinal capsulotomy was performed in the proximal end of longitudinal incision.

2.3.4. Acetabuloplasty and Labrum Repair

After the bilateral hip traction was performed, the space of hip joint was increased to approximately 1 cm, so that the arthroscopy can enter the central compartment and the acetabular labrum can expose satisfactorily. After the acetabuloplasty was performed appropriately, if necessary, the acetabular labrum was checked out carefully with probe to identify the torn area. Then 1–2 suture anchors were inserted in the acetabular rim according to the torn size. The torn labrum was fix by mattress suture every 0.5 cm apart.

2.3.5. Femoroplasty

When the management in central compartment completed, the hip traction was released and the arthroscopy entered the peripheral compartment. The perineal post was removed and the operative hip was positioned at 40° of flexion, neutral rotation and adduction/abduction. The modified longitudinal capsulotomy can provide a complete exposure of the femoral head–neck junction and directly identify the location and size of the cam deformity. Then, a 4.0-mm burr was used to demarcate the medial border and extended to the lateral synovial fold (12 o'clock) and the medial synovial fold (6 o'clock). The femoral neck was well visualized and the femoroplasty was performed to provide a smooth transition to the anterior femoral neck. After femoroplasty, impingement tests were performed to check the complete removal of cam deformity. A 45° abduction test is performed in both extension and in 90° of flexion to evaluate possible superolateral impingement. Then, an anterior impingement test is performed by positioning the hip into flexion with maximal internal rotation.

2.3.6. Capsular Closure

At the end of the arthroscopic procedures, the hip capsule was repaired using nonabsorbable, high-tensile strength sutures in a simple side-to-side or shoelace stitches. A total of 2 to 3 stitches were placed to repair the medial and lateral leaflets of the iliofemoral ligament and complete the capsular closure.

2.4. Postoperative Rehabilitation

All patients followed the standard protocol of postoperative rehabilitation. Rehabilitation exercises were initiated day 1 postoperatively. Lower extremity resistance exercises were used to begin restoring neuromuscular control and isometric strengthening of the surrounding hip musculature, such as hip abductors and quadriceps. Patients were encouraged to weight-bear as tolerated with crutches after 2 weeks postoperatively. Patients who received labral refixation or/and femoroplasty were ambulated with crutches for 4 weeks and then progressed to full weight-bearing. Range of motion was performed with a continuous passive motion machine, limiting hip rotation and abduction to below 20° and flexion to below 90°.

2.5. Data Collection and Statistical Analysis

During the surgical procedures, the capsulotomy time, traction time and overall surgical time were collected. After surgery, each patient underwent the outcome assessment both clinically and radiologically and compared with the preoperative data. The clinical outcomes included mHHS and VAS, as well as postoperative complications in 3 months, 6 months and 12 months' follow-up. The radiological outcomes included alpha angle and LCEA in X-rays (anteroposterior view, frog view), and the cam deformity was evaluated in 3D-CT.

All data were analyzed using the Stata software (version 13.0; Stata Corp., College Station, TX, USA). Continuous variables were summarized with mean ± standard deviation or median and interquartile range. Continuous variables with normal distribution including alpha angle, LCEA and mHHS were compared using the analysis of variance (ANOVA) and two-sample paired t-test. Quantitative data (VAS) which were not normally distributed were compared by the χ^2 test and two-sample paired Wilcoxon rank-sum test. Statistical significance level was set at $p < 0.05$.

3. Results

3.1. General Results

Twenty-two postoperative patients who underwent hip arthroscopy in our hospital from January 2019 to December 2021 were involved in this study. The patients (14 females and 8 males) had a mean age of 38.26 ± 12.82 years old. All patients were diagnosed cam deformity and labrum tear in the operation and underwent arthroscopic femoroplasty and labrum repair by the modified longitudinal capsulotomy.

3.2. Surgical Results and Radiological Outcomes

The mean capsulotomy time was 12.7 ± 3.5 min, the mean traction time was 36.2 ± 7.2 min and the overall surgical time was 123.6 ± 16.4 min. After surgery, all patients had an alpha angle < 55° and LCEA < 40° in X ray of frog view and anteroposterior view. And the cam deformity was no longer appeared in 3D-CT.

3.3. Clinical Outcomes

The mean follow-up time was 10.4 months with a range of 6–12 months. There were no major complications, including infection, neurapraxias, hip instability or revision appeared in any patients. The average mHHS were 74.4 ± 15.2, 78.2 ± 13.7 and 85.7 ± 14.5 in 3 months, 6 months and 12 months after surgery, respectively, which were all better than that before surgery (44.9 ± 8.6) ($p < 0.05$) (Figure 2A). The average VAS were 2.8 ± 1.2, 1.5 ± 0.6 and 1.2 ± 0.7 in 3 months, 6 months and 12 months after surgery, respectively, which were all lower than that before surgery (5.5 ± 2.0) ($p < 0.05$) (Figure 2B). The value of mHHS increased and the value of VAS decreased gradually with the time after surgery.

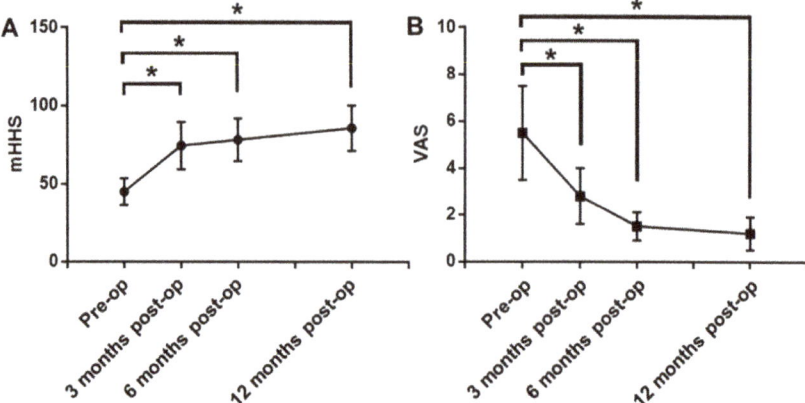

Figure 2. The results of mHHS and VAS. (**A**): The mHHS in 3 months, 6 months and 12 months after surgery were all better than that before surgery ($p < 0.05$). (**B**): The VAS in 3 months, 6 months and 12 months after surgery were all lower than that before surgery ($p < 0.05$). The mHHS increased and the VAS decreased gradually with the time after surgery. *: $p < 0.05$.

4. Discussion

The modified longitudinal capsulotomy by outside-in approach showed a satisfactory result in this study. Surgeons can complete all of the arthroscopic procedures conveniently after the capsulotomy by this approach. The postoperative mHHS and VAS were both better than before surgery, and patient reported outcomes became better gradually with the time after surgery with no infection, neurapraxias, hip instability or revision appeared in all patients. In spite of the short follow-up time and no control group in this study, the modified longitudinal capsulotomy by outside-in approach was indicated to be a promising method in hip arthroscopy referencing the similar studies previously [6,7]. Moreover, the radiation exposure of surgeons and patients can be avoided because this method did not need intraoperative fluoroscopy.

The outside-in approach was first proposed by Denist et al. in 2005 and proved to be a feasible method in the surgical practice [20]. This approach took the place of puncture approach by seldinger technique in traditional hip arthroscopy. In recent years, studies of hip arthroscopy using the outside-in approach has increased gradually [4,7–11]. This approach can make the operation process quite easy for surgeons performing hip arthroscopy, and all surgical procedures can be achieved without special surgical instruments for hip arthroscopy, or the intraoperative fluoroscopy. The simple procedures make this approach easy to learn and friendly for the beginner of hip arthroscopy. Furthermore, this approach is the best choice for patients with massive pincer deformity, in which the puncture approach can hardly enter the hip joint.

Capsulotomy was a milepost technique in the development of hip arthroscopy, which solved the problems of poor view and difficult procedures in hip arthroscopy [21]. For the different kinds of capsulotomy in previous studies, a systematic review showed 55% performed an interportal capsulotomy while 24% performed a T-capsulotomy [6]. Recently, some surgeons performed the longitudinal capsulotomy and obtained a satisfactory arthroscopic view for the consequent surgical procedures [7,11]. Based on this capsulotomy, we modified the technique by adding a small incision vertical to the longitudinal capsulotomy proximally. This improvement can expose the lesions deep in the hip joint, which help surgeons obtain a good view to observe and a sufficient space to perform the femoroplasty and labrum repair.

The security of capsulotomy is one of the most concerning problems in hip arthroscopy. Therefore, the capsulotomy was conservative and tried carefully when it proposed. After the capsulotomy technique widely used in hip arthroscopy and the development of capsule suture technique, many studies have proved the security of capsulotomy [22–26]. As for the outside-in approach, it avoided the damage of cartilage and labrum caused by puncture in traditional inside-out approach. In the current study, no complication appeared after the hip arthroscopy. On the one hand, the capsulotomy by outside-in approach provided sufficient view and convenient for surgical procedures. On the other hand, the capsulotomy by outside-in approach did not need hip traction and the overall traction time can significantly decrease. Thus, the iatrogenic cartilage or labrum injury and traction-related complications were successfully avoided in this approach.

After the surgical procedures in hip joint, repair of the incised capsule is suggested to avoid postoperative hip instability [22–25]. By the outside-in approach, an extracapsular space anterior to hip joint is established, which is just convenient for suturing the capsule. Due to the incising direction vertical to iliofemoral ligament, the interportal capsulotomy and T-capsulotomy can injure the iliofemoral ligament and lead to hip instability if the incised capsule not repaired [26–29]. The modified longitudinal capsulotomy can decrease this injury because the incising direction is paralleled to the iliofemoral ligament. In the present study, the capsular closure was performed in all patients and none of them appeared hip instability after surgery. Therefore, the postoperative rehabilitation processes can be accelerated appropriately after the hip arthroscopy using modified longitudinal capsulotomy.

Considering the feasibility, efficacy and security of the new method, the modified longitudinal capsulotomy by outside-in approach is proved to be a safe and feasible method for hip arthroscopy. This method is easy to perform without special surgical instruments or intraoperative fluoroscopy, and is also quite friendly to beginners of hip arthroscopy. Thus, this new approach is promising and suggested to be widely used clinically.

There were some limitations in this study. Firstly, it is a retrospective cohort study with a relatively small sample size. Secondly, there was no control group of the longitudinal capsulotomy or traditional inside-out approach. Finally, the follow-up time is relatively short. Even though it was found that most patients achieved minimal clinically important difference in 6 months after hip arthroscopy in previous studies [30,31], these limitations above unavoidably decreased the generalizability of the study results. Thus, further study with control group, more sample size and longer follow-up time is needed to check the efficacy of the modified longitudinal capsulotomy.

5. Conclusions

The modified longitudinal capsulotomy by outside-in approach is proved to be a safe and feasible method for hip arthroscopy considering to the feasibility, efficacy and security. The arthroscopic femoroplasty and labrum repair can be performed conveniently by this approach and the patient reported outcomes after surgery were better that before surgery in short-term follow-up. This new method is promising and suggested to be widely used clinically.

Author Contributions: Conceptualization, C.Z.; Data curation, J.P.; Investigation, G.H.; Methodology, C.Z.; Writing–original draft, S.C.; Writing–review and editing, D.X. All authors have read and agreed to the published version of the manuscript.

Funding: This research received no external funding.

Informed Consent Statement: Informed consent was obtained from all subjects involved in the study.

Data Availability Statement: Data are available upon reasonable request from the corresponding author.

Conflicts of Interest: The authors declare no conflict of interest.

References

1. Weinberg, D.S.; Gebhart, J.J.; Liu, R.W.; Salata, M.J. Radiographic Signs of Femoroacetabular Impingement Are Associated with Decreased Pelvic Incidence. *Arthroscopy* **2016**, *32*, 806–813. [CrossRef] [PubMed]
2. Cong, S.; Liu, S.; Xie, Y.; Luo, Z.; Chen, J. Evaluation of Cam Deformity on 3-Dimensional Computed Tomography with the Best-Fit Sphere Technique and the Alpha Angle Marking Method. *Am. J. Sports Med.* **2021**, *49*, 1023–1030. [CrossRef] [PubMed]
3. Atkins, P.R.; Aoki, S.K.; Whitaker, R.T.; Weiss, J.A.; Peters, C.L.; Anderson, A.E. Does Removal of Subchondral Cortical Bone Provide Sufficient Resection Depth for Treatment of Cam Femoroacetabular Impingement? *Clin. Orthop. Relat. Res.* **2017**, *475*, 1977–1986. [CrossRef] [PubMed]
4. Sandoval, E.; Martín-Ríos, M.D.; Cimas, D.; Masegosa, A.; Calvo, E. Hip arthroscopy for the treatment of femoroacetabular impingement: A comparative study between the classic and the outside-in access. *Hip Int.* **2016**, *26*, 290–294. [CrossRef]
5. Philippon, M.J.; Stubbs, A.J.; Schenker, M.L.; Maxwell, R.B.; Ganz, R.; Leunig, M. Arthroscopic management of femoroacetabular impingement: Osteoplasty technique and literature review. *Am. J. Sports Med.* **2007**, *35*, 1571–1580. [CrossRef]
6. Ekhtiari, S.; De Sa, D.; Haldane, C.E.; Larson, C.M.; Safran, M.R.; Ayeni, O.R. Hip arthroscopic capsulotomy techniques and capsular management strategies: A systematic review. *Knee Surg. Sports Traumatol. Arthrosc.* **2017**, *25*, 9–23. [CrossRef]
7. Yin, Q.F.; Wang, L.; Liang, T.; Zhao, H.; Wang, X. Longitudinal Capsulotomy in Hip Arthroscopy: A Safe and Feasible Procedure for Cam-Type Femoroacetabular Impingement. *Orthop. Surg.* **2021**, *13*, 1793–1801. [CrossRef]
8. Narvaez, M.V.; Cady, A.; Serrano, B.; Youssefzadeh, K.; Banffy, M. Outside-In Capsulotomy of the Hip for Arthroscopic Pincer Resection. *Arthrosc. Tech.* **2021**, *10*, e615–e620. [CrossRef]
9. Salas, A.P.; Brizuela-Ventura, M.; Velasco-Vazquez, H.; Mazek, J. The Outside-In Technique for Slipped Capital Femoral Epiphysis: A Safe and Reproducible Approach in Hip Arthroscopy. *Arthrosc. Tech.* **2020**, *9*, e493–e497. [CrossRef]
10. Moreta, J.; Cuéllar, A.; Aguirre, U.; Casado-Verdugo, L.; Sánchez, A.; Cuéllar, R. Outside-in arthroscopic psoas release for anterior iliopsoas impingement after primary total hip arthroplasty. *Hip Int.* **2021**, *31*, 649–655. [CrossRef]
11. Thaunat, M.; Sarr, S.; Georgeokostas, T.; Azeem, A.; Murphy, C.G.; Kacem, S.; Clowez, G.; Roberts, T. Femoroacetabular impingement treatment using the arthroscopic extracapsular outside-in approach: Does capsular suture affect functional outcome? *Orthop. Traumatol. Surg. Res.* **2020**, *106*, 569–575. [CrossRef] [PubMed]
12. Price, D.D.; Mcgrath, P.A.; Rafii, A.; Buckingham, B. The validation of visual analogue scales as ratio scale measures for chronic and experimental pain. *Pain* **1983**, *17*, 45–56. [CrossRef]
13. Samim, M.; Eftekhary, N.; Vigdorchik, J.M.; Elbuluk, A.; Davidovitch, R.; Youm, T.; Gyftopoulus, G. 3D-MRI versus 3D-CT in the evaluation of osseous anatomy in femoroacetabular impingement using Dixon 3D FLASH sequence. *Skelet. Radiol.* **2019**, *48*, 429–436. [CrossRef]
14. Fadul, D.A.; Carrino, J.A. Imaging of femoroacetabular impingement. *J. Bone Jt. Surg.* **2009**, *91* (Suppl. 1), 138–143. [CrossRef] [PubMed]
15. Yamasaki, T.; Yasunaga, Y.; Shoji, T.; Izumi, S.; Hachisuka, S.; Ochi, M. Inclusion and Exclusion Criteria in the Diagnosis of Femoroacetabular Impingement. *Arthroscopy* **2015**, *31*, 1403–1410. [CrossRef] [PubMed]
16. Notzli, H.P.; Wyss, T.F.; Stoecklin, C.H.; Schmid, M.R.; Hodler, J. The contour of the femoral head-neck junction as a predictor for the risk of anterior impingement. *J. Bone Jt. Surg. Br. Vol.* **2002**, *84*, 556–560. [CrossRef]
17. Peelle, M.W.; Della Rocca, G.J.; Maloney, W.J.; Curry, M.C.; Clohisy, J.C. Acetabular and femoral radiographic abnormalities associated with labral tears. *Clin. Orthop. Relat. Res.* **2005**, *441*, 327–333. [CrossRef]
18. Peters, S.; Laing, A.; Emerson, C.; Mutchler, K.; Joyce, T.; Thorborg, K.; Hölmich, P.; Reiman, M. Surgical criteria for femoroacetabular impingement syndrome: A scoping review. *Br. J. Sports Med.* **2017**, *51*, 1605–1610. [CrossRef]
19. Beaule, P.E.; Zaragoza, E.; Motamedi, K.; Copelan, N.; Dorey, F.J. Three-dimensional computed tomography of the hip in the assessment of femoroacetabular impingement. *J. Orthop. Res.* **2005**, *23*, 1286–1292. [CrossRef]
20. Dienst, M.; Seil, R.; Kohn, D.M. Safe arthroscopic access to the central compartment of the hip. *Arthroscopy* **2005**, *21*, 1510–1514. [CrossRef]
21. Thaunat, M.; Murphy, C.G.; Chatellard, R.; Sonnery-Cottet, B.; Graveleau, N.; Meyer, A.; Laude, F. Capsulotomy first: A novel concept for hip arthroscopy. *Arthrosc. Tech.* **2014**, *3*, e599–e603. [CrossRef] [PubMed]
22. Bolia, I.K.; Fagotti, L.; Briggs, K.K.; Philippon, M.J. Midterm Outcomes Following Repair of Capsulotomy Versus Nonrepair in Patients Undergoing Hip Arthroscopy for Femoroacetabular Impingement with Labral Repair. *Arthroscopy* **2019**, *35*, 1828–1834. [CrossRef] [PubMed]
23. Hewitt, J.D.; Glisson, R.R.; Guilak, F.; Vail, T. The mechanical properties of the human hip capsule ligaments. *J. Arthroplast.* **2002**, *17*, 82–89. [CrossRef]
24. Khair, M.M.; Grzybowski, J.S.; Kuhns, B.D.; Wuerz, T.H.; Shewman, M.S.; Nho, S.J. The Effect of Capsulotomy and Capsular Repair on Hip Distraction: A Cadaveric Investigation. *Arthroscopy* **2017**, *33*, 559–565. [CrossRef] [PubMed]
25. Chahla, J.; Mikula, J.D.; Schon, J.M.; Dean, C.S.; Dahl, K.; Menge, T.J.; Soares, E.; Turnbull, T.L.; Laprade, R.F.; Philippon, M.J. Hip Capsular Closure: A Biomechanical Analysis of Failure Torque. *Am. J. Sports Med.* **2017**, *45*, 434–439. [CrossRef] [PubMed]
26. Weber, A.E.; Neal, W.H.; Mayer, E.N.; Kuhns, B.D.; Shewman, E.; Salata, M.J.; Mather, R.C.; Nho, S.J. Vertical Extension of the T-Capsulotomy Incision in Hip Arthroscopic Surgery Does Not Affect the Force Required for Hip Distraction: Effect of Capsulotomy Size, Type, and Subsequent Repair. *Am. J. Sports Med.* **2018**, *46*, 3127–3133. [CrossRef]

27. Fagotti, L.; Utsunomiya, H.; Philippon, M.J. An Anatomic Study of the Damage to Capsular Hip Stabilizers During Subspine Decompression Using a Transverse Interportal Capsulotomy in Hip Arthroscopy. *Arthroscopy* **2020**, *36*, 116–123. [CrossRef]
28. Wuerz, T.H.; Song, S.H.; Grzybowski, J.S.; Martin, H.D.; Mather, R.C.; Salata, M.J.; Orías, A.A.E.; Nho, S.J. Capsulotomy Size Affects Hip Joint Kinematic Stability. *Arthroscopy* **2016**, *32*, 1571–1580. [CrossRef]
29. Van Arkel, R.J.; Amis, A.A.; Cobb, J.P.; Jeffers, J.R.T. The capsular ligaments provide more hip rotational restraint than the acetabular labrum and the ligamentum teres: An experimental study. *Bone Jt. J.* **2015**, *97*, 484–491. [CrossRef]
30. Nwachukwu, B.U.; Chang, B.; Adjei, J.; Schairer, W.W.; Ranawat, A.S.; Kelly, B.T.; Nawabi, D.H. Time Required to Achieve Minimal Clinically Important Difference and Substantial Clinical Benefit After Arthroscopic Treatment of Femoroacetabular Impingement. *Am. J. Sports Med.* **2018**, *46*, 2601–2606. [CrossRef]
31. Wolfson, T.S.; Ryan, M.K.; Begly, J.P.; Youm, T. Outcome Trends After Hip Arthroscopy for Femoroacetabular Impingement: When Do Patients Improve? *Arthroscopy* **2019**, *35*, 3261–3270. [CrossRef] [PubMed]

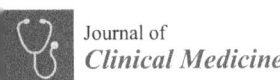

Article

Clinical Outcomes following Biologically Enhanced Demineralized Bone Matrix Augmentation of Complex Rotator Cuff Repair

Ian J. Wellington [1,*], Lukas N. Muench [2], Benjamin C. Hawthorne [1], Colin L. Uyeki [3], Christopher L. Antonacci [1], Mary Beth McCarthy [1], John P. Connors [1], Cameron Kia [1], Augustus D. Mazzocca [4] and Daniel P. Berthold [2]

1. Department of Orthopedic Surgery, University of Connecticut Health Center, Farmington, CT 06032, USA; bhawthorne@uchc.edu (B.C.H.); antonacci@uchc.edu (C.L.A.); mccarthy@uchc.edu (M.B.M.); jconnors@uchc.edu (J.P.C.); ckia@uchc.edu (C.K.)
2. Department of Orthopedic Surgery, Technical University of Munich, 80333 Munich, Germany; lukas.muench@gmail.com (L.N.M.); daniberthold@gmail.com (D.P.B.)
3. Frank H. Netter School of Medicine, Quinnipiac University, Hamden, CT 06518, USA; uyeki@uchc.edu
4. Massachusetts General Hospital, Massachusetts General Brigham, Harvard Medical School, Boston, MA 02115, USA; amazzocca@mgh.harvard.edu
* Correspondence: iwellington@uchc.edu; Tel.: +1-201-290-7306

Abstract: Complex rotator cuff tears provide a significant challenge for treating surgeons, given their high failure rate following repair and the associated morbidity. The purpose of this study is to evaluate the clinical outcomes of patients who underwent biologically enhanced demineralized bone matrix augmentation of rotator cuff repairs. Twenty patients with complex rotator cuff tears underwent arthroscopic rotator cuff repair by a single surgeon with demineralized bone matrix (DBM) augmentation that was biologically enhanced with platelet-rich plasma and concentrated bone marrow aspirate. Post-operative MRI was used to determine surgical success. Patient reported outcome measures and range of motion data were collected pre-operatively and at the final post-operative visit for each patient. Ten patients (50%) with DBM augmentation of their arthroscopic rotator cuff repair were deemed non-failures. The failure group had less improvement of visual analogue pain scale ($p = 0.017$), Simple Shoulder Test ($p = 0.032$), Single Assessment Numerical Evaluation ($p = 0.006$) and abduction ($p = 0.046$). There was no difference between the groups for change in American Shoulder and Elbow Society score ($p = 0.096$), Constant-Murley score ($p = 0.086$), forward elevation ($p = 0.191$) or external rotation ($p = 0.333$). The present study found that 50% of patients who underwent biologically enhanced DBM augmentation of their rotator cuff repair demonstrated MRI-determined failure of supraspinatus healing.

Keywords: shoulder; rotator cuff; allografts; demineralized bone matrix; biologics

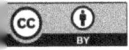

1. Introduction

Mechanical augmentation using extracellular matrix (ECM) materials—namely in the form of a graft of tissue or synthetic material presents an opportunity for optimizing the healing potential of complex rotator cuff pathologies [1]. These grafts can provide a scaffold for delivering biologic therapies (e.g., platelet-rich plasma (PRP) or concentrated bone marrow aspirate (cBMA)) to augment tendon healing at the operative site while also providing a load-sharing device. This load-sharing and more organized healing environment is thought to prevent scar tissue formation at the tendon-bone interface and encourage the growth of functional tissue comprised of tenocytes, chondrocytes, and osteocytes [1,2].

As a result of the large number of rotator cuff repairs (RCR) performed annually and the high rate of structural failure, considerable efforts have been devoted to developing grafts that augment the RCR site by mechanically reinforcing it as well as providing a biological scaffold that can enhance the rate and quality of the healing process [3]. Because the ECM of the graft directly interacts with tissue microenvironments for stem cell proliferation, it is necessary to consider the design of the patch and how it affects cell differentiation [2]. Prior studies have shown that the composition of microenvironments alters cellular adhesion, differentiation, and morphology [2,4–8]. Since Neviaser et al.'s first use of the interposition allograft for RCR, various graft types have expanded to include synthetic polymers, allograft, autograft, and xenograft materials with varying degrees of clinical success [9]. Common disadvantages to these efforts have included fibrous cartilage formation, strong inflammatory reactions, or rapid degradation of the graft.

Demineralized bone matrix (DBM) is composed of cancellous bone with both osteoinductive and osteoconductive properties. Previous work demonstrated that DBM scaffolding shows excellent adhesion, proliferation, and differentiation of mesenchymal stem cells [10]. Adhesion of these cells to the DBM was maintained even after a simulated arthroscopic mechanical washout stress test. While in vitro testing has shown this material to be an excellent scaffold for biologic augmentation of rotator cuff repairs, few studies have investigated its in vivo efficacy.

Thus, the purpose of the present study was to evaluate the clinical outcomes of patients who underwent biologically enhanced demineralized bone matrix augmentation of rotator cuff repair. It was hypothesized that biologically enhanced demineralized bone matrix augmentation repair would significantly improve shoulder function.

2. Materials and Methods

This was a retrospective study. All patients included were older than 18 years of age. Each underwent arthroscopic repair of a complex rotator cuff tear using a DBM scaffold (Flexigraft, Arthrex, Naples, FL, USA) augmented with autogenous PRP and cBMA harvested from the proximal humerus. Surgeries were performed by a single, shoulder fellowship-trained surgeon from September 2015 to December 2017. Institutional review board approval was obtained before the initiation of the study. Patients with RC tear arthropathy (Hamada grade > 3), irreparable massive tears, previous RC surgery requiring tendon transfers, nerve injuries, or pre-operative pseudoparalysis were excluded. Additionally, vulnerable patient populations such as pregnant women and prisoners, as well as individuals with a history of systemic infectious disease (e.g., hepatitis or human immunodeficiency virus) were excluded. All alternative treatment options were discussed with the patient, including continued conservative treatment. Basic demographic information (age, sex, and body mass index) and a thorough medical and surgical history were obtained for each patient.

2.1. Imaging

All patients undergoing surgery had a pre-operative magnetic resonance imaging (MRI) of the involved shoulder. On MRI, tendon retraction was quantified on coronal T2 fat-saturated images using the classification system of Patte (A. minimal retraction, B. retraction to humeral head, C. retraction to glenoid) [11]. Fatty infiltration was assessed on T1 sagittal oblique views based on the presence of fatty streaks within the supraspinatus muscle belly using Goutallier's grading system, which was originally described on computed tomography but is now commonly applied to MRI [12,13].

2.2. Surgical Technique

Patients received an interscalene block prior to induction via general anesthesia. Patients were positioned in the beach chair position. First, diagnostic arthroscopy was performed to evaluate the rotator cuff tear and to assess the mobility of the torn edge. For patients that had previously undergone RCR, loose suture material and/or anchors were removed. The graft was prepared by first being soaked in saline at room temperature for at least 30 min prior to use. The 2–3 cc's of concentrated BMA (cBMA) combined with 2–3 cc's of PRP were added to the graft.

2.3. Bone Marrow Aspirate

Aspiration was performed at the proximal humerus using the Bone Marrow Aspiration Kit (Arthrex) using previously described methods [14]. Four 12-mL double syringes were filled with 2 mL of 1000 U sodium heparin and 9 mL of saline. An 11-gauge non-fenestrated bone marrow aspiration trocar was inserted into the planned site for the first suture anchor at the tendon footprint. The four 12-mL syringes were then used to sequentially aspirate bone marrow from the trocar. Aspirate underwent centrifugation at 800 rpm for 4 min. The upper fractionated layer containing the concentrated bone marrow stromal cells was drawn into the inner syringe. The resulting cBMA from each of the 4 syringes were combined into one syringe.

2.4. PRP Concentration

Using the Autologous Conditioned Plasma (ACP) kit (Arthrex, Naples, FL, USA), blood was collected from each patient and then centrifuged at 1500 rpm for 5 min. The concentrated plasma layer was then drawn into a syringe and mixed with the cBMA.

2.5. DBM Preparation

The DBM (15 mm × 40 mm × 2 mm) was allowed to soak in saline for a minimum of 30 min prior to use. The cBMA/PRP mixture was then injected into the DBM using a tuberculin syringe. The patch was then soaked for a minimum of 30 min in excess biologic adjuvants.

2.6. Repair and Augmentation

After removal of the bone marrow aspiration trocar, the first medial anchor was inserted in its place. Additional anchors were placed as needed. A #2 Fiberwire (Arthrex, Naples, FL, USA) horizontal mattress suture was placed through the DBM graft, the ends of this suture were then passed from the articular side to the bursal side of the torn tendon edge using SutureLasso (Arthrex, Naples, FL, USA). The limbs or the suture were then pulled while the graft was guided into position on the articular side of the torn tendon. Once the DBM was in the proper position, the rotator cuff was repaired in the standard fashion using a double-row technique. Approximately 2 to 5 cc of excess cBMA and PRP were injected into the surrounding tendon. Biceps tenodesis was performed in patients who had pre-operative subpectoral pain. Additionally, subacromial decompression was performed in patients with either a curved or hooked acromion on pre-operative radiographs.

Post-operatively, patients were placed in a 30° abduction sling for 6 weeks. 28 days post-operatively, patients were advanced to 60° active assistive range of motion in external rotation at 30° of abduction and forward elevation from 30° to 180° during physical therapy. Patients were allowed to initiate an active assistive range of motion in external rotation and forward elevation without limitations until 12 weeks post-operatively. At 12 weeks, patients began isometric strengthening of the rotator cuff muscles with progression to isotonic strengthening at 18 weeks.

2.7. Clinical Outcome Measures

Simple Shoulder Test (SST), American Shoulder and Elbow Surgeons (ASES), Single Assessment Numerical Evaluation (SANE), visual analog pain scale (VAS), and Constant-Murley (CM) scores were collected pre-operatively and at the final post-operative visit for each patient. The change in these scores was calculated for each patient.

2.8. Determination of Surgical Outcome

Patients were divided into either surgical success or surgical failure groups for data analysis. To accomplish this, a one-year post-operative MRI was used to determine if the supraspinatus tendon successfully healed. For some patients, an earlier post-operative MRI was ordered if there was a concern of surgical failure. Five patients did not have

MRIs post-operatively due to their high degree of clinical improvement. These five were considered surgical successes.

2.9. Statistical Methods

Descriptive statistics were calculated as a mean and standard deviation or frequency and proportion for each group. Independent values student's t-tests were used to compare numerical data, and chi-square analysis with Fischer's exact tests was used to compare categorical data. 95% confidence intervals (CIs) were calculated. Missing data were excluded from the analysis. A *p*-value of less than 0.05 was considered to be statistically significant. All studies were performed using SPSS (version 28, IBM, Armonk, NY, USA) statistical software.

3. Results

Twenty total patients underwent RCR with DBM. Of the 20, 10 patients demonstrated failure of their repair on post-operative MRI, 5 patients demonstrated an intact repair on the post-operative MRI and 5 did not receive a postoperative MRI given their excellent clinical improvements (Figure 1). The five subjects that did not have a post-operative MRI were considered non-failures.

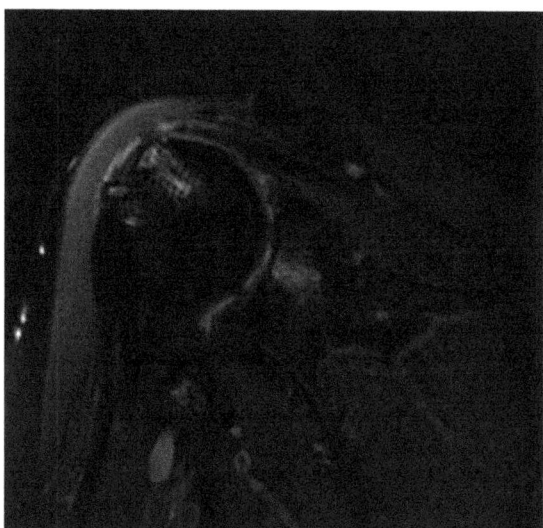

Figure 1. T2-weighted sagittal MRI of a shoulder following successful healing of a supraspinatus tear with DBM, PRP, and cBMA augmentation.

There were no differences between the success and failure groups for age, gender, body mass index (BMI), or diabetes status (Table 1). There were no patients with rheumatologic conditions or a history of cancer. There were no statistically significant differences between groups on handedness, surgical side, Patte Classification (tendon retraction), Goutallier Stage (fatty infiltration), history of prior shoulder surgery of any type, or history of prior rotator cuff repair (Table 1). Of the 10 non-failure patients, 1 had an acute tear while 9 were chronic. All the failed patients had chronic tears. Biceps tenodesis was performed concomitantly with the DBM repair in 10% of the non-failure group and 80% of the failure group, which was significantly different. Subacromial decompression was performed in 20% of non-failure patients and 30% of failure patients, which was not significantly different (Table 1).

Table 1. Demographic and Injury Information for Non-Failure and Failure Patients.

		Non-Failure (n = 10)	Failure (n = 10)	p-Value	95% CI Lower	95% CI Upper
Age (years ± SD)		58.6 ± 4.9	51.3 ± 10.2	0.056	−0.2	14.8
Gender (% Female)		40	40	1		
BMI (kg/m^2 ± SD)		27.6 ± 3.6	28.1 ± 3.7	0.754	−3.9	2.9
Smoking (%)		10	30	0.582		
Diabetes Mellitus (%)		30	10	0.582		
Rheumatologic Condition		0	0			
Cancer		0	0			
Handedness (% RHD)		90	100	0.305		
Surgical Side (% Right side)		60	70	0.639		
Chronic Tear (% Chronic)		90	100	0.305		
Primary Repair (% Primary)		40	30	0.639		
Patte Classification	A	5	4	0.637		
	B	3	5			
	C	0	0			
	NC	2	1			
Goutallier Classification	0	0	0	0.134		
	1	5	2			
	2	3	4			
	3	0	2			
	4	0	1			
	NC	2	1			
Previous Shoulder Surgery	0	4	2	0.281		
	1	6	4			
	2	0	2			
	3	0	1			
	4	0	1			
Previous RCR	0	4	3	0.315		
	1	6	4			
	2	0	1			
	3	0	2			
Biceps Tenodesis (%)		10	80	0.005 *		
SAD (%)		20	30	0.606		

BMI = body mass index; NC = not classified; RCR = rotator cuff repair, SAD = subacromial decompression; CT = Confidence Interval; * = $p < 0.05$.

There was no difference between the failure and non-failure groups for pre-operative VAS, ASES, SST, SANE, or CM scores. Additionally, there was no difference between groups for pre-operative forward elevation, abduction, or external rotation (Table 2).

The non-failure group had a greater post-operative decrease in pain (p = 0.017; CI: −5.4 to −6.1) compared to the failure group. The failure group also showed significantly worse post-operative improvements in SST (p = 0.032; CI: 0.2 to 5) and SANE (p = 0.006; CI: 15.8 to 79.6) (Table 3). There was no difference between the two groups for change in ASES (p = 0.096; CI: −3.7 to 41.6) and CM score (p = 0.086; CI: −3.5 to 46.3) though these approached significance. The non-failure group had a significantly greater improvement in abduction (p = 0.046; CI: 1 to 84), but there was no difference in forward elevation (p = 0.191; CI: −15 to 69) or external rotation (p = 0.333; CI: −9 to 26) (Table 3). There was no difference in follow up between the non-failure group (13.1 ± 6.3 months) and the failure group (13.5 ± 6.9 months) (p = 0.894; CI −6.6, 5.8).

Table 2. Pre-operative Pain and Functional Measurements.

	Non-Failure (n = 10)	Failure (n = 10)	p-Value	95% CI	
				Lower	Upper
VAS	5.8 ± 2.5	6.9 ± 2.1	0.302	−3.3	1.1
ASES	30.5 ± 19.3	29.6 ± 14.4	0.17	−5.1	26.9
SST	4.2 ± 3.3	2.5 ± 2.1	0.187	−0.9	4.3
SANE	8.3 ± 5.9	8.0 ± 7.4	0.921	−6	6.6
CM	43.0 ± 19.1	35.8 ± 8.4	0.289	−6.6	21
Forward Elevation	133 ± 44	119 ± 26	0.403	−20	48
Abduction	123 ± 46	100 ± 29	0.336	−19	53
External Rotation	42 ± 21	35 ± 8	0.341	−8	22

VAS = visual analogue scale; ASES = American Shoulder and Elbow Surgeons Shoulder Score; SST = Simple Shoulder Test; SANE = Single Assessment Numeric Evaluation; CM = Constant-Murley; CI = Confidence Interval.

Table 3. Post-operative Change in Pain and Function Scores.

	Non-Failure (n = 10)	Failure (n = 10)	p-Value	95% CI	
				Lower	Upper
VAS (n = 10,10)	−3.6 ± 3.1	−0.06 ± 1.9	0.017 *	−5.4	−0.6
ASES (n = 8,9)	29.6 ± 23.4	10.8 ± 20.3	0.096	−3.7	41.4
SST (n = 10,10)	3.7 ± 3.1	1.1 ± 1.8	0.032 *	0.2	5
SANE (n = 10,10)	68.0 ± 28.9	20.3 ± 38.5	0.006 *	15.8	79.6
CM (n = 5,9)	16.4 ± 16.3	−5.0 ± 22.3	0.086	−3.5	46.3
Forward Elevation (n = 10,10)	22 ± 29	−5 ± 56	0.191	−15	69
Abduction (n = 10,10)	26 ± 26	−16 ± 57	0.046 *	1	84
External Rotation (n = 10,10)	12 ± 13	3 ± 24	0.333	−9	26

VAS = visual analogue scale; ASES = American Shoulder and Elbow Surgeons Shoulder Score; SST = Simple Shoulder Test; SANE = Single Assessment Numeric Evaluation; CM = Constant-Murley; CI = Confidence Interval; * = $p < 0.05$.

4. Discussion

In the present study, patients treated with DBM augmented with cBMA and PRP for complex rotator cuff tears had a failure rate of 50%. There were no pre-operative differences in comorbidities or patient-reported outcome measures (PROM) between those with clinical rotator cuff repair failure and those who did not fail. However, there was a difference in rates of concomitant biceps tenodesis, with those in the failure group having undergone more of this procedure. The patients who did suffer failure expectedly had less improvement of PROMs than those who did not fail. All patients that failed repair ultimately required further revision surgery or went on to reverse shoulder arthroplasty.

Failure after rotator cuff repair is a common problem that complicates the treatment of this pathology. This is particularly true for chronic tears, revision surgeries, and complex-massive tears for which failure of repair is between 39.8 and 70% [15–20]. Biologic augmentation of these complex cases presents a possible option for decreasing the risk of this poor outcome [21–23]. Thon et al. found high rates of healing with the use of a bio-inductive collagen patch scaffold during the repair of massive rotator cuff tears [23]. Recent studies have also found lower failure rates in small and medium-sized tears augmented with PRP during the repair [24,25]. Additionally, cBMA has been found to significantly decrease rotator cuff repair failure rates [26–28].

In animal models, DBM augmentation for bone-tendon healing has shown promising results. Sundar et al. demonstrated the DBM augmented patellar tendon repair in an ovine model showed fewer failures when compared to non-augmented repairs at 12 weeks [29]. Mouse and rabbit models for rotator cuff repair have shown similar efficacy in DBM augmentation [30,31]. Smith et al. demonstrated that DBM augmented with PRP showed improved tendon-to-bone healing in large, retracted rotator cuff tears at 12 weeks [32]. The failure rate observed in our study is similar to the rates previously described for complex rotator cuff repairs, it is unclear to what degree this was impacted by the use of DBM [15–20]. This may draw concern that DBM and similar constructs may not significantly improve the healing of rotator cuff tears in humans.

While complex rotator cuff repair augmentation with DBM may have decreased the failure rate for this procedure, it is difficult to draw definitive conclusions regarding the impact of DBM on these repairs. This study was limited by its limited sample size and a lack of a comparison group who underwent standard repair without DBM augmentation. It is impossible to determine how this augmentation system impacts healing rates without utilizing a randomized-control methodology. Furthermore, there may have been selection bias in choosing patients who would be treated with DBM augmentation. Another limitation is the concomitant use of cBMA and PRP in these repairs. These additional augments were used as this is the current practice of the treating surgeon. As such, this case series addresses the success rate for DBM augmented with PRP and cBMA rather than the success rate of DBM alone. Furthermore, post-operative ASES scores were not available for three patients (one failure, two non-failure) and CM scores were not available for six patients (one failure, five non-failure). However, the pre-operative patient-reported measures, rather than the post-operative measures, are more meaningful for this study to ensure that there were no pre-operative differences between the failure and the non-failure groups. Finally, post-operative MRIs were not available for every patient, with five patients missing these. These five patients all showed significant clinical improvement post-operatively, and as such, an MRI was not obtained. These patients were deemed successes for the purpose of this study, though it is possible that some of these patients had asymptomatic retears. Ultimately, as full determination of the efficacy of biologically enhanced DBM as an augment for rotator cuff repairs is difficult with a retrospective case series, a prospective study, ideally, a randomized control trial, comparing those treated with this form of augmentation compared to those treated without would be ideal.

5. Conclusions

The present study found that 50% of patients who underwent biologically enhanced DBM augmentation of their rotator cuff repair demonstrated MRI-determined failure of supraspinatus healing. While this failure rate is similar to rates previously reported for similar tears it is difficult to conclude how much of an impact DBM augmentation had on overall healing. Further investigation, ideally with a randomized control study, is needed to determine the true impact of biologically enhanced DBM for the augmentation of rotator cuff repairs.

Author Contributions: Conceptualization, D.P.B., A.D.M., L.N.M. and M.B.M.; methodology, A.D.M., D.P.B., C.L.A., I.J.W. and J.P.C.; validation, M.B.M., C.K., L.N.M. and D.P.B.; formal analysis, I.J.W., J.P.C. and C.L.A.; investigation, I.J.W., B.C.H., L.N.M., D.P.B. and A.D.M.; resources, A.D.M.; data curation, L.N.M. and D.P.B.; writing—original draft preparation, I.J.W., B.C.H., C.K., J.P.C. and C.L.A.; writing—review and editing, I.J.W., L.N.M., C.L.U., M.B.M., A.D.M. and D.P.B.; supervision, M.B.M., L.N.M., D.P.B. and A.D.M.; project administration, D.P.B. and A.D.M. All authors have read and agreed to the published version of the manuscript.

Funding: This research received no external funding.

Institutional Review Board Statement: This study received approval from our institutional review board prior to initiation (IRB #20x-08101).

Informed Consent Statement: Informed consent was obtained from all subjects involved in the study.

Data Availability Statement: Not applicable.

Conflicts of Interest: Author A.D.M. serves as a consultant for Arthrex Inc.

References

1. Carr, J.B., II; Rodeo, S.A. The role of biologic agents in the management of common shoulder pathologies: Current state and future directions. *J. Shoulder Elb. Surg.* **2019**, *28*, 2041–2052. [CrossRef] [PubMed]
2. Voss, A.; McCarthy, M.B.; Hoberman, A.; Cote, M.P.; Imhoff, A.B.; Mazzocca, A.D.; Beitzel, K. Extracellular matrix of current biological scaffolds promotes the differentiation potential of mesenchymal stem cells. *Arthrosc. J. Arthrosc. Relat. Surg.* **2016**, *32*, 2381–2392. [CrossRef] [PubMed]
3. Amini, M.H.; Ricchetti, E.T.; Iannotti, J.P.; Derwin, K.A. Rotator cuff repair: Challenges and solutions. *Orthop. Res. Rev.* **2015**, *7*, 57–69.
4. Chowdhury, F.; Na, S.; Li, D.; Poh, Y.-C.; Tanaka, T.S.; Wang, F.; Wang, N. Material properties of the cell dictate stress-induced spreading and differentiation in embryonic stem cells. *Nat. Mater.* **2010**, *9*, 82–88. [CrossRef]
5. Dalby, M.J.; Gadegaard, N.; Tare, R.; Andar, A.; Riehle, M.O.; Herzyk, P.; Wilkinson, C.D.W.; Oreffo, R.O.C. The control of human mesenchymal cell differentiation using nanoscale symmetry and disorder. *Nat. Mater.* **2007**, *6*, 997–1003. [CrossRef]
6. Engler, A.J.; Sen, S.; Sweeney, H.L.; Discher, D.E. Matrix elasticity directs stem cell lineage specification. *Cell* **2006**, *126*, 677–689. [CrossRef]
7. Gentleman, E.; Swain, R.J.; Evans, N.D.; Boonrungsiman, S.; Jell, G.; Ball, M.D.; Shean, T.A.V.; Oyen, M.L.; Porter, A.; Stevens, M.M. Comparative materials differences revealed in engineered bone as a function of cell-specific differentiation. *Nat. Mater.* **2009**, *8*, 763–770. [CrossRef]
8. McMurray, R.J.; Gadegaard, N.; Tsimbouri, P.M.; Burgess, K.V.; McNamara, L.E.; Tare, R.; Murawski, K.; Kingham, E.; Oreffo, R.O.C.; Dalby, M.J. Nanoscale surfaces for the long-term maintenance of mesenchymal stem cell phenotype and multipotency. *Nat. Mater.* **2011**, *10*, 637–644. [CrossRef]
9. Neviaser, J.S.; Neviaser, R.J.; Neviaser, T.J. The repair of chronic massive ruptures of the rotator cuff of the shoulder by use of a freeze-dried rotator cuff. *J. Bone Jt. Surg. Am.* **1978**, *60*, 681–684. [CrossRef]
10. Hoberman, A.R.; Cirino, C.; McCarthy, M.B.; Cote, M.P.; Pauzenberger, L.; Beitzel, K.; Mazzocca, A.D.; Dyrna, F. Bone Marrow-Derived Mesenchymal Stromal Cells Enhanced by Platelet-Rich Plasma Maintain Adhesion to Scaffolds in Arthroscopic Simulation. *Arthrosc. J. Arthrosc. Relat. Surg.* **2018**, *34*, 872–881. [CrossRef]
11. Patte, D. Classification of rotator cuff lesions. *Clin. Orthop. Relat. Res.* **1990**, *254*, 81–86. [CrossRef]
12. Lippe, J.; Spang, J.T.; Leger, R.R.; Arciero, R.A.; Mazzocca, A.D.; Shea, K.P. Inter-Rater Agreement of the Goutallier, Patte, and Warner Classification Scores Using Preoperative Magnetic Resonance Imaging in Patients with Rotator Cuff Tears. *Arthrosc. J. Arthrosc. Relat. Surg.* **2012**, *28*, 154–159. [CrossRef] [PubMed]
13. Goutallier, D.; Postel, J.; Bernageau, J.; Lavau, L.; Voisin, M. Fatty muscle degeneration in cuff ruptures. Pre- and postoperative evaluation by CT scan. *Clin. Orthop. Relat. Res.* **1994**, *304*, 78–83. [CrossRef]
14. Mazzocca, A.D.; McCarthy, M.B.R.; Chowaniec, D.M.; Cote, M.P.; Arciero, R.A.; Drissi, H. Rapid isolation of human stem cells (connective tissue progenitor cells) from the proximal humerus during arthroscopic rotator cuff surgery. *Am. J. Sports Med.* **2010**, *38*, 1438–1447. [CrossRef]
15. Ricchetti, E.T.; Aurora, A.; Iannotti, J.P.; Derwin, K.A. Scaffold devices for rotator cuff repair. *J. Shoulder Elb. Surg.* **2012**, *21*, 251–265. [CrossRef]
16. George, M.S.; Khazzam, M. Current concepts review: Revision rotator cuff repair. *J. Shoulder Elb. Surg.* **2012**, *21*, 431–440. [CrossRef]
17. Meyer, D.C.; Wieser, K.; Farshad, M.; Gerber, C. Retraction of Supraspinatus Muscle and Tendon as Predictors of Success of Rotator Cuff Repair. *Am. J. Sports Med.* **2012**, *40*, 2242–2247. [CrossRef]
18. Muench, L.N.; Kia, C.; Williams, A.A.; Avery, D.M.; Cote, M.P.; Reed, N.; Arciero, R.A.; Chandawarkar, R.; Mazzocca, A.D. High Clinical Failure Rate After Latissimus Dorsi Transfer for Revision Massive Rotator Cuff Tears. *Arthrosc. J. Arthrosc. Relat. Surg.* **2020**, *36*, 88–94. [CrossRef]
19. Rashid, M.S.; Cooper, C.; Cook, J.; Cooper, D.; Dakin, S.G.; Snelling, S.; Carr, A.J. Increasing age and tear size reduce rotator cuff repair healing rate at 1 year: Data from a large randomized controlled trial. *Acta Orthop.* **2017**, *88*, 606–611. Available online: http://www.tandfonline.com/action/authorSubmission?journalCode=iort20&page=instructions (accessed on 12 January 2022). [CrossRef]
20. Chung, S.W.; Kim, J.Y.; Kim, M.H.; Kim, S.H.; Oh, J.H. Arthroscopic Repair of Massive Rotator Cuff Tears: Outcome and Analysis of Factors Associated with Healing Failure or Poor Postoperative Function. *Am. J. Sports Med.* **2013**, *41*, 1674–1683. [CrossRef]
21. Bailey, J.R.; Kim, C.; Alentorn-Geli, E.; Kirkendall, D.T.; Ledbetter, L.; Taylor, D.C.; Toth, A.P.; Garrigues, G.E. Rotator Cuff Matrix Augmentation and Interposition: A Systematic Review and Meta-analysis. *Am. J. Sports Med.* **2018**, *47*, 1496–1506. [CrossRef] [PubMed]
22. Duchman, K.R.; Mickelson, D.T.; Little, B.A.; Hash, T.W.; Lemmex, D.B.; Toth, A.P.; Garrigues, G.E. Graft use in the treatment of large and massive rotator cuff tears: An overview of techniques and modes of failure with MRI correlation. *Skelet. Radiol.* **2018**, *48*, 47–55. [CrossRef] [PubMed]
23. Thon, S.G.; O'Malley, L.; O'Brien, M.J.; Savoie, F.H., III. Evaluation of Healing Rates and Safety with a Bioinductive Collagen Patch for Large and Massive Rotator Cuff Tears: 2-Year Safety and Clinical Outcomes. *Am. J. Sports Med.* **2019**, *47*, 1901–1908. [CrossRef] [PubMed]

24. Chiapparelli, E.; Bowen, E.; Okano, I.; Salzmann, S.N.; Reisener, M.-J.; Shue, J.; Sama, A.A.; Cammisa, F.P.; Girardi, F.P.; Hughes, A.P. Spinal Cord Medial Safe Zone for C2 Pedicle Instrumentation: An MRI Measurement Analysis. *Spine* **2022**, *47*, E101–E106. [CrossRef] [PubMed]
25. Warth, R.J.; Dornan, G.J.; James, E.W.; Horan, M.P.; Millett, P.J. Clinical and Structural Outcomes after Arthroscopic Repair of Full-Thickness Rotator Cuff Tears with and without Platelet-Rich Product Supplementation: A Meta-analysis and Meta-regression. *Arthrosc. J. Arthrosc. Relat. Surg.* **2015**, *31*, 306–320. [CrossRef]
26. Imam, M.A.; Holton, J.; Horriat, S.; Negida, A.S.; Grubhofer, F.; Gupta, R.; Narvani, A.; Snow, M. A systematic review of the concept and clinical applications of bone marrow aspirate concentrate in tendon pathology. *SICOT J.* **2017**, *3*, 58. [CrossRef]
27. Havlas, V.; Kotaška, J.; Koníček, P.; Trč, T.; Konrádová, Š.; Kočí, Z.; Syková, E. Use of cultured human autologous bone marrow stem cells in repair of a rotator cuff tear: Preliminary results of a safety study. *Acta Chir. Orthop. Traumatol. Cech.* **2015**, *82*, 229–234.
28. Hernigou, P.; Flouzat Lachaniette, C.H.; Delambre, J.; Zilber, S.; Duffiet, P.; Chevallier, N.; Rouard, H. Biologic augmentation of rotator cuff repair with mesenchymal stem cells during arthroscopy improves healing and prevents further tears: A case-controlled study. *Int. Orthop.* **2014**, *38*, 1811–1818. [CrossRef]
29. Sundar, S.; Pendegrass, C.J.; Blunn, G.W. Tendon bone healing can be enhanced by demineralized bone matrix: A functional and histological study. *J. Biomed. Mater. Res. Part B* **2009**, *88*, 115–122. [CrossRef]
30. Thangarajah, T.; Henshaw, F.; Sanghani-Kerai, A.; Lambert, S.M.; Blunn, G.W.; Pendegrass, C.J. The effectiveness of demineralized cortical bone matrix in a chronic rotator cuff tear model. *J. Shoulder Elb. Surg.* **2017**, *26*, 619–626. [CrossRef]
31. Lee, W.-Y.; Kim, Y.-M.; Hwang, D.-S.; Shin, H.-D.; Joo, Y.-B.; Cha, S.-M.; Kim, K.-H.; Jeon, Y.-S.; Lee, S.-Y. Does demineralized bone matrix enhance tendon-to-bone healing after rotator cuff repair in a rabbit model? *Clin. Orthop. Surg.* **2021**, *13*, 216. [CrossRef] [PubMed]
32. Smith, M.J.; Pfeiffer, F.M.; Cook, C.R.; Kuroki, K.; Cook, J.L. Rotator cuff healing using demineralized cancellous bone matrix sponge interposition compared to standard repair in a preclinical canine model. *J. Orthop. Res.* **2018**, *36*, 906–912. [CrossRef] [PubMed]

MDPI
St. Alban-Anlage 66
4052 Basel
Switzerland
Tel. +41 61 683 77 34
Fax +41 61 302 89 18
www.mdpi.com

Journal of Clinical Medicine Editorial Office
E-mail: jcm@mdpi.com
www.mdpi.com/journal/jcm

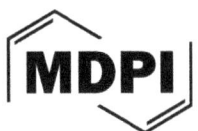

www.ingramcontent.com/pod-product-compliance
Lightning Source LLC
LaVergne TN
LVHW070623100526
838202LV00012B/713